Management of Breast Canc

Malcolm W. R. Reed · Riccardo A. Audisio
Editors

Management of Breast Cancer in Older Women

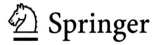 Springer

Editors
Malcom W.R. Reed, MB ChB BMedSci,
MD, FRCS(Eng)
Academic Unit of Surgical Oncology
University of Sheffield and Sheffield
Teaching Hospitals NHS Trust
Sheffield
UK

Riccardo A. Audisio, MD FRCS(Engl)
University of Liverpool
St Helens Teaching Hospital
St Helens
UK

ISBN 978-0-85729-515-6 (PB)
ISBN 978-1-84800-264-7 (HB)   e-ISBN 978-1-84800-265-4
DOI 10.1007/978-1-84800-265-4
Springer London Dordrecht Heidelberg New York

British Library Cataloguing in Publication Data
A catalogue record for this book is available from the British Library

Library of Congress Control Number: 2009942232

Springer is part of Springer Science+Business Media (www.springer.com)

Foreword

I was looking at Mrs T – all 45 kilos of her – with somewhat puzzled thoughts. I had prescribed her capecitabine at very prudent doses, in view of her 91-year-old kidneys and physiology. She had reduced my treatment even further, "because it was making her tired." As a result, she was taking a grand total of 500 mg of capecitabine a day. Yet, her metastatic, ER/PR-negative, Her2-positive breast cancer was undoubtedly responding. Her pain was improving and her chest mass was shrinking, as were her lung metastases… What was the secret of that response? Were Mrs T's kidneys eliminating even less drug than predicted by her creatinine clearance? Was her sarcopenia altering drug distribution? Was she absorbing more drug than average? Or was her tumor exquisitely sensitive to fluoropyrimidines? "Physicians," said Voltaire, "pour drugs they know little for diseases they know even less into patients they know nothing about." Medicine has made tremendous progress since the eighteenth century. Yet, there are fields where quite a lot remains to be learned. In developed countries, 25% of breast cancers occur in patients aged 75 years and older. Yet, these patients represent only 4% of the population of traditional clinical trials. That ought to let us wonder how relevant data acquired in patients in their 60s are to a nonagenarian. Fortunately, geriatric oncologists have been stepping up to the task and have generated data to help us to treat such patients.

Drs. Reed and Audisio have assembled in this book the results of their work. The readers will find in a condensed format data to help them to treat this important subgroup of breast cancer patients. They will find in this book data ranging from the impact of age on the biology of breast cancer to the psychosocial considerations. Two well-developed treatment sections will help the readers to practice personalized cancer care for our senior patients. The editors have assembled a remarkable panel of experts in breast cancer and geriatric oncology to contribute their knowledge in their respective field of expertise. This book will no doubt earn a well-deserved place as a reference in the office of oncologists treating older women with breast cancer. May it help us to know more about the drugs, the diseases, and the patients we treat.

Martine Extermann
Florida, USA

Preface

The aim of this book is to provide the readers with a comprehensive review of the important topic of the management of breast cancer in elderly women. The increasing prevalence of breast cancer in the aging population and the extended availability of screening have huge implications for health care services around the world. In the United Kingdom alone, these factors will contribute to an increased incidence of breast cancer of 20% over the next 10 years, representing a huge challenge for clinicians and researchers alike.

Although over half of the patients diagnosed with breast cancer are over the age of 70, there is a major lack of evidence based on randomised clinical trials to guide clinicians and patients in the selection of the best treatment options. Largely because of this failure to include these patients in clinical trials, there are very few evidence-based guidelines to guide treatment. All too often, older patients are managed in accordance with guidelines based on research trials that incorporated exclusively younger women. This deficiency often results in older patients failing to receive appropriate management in all aspects of their care, from screening through diagnosis, therapy, and follow-up.

Despite the real and recognised changes in physiology and functional status with age, assumptions are often made about treatments based on misconceptions in relation to patient's preferences and suitability for such therapies. This can result in under staging and inappropriate under- ,or in some cases, overzealous treatment.

In the face of this background, there is increasing recognition that this issue needs to be addressed and that there exists within the field of geriatrics the appropriate specialist skills to help oncologists to select the appropriate treatment for patients. The editors have an established research and clinical interest in this topic and have brought together a multidisciplinary team of contributors from the fields of epidemiology, oncology, and geriatrics to provide the readers with a comprehensive review of the field. The editors' and contributors' aim is to provide a detailed background to each topic along with clear and useful guidance based on the best available evidence. All the contributors are acknowledged experts in their field and the editors are grateful to them for the time and effort they have committed to this project. We have included relatively new areas such as breast reconstruction and the interpolation between age and race/ethnicity in order to cover the subject area comprehensively.

The editors acknowledge the support of SIOG (International Society of Geriatric Oncology) and the efficient and enthusiastic editorial support from Barbara Lopez-Lucio and our publisher, Springer.

Malcolm W.R. Reed
Sheffield, UK
Riccardo A. Audisio
St. Helens, UK

Contents

Part III Therapeutics

Part IV Psychosocial Considerations

Contributors

Sam H. Ahmedzai
School of Medicine and Biomedical Sciences, The University of Sheffield,
Sheffield, South Yorkshire, UK

Riccardo A. Audisio
Department of Surgery, St. Helens and Knowsley University Hospitals,
St. Helens, UK

Valerie Beral
Cancer Epidemiology Unit, University of Oxford,
Oxford, OX1 2JD, UK

Laura Biganzoli
Department of Oncology, Hospital of Prato – Instituto Toscano Tumori,
Prato, Italy

Ruth V. Broadhurst
Department of Palliative Medicine, Sheffield Teaching Hospitals NHS Foundation
Trust, Sheffield, UK

Elaine Cachia
Department of Palliative Medicine, Sheffield Teaching Hospitals NHS Foundation
Trust, Sheffield, UK

Christopher M. Caddy
Department of Plastic Surgery, Sheffield Teaching Hospitals NHS Foundation
Trust (Northern General Hospital), Sheffield, UK

Jan Willem W. Coebergh
Department of Public Health, Erasmus Medical Centre, Rotterdam,
The Netherlands

Robert E. Coleman
Academic Unit of Clinical Oncology, Weston Park Hospital,
Sheffield, UK

Maja J.A. de Jonge
Department of Medical Oncology, Erasmus MC – Daniel den Hoed, Rotterdam,
The Netherlands

Claudia Di Bartolomeo
Department of Oncology, INRCA-IRCCS, Rome, Italy

Virginie Durbecq
Pathology Department, Jules Bordet Institute, Brussels, Belgium

Martine Extermann
Senior Adult Oncology Program, H. Lee Moffitt Cancer Center and Research
Institute, Tampa, Florida, USA

Lindsay J.L. Forbes
Adamson Centre for Mental Health, St. Thomas' Hospital,
King's College London, London, UK

Toral Gathani
Cancer Epidemiology Unit, University of Oxford, Oxford, UK

Margot A. Gosney
Institute of Health Sciences, University of Reading, Reading, UK

Paul Hamberg
Department of Medical Oncology, Erasmus MC – Daniel den Hoed, Rotterdam,
The Netherlands

Daniel Hind
Clinical Trials Research Unit, School of Health and Related Research (ScHARR),
University of Sheffield, Sheffield, UK

Arti Hurria
Division of Medical Oncology and Therapeutics Research, City of Hope, Duarte,
California, USA

Irmgard Irminger-Finger
Department of Gynecology and Obstetrics and, Department of Medical Genetics
and Laboratories, University Hospitals Geneva, Geneva, Switzerland

Giovanni Battista Ivaldi
Department of Radiation Oncology, European Institute of Oncology, Milan, Italy

Siri Rostoft Kristjansson
Department of Geriatric Medicine, Oslo University Hospital, Ullevål, Oslo,
Norway

Denis Larsimont
Pathology Department, Jules Bordet Institute, Brussels, Belgium

Maria Cristina Leonardi
Department of Radiotherapy, European Institute of Oncology, Milan, Italy

Marieke J. Louwman
Research Department, Comprehensive Cancer Centre South, Eindhoven,
The Netherlands

Helen L. Neville-Webbe
Academic Unit of Clinical Oncology, Weston Park Hospital, University
of Sheffield, Sheffield, South Yorkshire, UK

Roberto Orecchia
Department of Radiation Oncology, European Institute of Oncology,
University of Milan, Milan, Italy

Sumanta Kumar Pal
Department of Medical Oncology and Experimental Therapeutics, City of Hope
Comprehensive Cancer Center, Duarte, CA, USA

Robert S. Pretorius
Departments of Anaesthesia, Critical Care, and Pain Management, Glenfield
Hospital, University Hospitals of Leicester NHS Trust, Leicester, UK

Amanda J. Ramirez
Cancer Research UK/London, London Psychosocial Group,
King's College London, London, UK

Malcolm W.R. Reed
Academic Unit of Surgical Oncology, University of Sheffield and Sheffield
Teaching Hospitals NHS Trust, Sheffield, UK

Lazzaro Repetto
Department of Oncology, INRCA-IRCCS, Rome, Italy

Thompson G. Robinson
Department of Cardiovascular Sciences, University of Leicester,
University Hospitals of Leicester NHS Trust, Leicester, UK

Pierre G.M. Scalliet
Department Radiation Oncology, Cliniques Universitaires Saint Luc, Brussels,
Belgium

Caroline M. Seynaeve
Department of Medical Oncology, Erasmus MC – Daniel den Hoed, Rotterdam,
The Netherlands

Marjorie Kagawa Singer
Community Health Sciences Department, and, Department of Asian American
Studies, University of California Los Angeles, School of Public Health,
Los Angeles, CA, USA

Anne Stotter
Department of Breast/General Surgery, University Hospitals Leicester NHS Trust,
Glenfield Hospital, Leicester, UK

Antonella Surbone
Department of Medicine, New York University, New York, NY, USA

Mohammad Tahir
Department of Breast Surgery, Glenfield Hospital,
University Hospitals of Leicester NHS Trust, Leicester, UK

Bernadette Th. Veering
Department of Anesthesiology, Leiden University Medical Center, Leiden,
The Netherlands

Adri C. Voogd
Department of Epidemiology, Maastricht University Medical Centre, Maastricht,
The Netherlands

Nilesh L. Vora
Departments of Medical Oncology and Experimental Therapeutics,
City of Hope Comprehensive Cancer Center, Duarte, CA, USA

Marcus J.D. Wagstaff
Department of Plastic Surgery, Sheffield Teach Hospitals NHS Trust, Sheffield,
UK

Hans P.M.W. Wildiers
Department of General Medical Oncology, Uz Leuven – Gasthuisberg, Leuven,
Belgium

Matthew C. Winter
Academic Unit of Clinical Oncology, Weston Park Hospital, The University
of Sheffield, Sheffield, South Yorkshire, UK

Lynda Wyld
Academic Unit of Surgical Oncology, University of Sheffield, Sheffield, South
Yorkshire, UK

Part I
Background and Epidemiology

Chapter 1
Basic Science of Breast Cancer in Older Patients

Irmgard Irminger-Finger

1.1 Introduction

Breast cancer is the leading cancer for females in North America and Europe. Although the environment and cultural and ethical backgrounds have an impact on breast cancer frequency, two major risk factors arise above all doubt, namely, increasing age and estrogen exposures. It seems that a cumulative effect of both is leading to the peak of breast cancer incidence in postmenopausal women. In addition, molecular signaling pathways that change with aging might be involved in the predisposition setting. These aging-related signaling pathways and their relation to cancer-related signaling pathways will be discussed here. A second theme will be highlighted in different ways, namely the involvement of the breast cancer predisposition genes in age-dependent incidence of breast cancer.

1.2 Breast Cancer Risk Factors and the Biology of Breast Cancer

Breast cancer incidence and death rates increase with age (Fig. 1.1). About 95% of breast cancer cases in the US occurred in women aged 40 and older. The observed decrease in women aged 80 years and older might reflect the reduced rates of screening and incomplete detection. Today a woman's risk of developing breast cancer during her lifetime is 12.3%, or 1 in 8, while it was 1 in 11 in the 1970s. Mostly, this increase is thought to be due to increased life expectancy.

Hormone exposure is another risk factor, since early menarche, late menopause, and hormone replacement therapy are accepted risk factors (Hulka and Moorman 2001).

I. Irminger-Finger (✉)
Department of Gynecology and Obstetrics and Department of Medical Genetics
and Laboratories, University Hospitals Geneva, Geneva, Switzerland
e-mail: Irmgard.irminger@hcuge.ch

M.W. Reed and R.A. Audisio (eds.), *Management of Breast Cancer in Older Women*,
DOI 10.1007/978-1-84800-265-4_1, © Springer-Verlag London Limited 2011

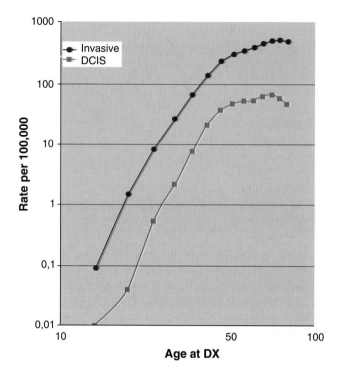

Fig. 1.1 Breast cancer incidence is correlated with age of patient at diagnosis. Breast cancer incidence rate at age of diagnosis (DX) is indicated for invasive and in situ cancers

Indeed, hormone replacement therapy prescription was reduced in the 1990s and led to a decline of breast cancer incidence in the US (Collaborative Group on Hormonal Factors in Breast Cancer 1997).

Interestingly, multiple pregnancies and breastfeeding are factors that decrease a woman's risk for breast cancer (Collaborative Group on Hormonal Factors in Breast Cancer 2002; Shantakumar et al. 2007). This suggests that changes in hormone profiles might be beneficial for protection against the development of breast cancer.

Breast density, an increase of glandular tissue versus fatty tissue, is a strong risk factor for breast cancer (Barlow et al. 2006). Another risk factor is obesity, specifically for postmenopausal women (Eliassen et al. 2006), since fat tissue produces estrogens thus increasing the level of circulating estrogens. Alcohol consumption is strongly associated with increased breast cancer risk (Hamajima et al. 2002), and the mechanism is also based on the generation of increased estrogen and androgen levels through conversion of alcohol (Singletary and Gapstur 2001).

Risk factors include thus behavioral, social, and nutritional factors. However, the differences in breast cancer risk of women of different ethnic origin can only partially be attributed to lifestyle and environment, and a genetic component cannot be excluded.

1.3   Genetic Predisposition to Breast Cancer

Genetic predisposition to breast cancer is clearly associated with mutations in breast cancer predisposition genes BRCA1 and BRCA2. Women with a family history of breast cancer in first degree relatives have a strongly increased risk of developing breast cancer. As much as 5 to 10% of breast cancer cases are estimated to result from mutations in the genes for BRCA1 and BRCA2 (Ford et al. 1998).

Today mutations in these genes can be identified, but the prediction of risk is complicated and might be a combination of genetic susceptibility and lifestyle. Furthermore, while mutations in the BRCA1 and BRCA2 genes are correlated with increased breast cancer risk, the status of factors or other gene products that modulate their function, such as the BRCA1-associated protein BARD1 (Irminger-Finger and Jefford 2006), might also be implicated in what makes up the combined genetic susceptibility.

Mutations in genes other than BRCA1 and BRCA2 have also been identified, although to a lesser extent, in breast cancer patients, namely, TP53, PTEN (Palacios et al. 2008). Indeed, mutations in predisposition genes lead to earlier onset of breast cancer than observed for sporadic cancers, a fact generally attributed to less efficient repair and cell cycle control functions in heterozygous cells, which then permit loss of heterozygosity and a rapid progression to malignant transformation. However, the steps that make a heterozygous cell with one deficient allele of BRCA1 or BRCA2 transform into a malignant cell are not understood, nor has it been investigated why the heterozygous condition leads to early-onset breast cancer with a certain probability.

Thus, other mechanisms than mutations might exist that could be initiating or supporting factors toward a malignant transformation of mammary gland cells. Overexpression of MDM2, the protein responsible for rapid turnover of p53 in normal cells, overexpression of cyclin D, a factor driving mitosis, or overexpression of HER2, are examples often found in association with breast cancer, but the mechanisms that explain their role in the development and propagation and age-related risk of breast cancer are not understood.

1.4   Biology of Aging

Other factors that contribute to breast cancer initiation and proliferation might be factors that are related to aging. To investigate how aging could drive breast cancer risk, it is important to understand the molecular pathways that drive aging and secondly to investigate how they interfere with pathways relevant for breast cancer.

1.4.1   Damage by Oxidative Stress

A fundamental mechanism of aging is based on the production of reactive oxygen species (ROS) and free radicals (Ramsey and Sharpless 2006). ROS and free radicals can be generated by environmental circumstances or can have inherent cellular origins, a consequence of cellular respiration, in summary termed oxidative stress. ROS can activate transcription of genes implicated in inflammatory and other disease-associated processes, or cause damage on DNA, proteins, and lipids (Langen et al. 2003). In response to this accumulation of damage, cells might undergo apoptosis or become senescence (Fig. 1.2), leading to a decrease in viable cells. Prevention of oxidative stress is therefore an important contribution to a general slowing of the aging process (Song et al. 2005). Evidently, oxidative stress production of ROS can be influenced by nutrition and lifestyle.

1.4.2   Replicative Senescence Controlled by Telomere Length

It is well-established that in vitro cells undergo a limited number of cell divisions dictated by the length of telomeres (Allsopp et al. 1995; Hayflick 1985). Critical shortening of telomeres leads to cell cycle arrest and cellular senescence (Fig. 1.2), a phenomenon termed replicative senescence. A causal relationship between reduction of replicative potential and induction of cellular senescence and the shortening of telomeres has been established in vitro, and the diminishing of telomere length during aging has been demonstrated in vivo (Artandi and DePinho 2000; Kajstura et al. 2000). Telomere shortening and loss has been associated with genetic changes, and experimental data in mouse models support the link between telomere length and cancer susceptibility (DePinho 2000; Ferron et al. 2004; Metcalfe et al. 1996).

1.4.3   Cellular Senescence and Apoptosis

Aging is thought to be the result of genetically programmed and environmentally inflicted accumulation of damage to tissues and cells. Mechanisms of decline of active cells are apoptosis and cellular senescence. Cellular senescence is the irreversible exit of the cell cycle and can be caused by various stimuli. Senescence occurring at the end of the proliferative life span of normal cells is a response to telomere shortening (Fig. 1.2).

Senescence therefore contributes to tumor suppression, but also to tissue insufficiency. Senescence does not happen in cancer cells, and so it does not deviate cancer cells (Campisi 2001).

Apoptosis, the induced, regulated cellular suicide is an important mechanism for tissue homeostasis and renewal. Apoptosis can be triggered by a variety of signals. These signals can be a response to genomic insults (Amundson et al. 1998; Jiang et al. 2005), to telomere erosion (Zhang et al. 1999), or to developmental or tissue regulatory signals.

Apoptosis signals might be important in all proliferative tissues and counterbalanced by replenishing with functional cells by tissue-specific stem cells (Rizo et al. 2006).

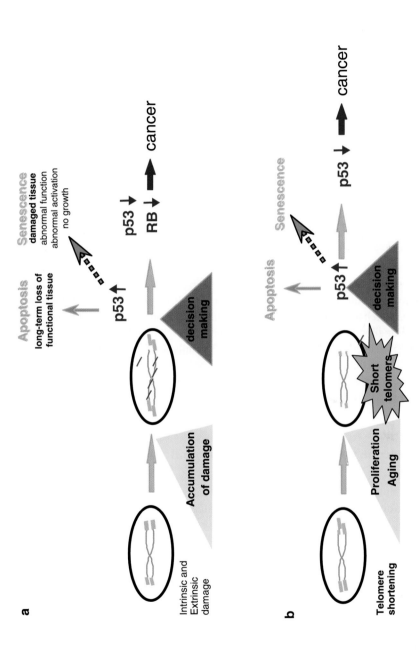

Fig. 1.2 Mechanisms contributing to aging and cancer. (**a**) DNA damage signaling requires p53 or retinoblastoma (RB) to induce cell cycle arrest and apoptosis or senescence. (**b**) Telomere shortening leads to a DNA damage response signal towards p53. Elimination of cells by apoptosis and reduction of functional cells by senescence leads to tissue aging

The pathways of apoptosis might be triggered by extracellular signals (Kari et al. 2003; Rizo et al. 2006; Smith et al. 2003), activating receptors, or intra cellular signals activating specific kinases (Watters 1999). A key player in apoptosis signaling is the tumor suppressor TP53. The p53 protein is stabilized by phophorylation by stress response kinases at various sites (Chao et al. 2006; Feki et al. 2005; Feng et al. 2006). In cells growing normally, p53 is rarely detectable, due to its rapid turnover controlled by MDM2 (Kubbutat et al. 1997; Yin et al. 2002).

Once p53 is stabilized and activated, it assumes tumor suppressor functions through its role as transcription factor, activating transcription of p21, to induce cell-cycle arrest, and bax, to induce apoptosis (Megyesi et al. 1996; Yamaguchi et al. 2004). The factors regulating the decision between these two pathways are not completely clear, but might involve a quantitative threshold mechanism (Moll and Zaika 2001) or implicate other posttranslational regulation, such as acetylation (Kaneshiro et al. 2007).

1.4.4 Tissue Aging Through Stem Cell Aging

Aging of stem cells can be influenced by extrinsic changes or by the accumulation of mutations or changes occurring in the *stem cell niche,* those cells nourishing the *stem cells,* which are responsible for replenishing an organ or tissue with functional cells. Tumor suppressor pathways, which comprise signaling from telomere shortening to p53 and p16/INK4a actions (Fig. 1.3), whilst important for the control of cancer cell growth, have the negative action of reducing the replicative function of stem cells. Indeed, with advancing age, p16 expression increases in stem cells (Janzen et al. 2006) suggesting that tissue aging is due to stem cell exhaustion.

1.5 Molecular Crossroads of Cancer and Aging

Telomere shortening could be an important cancer-predisposing mechanism in tissues with high proliferation, mostly of epithelial cells. Indeed, epithelial-cell-derived cancers happen to be frequent in old age and rare in children (DePinho 2000).

1.5.1 Cellular Senescence: A Double-Edged Sword

Aging is thought to be the result of genetically programmed and environmentally inflicted accumulation of damage to tissues and cells. Mechanisms that contribute to the decline of active cells are apoptosis and cellular senescence. Thus, senescence, like apoptosis, contributes to tumor suppression, but also to tissue insufficiency. Interestingly, oncogene-induced senescence is observed as a form of

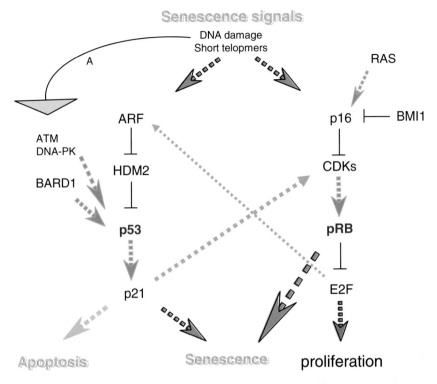

Fig. 1.3 Senescence signaling, a double edged sword: the p53-pRB pathway of senescence control. Senescence signaling induces ARF and p16. ARF inhibits HDM2, a down-regulator of p53. Activation of p53 by HDM inhibition or ATM, or DNA-PK and BARD1 (Feki et al. 2005) results in p21 induction and cell cycle arrest. Both p21 and p16 inhibit CDKs. Without phosphorylation of pRB by cyclins, E2F is repressed. Active E2F can induce transcription of ARF. RAS signaling can induce p16. BMI1 acts as inhibitor of p16-induced senescence signaling

response to excessive replicative stimuli. One example for an oncogene-inducing senescence is RAS (Serrano et al. 1997), suggesting that oncogenic events can finally lead to proliferation arrest (Fig. 3.3). Importantly, the senescence pathway can be activated in cells that are resistant to apoptosis, the programmed cell death. Furthermore, manipulating genes that are regulators of apoptosis can cause cells to undergo senescence and vice versa (Campisi 2003).

1.5.2   Actors at the Crossroads of Senescence and Cancer

A common regulator of apoptosis and senescence is p53. Senescence is associated with the expression of the cyclin-dependent kinase (CDK) inhibitors p21 and p16, components of the p53 and retinoblastoma (RB) tumor suppressor pathways, which are frequently disrupted in cancer. Both pathways can establish and maintain growth arrest and senescence (Fig. 3.3).

Upon damage signals, p53 is phosphorylated by DNA damage sensors, in particular ATM and DNA-PK, which results in its stabilization and activation. Activated p53 induces expression of p21, a CDK inhibitor. Inhibition of CDKs results in transient growth arrest (when accompanied by repair) or senescence. Alternatively, senescence signaling toward p53 is transmitted via ARF (Kamijo et al. 1999), an inhibitor of MDM2 (HDM2 in humans), which is a ubiquitin ligase targeting p53 for degradation and keeps p53 protein levels low in proliferating cells (Sherr and McCormick 2002).

The RB pathway of senescence is induced by p16. Since CDKs phosphorylate RB in a cell-cycle-dependent fashion, their inhibition leads to hypophosphorylation of RB. In its hypophosphorylated state RB halts cell proliferation by suppressing the activity of the transcription factor E2F, which stimulates expression of genes required for cell-cycle progression. Thus activation of p16 leads to cell-cycle arrest or senescence.

There is cross talk between the p53 and RB pathways. p21 action on CDKs inhibits RB phosphorylation. The RB pathway links to the p53 pathway through induction of ARF by E2F. An important regulator of senescence is BMI-1, an oncogene and a repressor of p16 (Park et al. 2004), with anti-aging activity in mice (Itahana et al. 2003). Interestingly, p16 expression in tissues increases with age. Mice without p16 live longer, show better tissue regeneration, but are more cancer prone (Janzen et al. 2006). Similarly, hyperactive p53 prevents cancer but provokes premature aging (Sharpless and DePinho 2002; Tyner et al., 2002). Thus the senescence pathways represent a trade-off between tumor suppression and aging. Importantly, some of the factors involved in these pathways are associated with and are targets for treatment of breast cancer.

1.6   Biomarkers for Breast Cancer Change with Age

Biomarkers of breast cancer are indicators of the number of mitosis or apoptosis in tissues, the mitotic index or Ki-67 positivity and apoptotic index thus reflecting tumor growth. Other markers are linked to the invasive potential and include VEGF, or proteases such as cathepsin D. Another generally used biomarker for breast cancer is p53 positivity, reflecting a stabilized aberrant p53 and suggesting a certain loss of cell-cycle control (Benz et al. 2003).

The estrogen receptor (ER) is probably the most powerful predictive marker in breast cancer management, both in determining prognosis and in predicting response to hormone therapies. Progesterone receptor (PR) is also a widely used marker, although its value is less well established. HER-2 status has become a routine prognostic and predictive factor for treatment in breast cancer.

Interestingly, biomarkers indicative of invasive behavior of breast cancers do not correlate with patient age at diagnosis, but hormone receptor status is correlated with age (Eppenberger-Castori et al. 2002; Quong et al. 2002). Factors that are indicative of tumor proliferation are in general inversely correlated with age (e.g., HER2); this observation is consistent with the observation of slower growth rates of breast tumors in older patients.

Importantly however, ER, but not PR, expression is correlated with patient age at diagnosis (Benz et al. 2003; Eppenberger-Castori et al. 2002; Quong et al. 2002). In summary, breast cancers in older women are more likely to be ER positive, but less likely to be HER2 or p53 positive.

ER has transcription activation function for a large variety of ER response genes, including PR, Bcl-2, cathepsin D, also expressed in normal and malignant mammary gland cells. Co-overexpression of ER and ER-response genes indicates an intact ER signaling pathway. Consequently, PR expression, when not co-expressed with ER, is indicative of defective ER signaling (Petz and Nardulli 2000). Thus, it is unclear whether inhibition of ER by anti-estrogens is an effective treatment of these types of cancer.

1.6.1 Oxidative Stress and Estrogen Receptor Pathways

Among several ER-α [alpha] response genes are the PR, Bcl2, and cathepsin D. Tumors that are overexpressing ER are thought to activate the full ER-response gene set. However, age-specific comparison of the expression levels of ER and ER-response genes showed, that, while ER upregulation in breast tumors is clearly correlated with increasing age, the expression levels of the respective response genes, namely PR, Bcl2, AP1, and the oxidative stress-activated kinase Erk5, are not (Quong et al. 2002). This is consistent with previous observations of ER-positive/PR-negative breast cancers increased with patient age. The results of this study suggest that age-dependent oxidative stress is a modulator of the responsiveness of ER-response genes.

1.6.2 Metabolism and Oxidative Stress

As discussed above, the generation of intracellular ROS through the metabolism of glucose and production of ATP is inevitable and can act as a constitutive tumor promoter by inducing mutations in genes and defects on proteins and lipids. However, tumor cells have also constitutively activated glycolysis and produce increased levels of lactic acid (Gatenby and Gillies 2007).

Although the glycolysis pathway is activated in tumors even in normoxia (Warburg effect), hypoxia could play a role in the initial switch to glycolysis. Stimulators other than hypoxia can be loss of p53 function or activation of the phosphoinositide-dependent kinase 1 (PDK1)/Akt pathway, which is an important regulator of multiple biological processes including cell growth, survival, and glucose metabolism (Young and Anderson 2008), and is negatively regulated by the tumor suppressor PTEN (Fig. 1.4).

These pathways might be of particular importance in breast cancer since PTEN is often mutated in breast cancer. Furthermore, epidermal growth factor (EGF) and human EGF receptor (HER2) downstream signaling pathways are via Raf/MEK/ERK and PI3K/PDK1/Akt (Schlessinger 2004). Thus nutrition and accumulation of damage, as an inevitable consequence are linked to pathways involved with breast cancer predisposition.

1.7 Drugs and their Molecular Targets for the Treatment of Breast Cancer

There are several molecular tools under investigation and a few already applied today in the treatment of breast cancer. The types of molecules that are being developed or tested and which target cellular signaling pathways are either small molecules, inhibitors of protein–protein interactions, kinase inhibitors, small molecules inhibiting specific kinases, histone deacetylase inhibitors acting on DNA and gene expression, or monoclonal antibodies.

Another class of treatments comprises cytotoxins acting on the microtubule cytoskeleton, as is the case for taxols, or on the structure and packaging of DNA with topoisomerase inhibitors. A third group of treatment tools are hormone or hormone-induced pathway inhibitors, such as somatostatin analogues for inhibition of somatostatin, aromatase inhibitors, or tamoxifen, an antiestrogen modulating ER activity.

Many targeted drugs in use for breast cancer treatment are directed against HER-2. HER-2 is a member of the (EGFR) family, composed of EGFR (ErbB1), HER-2 (ErbB2), HER-3 and HER-4. HER-2, overexpressed in many breast cancers, is targeted by either ectodomain-binding monoclonal antibodies (mAb) or by small molecule tyrosin kinase inhibitors (TKIs) competing with ATP for the cytoplasmic tyrosine kinase domain. The efficiency in anticancer treatment by the mAb transtuzumab and by the IKI lapatinib, both inhibiting HER-2 signaling, is investigated in many trials (Widakowich et al. 2007). Similarly, mAb cetuximab and TKIs gefitinib, canertinib, and erlotinib target the EGFR. Downstream effectors of this signaling pathway are also targets for inhibition, namely mTOR with rampamycin analogues (Fig. 1.4).

Interestingly, with the exception of aromatase inhibitors and tamoxifen and its analogues, none of the drugs in use or under trial have a functional link to estrogen or estrogen signaling pathways.

1.7.1 The Multi-Target Player Genistein

An important biological effect on the incidence of breast cancer is observed by the soy isoflavone genistein. The concentration of plasma genistein was inversely

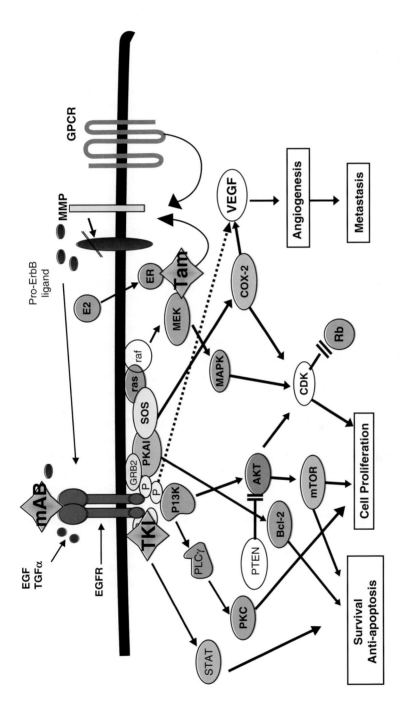

Fig. 1.4 Converging pathways of epidermal growth factor receptor (EGFR)/HER2 and estrogen signaling. Inhibitory drugs, such as mAB against the extracellular domain of EGFR or HER2, tyrosin kinase inhibitor (TKI) against the intracellular kinase domain, and Tamoxifen (Tam), inhibiting estrogen receptor (ER), are indicated. (Bianco et al. 2007)

correlated with the risk of developing breast cancer in Asian women (Lampe et al. 2007). Interestingly genistein has anticancer properties due to its antioxidant properties but also by interfering with signaling pathways that are activated in cancer and by activating apoptotic pathways.

Genistein binds to ER-α [alpha] and β [beta] and competes with more potent estrogens, such as β[beta]-estradiol. Interestingly, genistein inhibits the growth of both estrogen positive and negative breast cancer cells in vitro, presumably based on other interactions with cancer signaling pathways, namely by inhibiting protein-tyrosine kinase (PKT) and HER2 phosphorylation (Sakla et al. 2007). Importantly, genistein inhibits activation and nuclear localization of NF-KB (Davis et al. 1999) by inhibiting phosphorylation of the IkB, by IkB kinase a (IKKa) and b (IKKb), which when unphosphorylated sequesters NF-KB in the cytoplasm. Finally, genistein interferes with Akt signaling, which interferes with multiple survival pathways (El Touny and Banerjee 2007). Thus genistein acts by interfering with signaling in multiple ways, including those of inhibitory drug targets.

1.8   A Possible Link Between the Breast Cancer Predisposition Genes and Estrogen

The breast cancer predisposition genes BRCA1 and BRCA2 both collaborate in DNA repair and cell-cycle control. Both BRCA1 and BRCA2 bind to the repair protein RAD51, but, although linked to similar functions, BRCA1 and BRCA2 are structurally different and do not directly interact.

An important binding partner for BRCA1 is the BRCA1-associated protein BARD1 (Irminger-Finger and Jefford 2006). Indeed BARD1 stabilizes BRCA1, and most functions of BRCA1 depend on the formation of a BRCA1-BARD1 heterodimer, which has E3 ubiquitin ligase activity.

BARD1, although seemingly important in BRCA1-dependent tumor suppressor functions, is relatively rarely mutated in breast cancer. However, in all types of gynecological cancer isoforms of BARD1, derived from differential splicing, were detected (Li et al. 2007; Wu et al. 2006). These isoforms lack the BRCA1-interaction domain, are proproliferative, and their inhibition can block cancer cell growth, which defines them as oncogenic.

Since its cloning in 1994, research on BRCA1 has generated knowledge on its fundamental cellular functions involved in cell-cycle control and DNA repair, but the link between BRCA1 and estrogen signaling in breast tumorigenesis has remained uncertain.

Some studies indicate that BRCA1 physically interacts with ER-α [alpha] and inhibits its transcriptional activity (Fan et al. 2001) and inactivation of BRCA1 (by mutation or knockdown) confers activation of ER-α in the absence of ligand (Ma et al. 2006). It was thought for a long time that the presence of functional BRCA1 is important for keeping estrogen-signaling related cell proliferation under control. This thought is substantiated with the recent finding that the BRCA1–BARD1 heterodimer E3 ligase activity can target the ER-a, providing an explanation for a protective role of BRCA1 in breast cancer (Eakin et al. 2007).

Interestingly, BARD1 is an ER-response gene and induced by estrogen (Creekmore et al. 2007). However, the BRCA1 gene lacks a consensus estrogen response element (Hockings et al. 2008), but BRCA1 protein upregulation can be due to BARD1 up-regulation in response to estrogens.

The BRCA1 action on ER-α [alpha] requires BRCA1 binding to BARD1, but BARD1 expression is repressed in most breast and ovarian cancer and oncogenic isoforms, incapable of interacting with BRCA1 are expressed (Fig. 1.5). Since

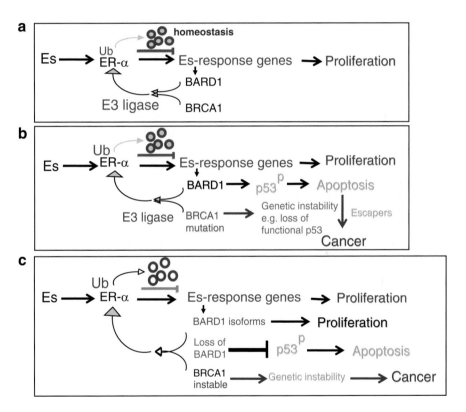

Fig. 1.5 Modulation of estrogen-ER signaling by BRCA1 and BARD1. (**a**) BARD1 and BRCA1 could act as E3 ligase in degradation of ER-α [alpha] (Eakin et al. 2007). BARD1 is induced by ER-α [alpha] (Creekmore et al. 2007), which could create a regulatory loop to control tissue homeostasis. (**b**) BRCA1 mutations lead to deficiency of E3 ligase function, but an increase of BARD1 over BRCA1, which could induce apoptosis (Irminger-Finger et al. 2001). However, genetic instability in the absence of BRCA1, permits cells to escape from apoptosis, consistent with loss of functional p53 in *BRCA1* knockout cells. (**c**) In breast and ovarian cancer loss of full length BARd1 and expression of isoform is observed, this should result in BRCA1 instability, loss of E3 ligase activity, loss of ER-α [alpha] degradation, loss of BARD1 apoptotic functions, increased expression of BARD1 isoforms, which are oncogenic (Li et al. 2007)

these isoforms are proproliferative, they might play an important role in ER-positive breast cancers.

A switch from FL BARD1 to BARD1 isoforms would lead to BRCA1 degradation, without affecting BRCA1 gene structure, upregulation of ER-α [alpha], in consequence up-regulation of PR, und proliferation.

This hypothesis puts in question genetic testing for BRCA1 mutations in tumors, which might be misleading. It also suggests that BARD1 isoforms might be important novel targets for treatment, since their inhibition provokes cell-proliferation arrest.

1.9   Conclusion

A strong link exists between breast cancer risk and estrogen exposure. As estrogens act as growth factors for hormone-dependent tissues, it is important to characterize the molecular signaling pathways involved. With increasing age and time of exposure to estrogen the associated breast cancer risk increases, but also the accumulating damage due to the exposure to oxidative stress. In addition, the biology of breast tissue itself changes with age, and the molecular pathways relevant for tissue aging will influence the impact of risk factors and might even represent additional risk factors.

Thus, what drives cancer might ultimately come down to a few genes, and what promotes cancer might be specific for the organ.

This was nicely shown with the comparison of specific breast cancer gene signatures that converge on signaling hubs (Shen et al. 2008). High concordance of several breast-cancer gene signatures for predicting disease recurrence despite minimal overlap of the gene lists was shown. Interestingly, the signatures did not identify the same set of genes but converged on the activation of a similar set of oncogenic and clinically relevant pathways. A clear and consistent pattern across the four breast cancer signatures is the activation of the estrogen-signaling pathway. Other common features include BRCA1-regulated pathway, extracellular matrix protease inhibitor (RECK) pathways, and insulin signaling associated with the ER-positive disease signatures, all providing possible explanations for the prediction concordance (Shen et al. 2008).

Finally, the notion of age-dependent differences is not integrated in these studies, but signaling pathways involved in aging are comprised in the common signature. Thus, analyses that pay attention to and integrate information for dissecting senescence/cancer pathways remain to be performed.

References

Allsopp RC, Chang E, Kashefi-Aazam M, Rogaev EI, Piatyszek MA, Shay JW, Harley CB (1995) Telomere shortening is associated with cell division in vitro and in vivo. Exp Cell Res 220: 194–200

Amundson SA, Myers TG, Fornace AJ Jr (1998) Roles for p53 in growth arrest and apoptosis: putting on the brakes after genotoxic stress. Oncogene 17:3287–3299

Artandi SE, DePinho RA (2000) Mice without telomerase: What can they teach us about human cancer? Nat Med 6:852–855

Barlow WE, White E, Ballard-Barbash R, Vacek PM, Titus-Ernstoff L, Carney PA, Tice JA, Buist DS, Geller BM, Rosenberg R et al (2006) Prospective breast cancer risk prediction model for women undergoing screening mammography. J Natl Cancer Inst 98:1204–1214

Benz CC, Thor AD, Eppenberger-Castori S, Eppenberger U, Moore D 3rd (2003) Understanding the age dependency of breast cancer biomarkers. Adv Gerontol 11:117–120

Bianco R, Gelardi T, Damiano V, Ciardiello F, Tortora G (2007) Rational bases for the development of EGFR inhibitors for cancer treatment. Int J Biochem Cell Biol 39:1416–1431

Campisi J (2001) Cellular senescence as a tumor-suppressor mechanism. Trends Cell Biol 11:S27–S31

Campisi J (2003) Cellular senescence and apoptosis: how cellular responses might influence aging phenotypes. Exp Gerontol 38:5–11

Chao C, Herr D, Chun J, Xu Y (2006) Ser18 and 23 phosphorylation is required for p53-dependent apoptosis and tumor suppression. Embo J 25:2615–2622

Collaborative Group on Hormonal Factors in Breast Cancer (1997) Breast cancer and hormone replacement therapy: collaborative reanalysis of data from 51 epidemiological studies of 52,705 women with breast cancer and 108,411 women without breast cancer. Lancet 350: 1047–1059

Collaborative Group on Hormonal Factors in Breast Cancer (2002) Breast cancer and breastfeeding: collaborative reanalysis of individual data from 47 epidemiological studies in 30 countries, including 50302 women with breast cancer and 96973 women without the disease. Lancet 360:187–195

Creekmore AL, Ziegler YS, Boney JL, Nardulli AM (2007) Estrogen receptor alpha regulates expression of the breast cancer 1 associated ring domain 1 (BARD1) gene through intronic DNA sequence. Mol Cell Endocrinol 267:106–115

Davis JN, Kucuk O, Sarkar FH (1999) Genistein inhibits NF-kappa B activation in prostate cancer cells. Nutr Cancer 35:167–174

DePinho RA (2000) The age of cancer. Nature 408:248–254

Eakin CM, Maccoss MJ, Finney GL, Klevit RE (2007) Estrogen receptor alpha is a putative substrate for the BRCA1 ubiquitin ligase. Proc Natl Acad Sci U S A 104:5794–5799

El Touny LH, Banerjee PP (2007) Akt GSK-3 pathway as a target in genistein-induced inhibition of TRAMP prostate cancer progression toward a poorly differentiated phenotype. Carcinogenesis 28:1710–1717

Eliassen AH, Colditz GA, Rosner B, Willett WC, Hankinson SE (2006) Adult weight change and risk of postmenopausal breast cancer. Jama 296:193–201

Eppenberger-Castori S, Moore DH Jr, Thor AD, Edgerton SM, Kueng W, Eppenberger U, Benz CC (2002) Age-associated biomarker profiles of human breast cancer. Int J Biochem Cell Biol 34:1318–1330

Fan S, Ma YX, Wang C, Yuan RQ, Meng Q, Wang JA, Erdos M, Goldberg ID, Webb P, Kushner PJ et al (2001) Role of direct interaction in BRCA1 inhibition of estrogen receptor activity. Oncogene 20:77–87

Feki A, Jefford CE, Berardi P, Wu JY, Cartier L, Krause KH, Irminger-Finger I (2005) BARD1 induces apoptosis by catalysing phosphorylation of p53 by DNA-damage response kinase. Oncogene 24:3726–3736

Feng L, Hollstein M, Xu Y (2006) Ser46 phosphorylation regulates p53-dependent apoptosis and replicative senescence. Cell Cycle 5:2812–2819

Ferron S, Mira H, Franco S, Cano-Jaimez M, Bellmunt E, Ramirez C, Farinas I, Blasco MA (2004) Telomere shortening and chromosomal instability abrogates proliferation of adult but not embryonic neural stem cells. Development 131:4059–4070

Ford D, Easton DF, Stratton M, Narod S, Goldgar D, Devilee P, Bishop DT, Weber B, Lenoir G, Chang-Claude J et al (1998) Genetic heterogeneity and penetrance analysis of the BRCA1 and

BRCA2 genes in breast cancer families. The Breast Cancer Linkage Consortium. Am J Hum Genet 62:676–689

Gatenby RA, Gillies RJ (2007) Glycolysis in cancer: a potential target for therapy. Int J Biochem Cell Biol 39:1358–1366

Hamajima N, Hirose K, Tajima K, Rohan T, Calle EE, Heath CW Jr, Coates RJ, Liff JM, Talamini R, Chantarakul N et al (2002) Alcohol, tobacco and breast cancer—collaborative reanalysis of individual data from 53 epidemiological studies, including 58, 515 women with breast cancer and 95, 067 women without the disease. Br J Cancer 87:1234–1245

Hayflick L (1985) The cell biology of aging. Clin Geriatr Med 1:15–27

Hockings JK, Degner SC, Morgan SS, Kemp MQ, Romagnolo DF (2008) Involvement of a specificity proteins-binding element in regulation of basal and estrogen-induced transcription activity of the BRCA1 gene. Breast Cancer Res 10:R29

Hulka B S, Moorman P G (2001) Breast cancer: hormones and other risk factors. Maturitas 38: 103–113; discussion 113–106

Irminger-Finger I, Jefford CE (2006) Is there more to BARD1 than BRCA1? Nat Rev Cancer 6:382–391

Irminger-Finger I, Leung WC, Li J, Dubois-Dauphin M, Harb J, Feki A, Jefford CE, Soriano JV, Jaconi M, Montesano R, Krause KH (2001) Identification of BARD1 as mediator between proapoptotic stress and p53-dependent apoptosis. Mol Cell 8:1255–1266

Itahana K, Zou Y, Itahana Y, Martinez JL, Beausejour C, Jacobs JJ, Van Lohuizen M, Band V, Campisi J, Dimri GP (2003) Control of the replicative life span of human fibroblasts by p16 and the polycomb protein Bmi-1. Mol Cell Biol 23:389–401

Janzen V, Forkert R, Fleming HE, Saito Y, Waring MT, Dombkowski DM, Cheng T, DePinho RA, Sharpless NE, Scadden DT (2006) Stem-cell ageing modified by the cyclin-dependent kinase inhibitor p16INK4a. Nature 443:421–426

Jiang H, Luo S, Li H (2005) Cdk5 activator-binding protein C53 regulates apoptosis induced by genotoxic stress via modulating the G2/M DNA damage checkpoint. J Biol Chem 280: 20651–20659

Kajstura J, Pertoldi B, Leri A, Beltrami CA, Deptala A, Darzynkiewicz Z, Anversa P (2000) Telomere shortening is an in vivo marker of myocyte replication and aging. Am J Pathol 156:813–819

Kamijo T, van de Kamp E, Chong MJ, Zindy F, Diehl JA, Sherr CJ, McKinnon PJ (1999) Loss of the ARF tumor suppressor reverses premature replicative arrest but not radiation hypersensitivity arising from disabled atm function. Cancer Res 59:2464–2469

Kaneshiro K, Tsutsumi S, Tsuji S, Shirahige K, Aburatani H (2007) An integrated map of p53-binding sites and histone modification in the human ENCODE regions. Genomics 89:178–188

Kari C, Chan TO, Rocha de Quadros M, Rodeck U (2003) Targeting the epidermal growth factor receptor in cancer: apoptosis takes center stage. Cancer Res 63:1–5

Kubbutat MH, Jones SN, Vousden KH (1997) Regulation of p53 stability by Mdm2. Nature 387:299–303

Lampe JW, Nishino Y, Ray RM, Wu C, Li W, Lin MG, Gao DL, Hu Y, Shannon J, Stalsberg H et al (2007) Plasma isoflavones and fibrocystic breast conditions and breast cancer among women in Shanghai, China. Cancer Epidemiol Biomarkers Prev 16:2579–2586

Langen RC, Korn SH, Wouters EF (2003) ROS in the local and systemic pathogenesis of COPD. Free Radic Biol Med 35:226–235

Li L, Ryser S, Dizin E, Pils D, Krainer M, Jefford CE, Bertoni F, Zeillinger R, Irminger-Finger I (2007) Oncogenic BARD1 isoforms expressed in gynecological cancers. Cancer Res 67:11876–11885

Ma Y, Katiyar P, Jones LP, Fan S, Zhang Y, Furth PA, Rosen EM (2006) The breast cancer susceptibility gene BRCA1 regulates progesterone receptor signaling in mammary epithelial cells. Mol Endocrinol 20:14–34

Megyesi J, Udvarhelyi N, Safirstein RL, Price PM (1996) The p53-independent activation of transcription of p21 WAF1/CIP1/SDI1 after acute renal failure. Am J Physiol 271:F1211–F1216

Metcalfe JA, Parkhill J, Campbell L, Stacey M, Biggs P, Byrd PJ, Taylor AM (1996) Accelerated telomere shortening in ataxia telangiectasia. Nat Genet 13:350–353

Moll UM, Zaika A (2001) Nuclear and mitochondrial apoptotic pathways of p53. FEBS Lett 493:65–69

Palacios J, Robles-Frias MJ, Castilla MA, Lopez-Garcia MA, Benitez J (2008) The molecular pathology of hereditary breast cancer. Pathobiology 75:85–94

Park IK, Morrison SJ, Clarke MF (2004) Bmi1, stem cells, and senescence regulation. J Clin Invest 113:175–179

Petz LN, Nardulli AM (2000) Sp1 binding sites and an estrogen response element half-site are involved in regulation of the human progesterone receptor A promoter. Mol Endocrinol 14:972–985

Quong J, Eppenberger-Castori S, Moore D 3rd, Scott GK, Birrer MJ, Kueng W, Eppenberger U, Benz CC (2002) Age-dependent changes in breast cancer hormone receptors and oxidant stress markers. Breast Cancer Res Treat 76:221–236

Ramsey MR, Sharpless NE (2006) ROS as a tumour suppressor? Nat Cell Biol 8:1213–1215

Rizo A, Vellenga E, de Haan G, Schuringa JJ (2006) Signaling pathways in self-renewing hematopoietic and leukemic stem cells: do all stem cells need a niche? Hum Mol Genet 15(2): R210–R219

Sakla MS, Shenouda NS, Ansell PJ, Macdonald RS, Lubahn DB (2007) Genistein affects HER2 protein concentration, activation, and promoter regulation in BT-474 human breast cancer cells. Endocrine 32:69–78

Schlessinger J (2004) Common and distinct elements in cellular signaling via EGF and FGF receptors. Science 306:1506–1507

Serrano M, Lin AW, McCurrach ME, Beach D, Lowe SW (1997) Oncogenic ras provokes premature cell senescence associated with accumulation of p53 and p16INK4a. Cell 88:593–602

Shantakumar S, Terry MB, Teitelbaum SL, Britton JA, Millikan RC, Moorman PG, Neugut AI, Gammon MD (2007) Reproductive factors and breast cancer risk among older women. Breast Cancer Res Treat 102:365–374

Sharpless NE, DePinho RA (2002) p53: good cop/bad cop. Cell 110:9–12

Shen R, Chinnaiyan AM, Ghosh D (2008) Pathway analysis reveals functional convergence of gene expression profiles in breast cancer. BMC Med Genomics 1:28

Sherr CJ, McCormick F (2002) The RB and p53 pathways in cancer. Cancer Cell 2:103–112

Singletary KW, Gapstur SM (2001) Alcohol and breast cancer: review of epidemiologic and experimental evidence and potential mechanisms. Jama 286:2143–2151

Smith KJ, Diwan H, Skelton H (2003) Death receptors and their role in dermatology, with particular focus on tumor necrosis factor-related apoptosis-inducing ligand receptors. Int J Dermatol 42:3–17

Song YS, Lee BY, Hwang ES (2005) Dinstinct ROS and biochemical profiles in cells undergoing DNA damage-induced senescence and apoptosis. Mech Ageing Dev 126:580–590

Tyner SD, Venkatachalam S, Choi J, Jones S, Ghebranious N, Igelmann H, Lu X, Soron G, Cooper B, Brayton C et al (2002) p53 mutant mice that display early ageing-associated phenotypes. Nature 415:45–53

Watters D (1999) Molecular mechanisms of ionizing radiation-induced apoptosis. Immunol Cell Biol 77:263–271

Widakowich C, de Azambuja E, Gil T, Cardoso F, Dinh P, Awada A, Piccart-Gebhart M (2007) Molecular targeted therapies in breast cancer: where are we now? Int J Biochem Cell Biol 39:1375–1387

Wu JY, Vlastos AT, Pelte MF, Caligo MA, Bianco A, Krause KH, Laurent GJ, Irminger-Finger I (2006) Aberrant expression of BARD1 in breast and ovarian cancers with poor prognosis. Int J Cancer 118:1215–1226

Yamaguchi H, Chen J, Bhalla K, Wang HG (2004) Regulation of Bax activation and apoptotic response to microtubule-damaging agents by p53 transcription-dependent and -independent pathways. J Biol Chem 279:39431–39437

Yin Y, Stephen CW, Luciani MG, Fahraeus R (2002) p53 Stability and activity is regulated by Mdm2-mediated induction of alternative p53 translation products. Nat Cell Biol 4:462–467

Young CD, Anderson SM (2008) Sugar and fat—that's where it's at: metabolic changes in tumors. Breast Cancer Res 10:202

Zhang X, Mar V, Zhou W, Harrington L, Robinson MO (1999) Telomere shortening and apoptosis in telomerase-inhibited human tumor cells. Genes Dev 13:2388–2399

Chapter 2
Tumor Biology and Pathology

Virginie Durbecq and Denis Larsimont

2.1 Introduction

Age is one of the most important risk factors for human malignancies, including breast cancer. Approximately 50% of all new breast cancers occur in women aged 65 years or more, a proportion which is likely to grow because of increased life expectancy and therefore increased proportion of elderly subjects in the general population. The 10-year probability of developing invasive breast cancer increases from less than 1.5% at age 40 to about 3% at age 50 and to more than 4% by age 70, resulting in a cumulative lifetime of 13.2% (1/8 of the women) (Smigal et al. 2006).

Age at diagnosis has been shown to be an independent indicator of breast cancer prognosis and despite the fact that breast cancer incidence increases with the age of the patient, it is generally stated that older women develop cancer with a relatively slower growth rate and that their prognosis is therefore better than that of the general population. Several publications have reported that advanced age is associated with favorable biological features, including a higher proportion of estrogen receptor (ER)-positive tumors.

Nevertheless, even if an increased incidence of cancers of favorable prognosis is observed among older women, tumors known to have an aggressive behavior occur in all age groups, especially ER-positive tumor with high histological grade (Durbecq et al. 2008).

2.2 Clinical Stage at Diagnosis

The majority of both young and old patients with breast cancer present with Stage I or II disease. Nevertheless, breast cancer in most elderly patients is commonly diagnosed at a more advanced clinical stage. The rationale is that women over the

V. Durbecq (✉)
Pathology Department, Jules Bordet Institute, 121 Boulevard de Waterloo,
1000, Brussels, Belgium
e-mail: virginie.durbecq@bordet.be

M.W. Reed and R.A. Audisio (eds.), *Management of Breast Cancer in Older Women*,
DOI 10.1007/978-1-84800-265-4_2, © Springer-Verlag London Limited 2011

age of 70 remain underrepresented in screening mammography populations resulting in a delayed breast cancer diagnosis. Importantly, the association between length of patient delay and late stage diagnosis was observed mainly among women with more aggressive poorly differentiated breast tumors.

Thus, older women represent a group in which considerable impact of the screening might still be made. Moreover, breast tissue becomes less dense with age, resulting in an improved positive predictive value of an abnormal mammogram in women over 65 years of age. In a well-organized, population-based breast cancer screening program, mammography screening up to the age of 75 years could then be appropriate (Table 2.1).

2.3   Distribution with Age of Pathological Subtype

Infiltrating ductal carcinoma remains the most common histologic subtype of breast cancer diagnosed regardless of the age of the patient. Several studies did not find a significant association between breast cancer tumor histology and increasing age of the patients. Nevertheless, tumors of the lobular subtype were almost absent in patients younger than 50 years and mucinous carcinomas were observed more frequently in the elderly (Durbecq et al. 2008; Evron et al. 2006). These results confirmed that lobular tumors are associated with less aggressive biological characteristics than the ductal ones (mostly estrogen receptor positive, less grade 3) (Durbecq et al. 2008). Moreover, tumors with mucinous or tubular histology are less likely associated with nodal invasion than breast cancer histological subtypes (Caywood et al. 2005).

2.4   Tumor Size

All but a few studies assessing the effect of age on tumor size have demonstrated that patients older than age 70 were more likely to have larger tumors (Molino et al. 2006). The main explanation is probably because of the delay in diagnosing cancer as a result of reduced screening mammography. Consequently, elderly patients were more likely to undergo mastectomy. These results were corroborated by the fact that no difference in tumor size was observed according to the age of diagnosis before the widespread use of mammography (therefore patients with clinically detected disease).

As mentioned above, the association between diagnostic delay and increasing tumor size is also associated with aggressive characteristics, i.e., higher proliferation rate, higher histological grade, as well as nodal invasion. Consequently, we observed that a significant number of the tumors developed by elderly women, even if they were ER-positive, presented aggressive biological characteristics (Durbecq et al. 2008). Some studies reported that these tumors are biologically less aggressive than the ER-negative breast tumors developed by young women (Molino et al. 2006) whereas others reported that breast carcinomas are not more indolent in the elderly than in younger patients.

Table 2.1 Breast cancer screening guidelines

Medicare	American Academy of Family Physicians	American College of Obstetricians and Gynecologists	American Cancer Society	American Medical Association	Canadian Task Force on Preventive Health Care	US preventive Services Task Force	Overall Recommendation
Yearly after 40 years	Every 1–2 years for women 50–69 years	Every 1–2 years after 50 years	Yearly after 40 years	Yearly after 50 years	Every 1–2 years for women 50–69 years	Every 1–2 years for women 50–69 years	After 70 years risk factor associated with BC should be explored every 1–2 years to discuss screening and to address the risks and benefits associated with screening as well as the individual's co-morbidities, life expectancy, health status, and quality of life.

There are numerous published recommendations for cancer screening among older adults. However, the recommendations established by the United States Preventive Services Task Force (USPSTF) are the only ones that are solely evidence-based. Recognizing the heterogeneity of older adults, it is critical to consider the overall health status of the individual. With permisison from Resnick and McLeskey 2008

2.5   Nodal Status and Vascular Invasion

No age relationship for nodal involvement or risk of distant metastasis was observed in breast cancer patients except for those patients before aged under 40 who developed more aggressive ER-negative tumors which were more likely to metastasize. Nevertheless, an increased incidence of node involvement was reported in patients older than 70 (Molino et al. 2006) associated with an increased incidence of ER-positive, high-grade tumors. This result was consistent with the fact that tumor size and histological grade were correlated with nodal invasion in older women (Durbecq et al. 2008). Actually, we observed that the metastatic potential of breast cancer in the elderly does not differ significantly from the one of the global population when stratified according to tumor size (Durbecq et al. 2008); a result which does not support the assumption that breast cancers are more indolent in elderly patients.

Elderly patients are ideal candidates for sentinel lymph node biopsy. This technique is now widely considered as an acceptable treatment option in patients of all ages with tumor size less than 2–3 cm and no clinical evidence of axillary involvement. Such biopsies could significantly affect subsequent treatment decision in older patients including adjuvant systemic treatment. Controversy exists regarding the need for complementary axillary dissection in case of sentinel lymph node positivity. As the risk of macroscopic disease is limited, the nomogram developed by Van Zee et al. (Van Zee et al. 2003) which predicts the risk of subsequent nodal metastasis on the basis of the sentinel lymph node status and of the tumor characteristics could be useful when deciding whether to do a completion axillary dissection in older patients.

2.6   Aging and Endocrine-Dependence of Breast Cancer

Almost all reported studies demonstrate that elderly women predominantly develop ER-positive breast cancers and therefore present a better prognosis compared to young patients. Nevertheless, some elderly patients develop ER-negative tumors or ER-positive and high-grade tumors.

When patient's age and menopausal status were analyzed together, age was found to be the primary determinant of increased ER concentration. This result was in agreement with the observation that no association was observed between tumor biology and the menopausal status (Durbecq et al. 2008). Actually, the natural peri-menopausal decline in ovarian-produced estrogen serum level does not fully account for the age-related change in ER-regulated mammary epithelial pathways. Indeed, the marked age-related increase in stromal and epithelial aromatase expression produces postmenopausal mammary gland estrogen levels comparable with those measured in pre-menopausal women.

ER inducible markers such as progesterone receptor (PR) pS2, Bc12 and cathepsin D are overexpressed in tumors. However, contrary to ER, they show no age-associated changes in their expression (Yau et al. 2007), suggesting a specific reduction in ER signaling in breast cancer from older patients. However, several groups reported that patients older than 40 years more frequently develop PR-positive tumors (Durbecq et al. 2008; Molino et al. 2006); a pronounced increase in PR content being found in patients older than 75 years. As a result, we observed a higher proportion of ER- and PR-positive tumors in the older patients in line with the inverse correlation observed between HER2 overexpression and PR positivity arising after age 40. On the other hand, we also observed a higher proportion of ER-positive but PR-negative tumors in patients older than 50 years (Yau et al. 2007). This last data may be explained by the fact that breast cancers from women older than 40 years old lose the SP1 DNA binding function necessary for PR gene expression.

Alongside the increase in ER-positive tumors with increased age, the percentage of ER- and PR-negative tumors decreased with increasing age as did the fraction of ER-negative but PR-positive tumors (Durbecq et al. 2008; Molino et al. 2006). These latter tumor types, considered as more aggressive and of worse prognosis than the ER & PR negative ones, represent 12% of the highly aggressive ER- and HER2-negative breast cancer.

Finally, two estrogen growth-regulating genes, GREB1 and AREG, known to induce cell proliferation upon ER activation, show lower expression in older cohort consistent with a recent study demonstrating a negative correlation between these estrogen inducible genes and age (Creighton et al. 2006).

In elderly women with hormone-sensitive breast cancer, hormone treatment decisions should be based on a risk–benefit analysis taking into account the low relapse rate within the first 10 years, the potential reduction in ipsilateral and contralateral breast cancer relapse, the patient's life expectancy, and treatment-related adverse events. Data show that there are no age-related differences in the efficacy of tamoxifen and aromatase inhibitors. Aromatase inhibitors are slightly more effective than tamoxifen but elderly patients are more vulnerable to some adverse events. Importantly, ageing has been shown to be related to alteration in the metabolism of tamoxifen, resulting in higher levels of tamoxifen and its metabolites in elderly women. However, a lower dose of tamoxifen might prove to be as useful as and potentially less toxic than standard doses.

Elderly patients with ER- and PR-negative tumors should not receive hormone treatment. Treatment with adjuvant chemotherapy should not be an age-based decision but should take into account individual patients' estimated absolute benefit, life expectancy, treatment tolerance, and preference, older patients with node-positive tumors potentially deriving the largest benefit in survival gain.

2.7 Aging and Growth Factor Receptors Dependence

Tissue ageing has a great influence on the molecular subtype of breast cancer developed as clearly illustrated by the fact that the growth factor receptors HER2 and EGFR are linearly correlated with the age of the patient at diagnosis (Durbecq et al. 2008; Molino et al. 2006). Consistent with the declining tumor growth rate, HER2 and EGFR expression declines significantly in tumors from patients older than 40 (Durbecq et al. 2008; Molino et al. 2006). The frequency of tumor co-positivity and the correlation between EGFR+ and HER2+ also declines continuously and significantly with age. In agreement with the results above, an age-related inverse correlation was reported between the hormonal receptors and HER2 after age 45.

Even though incidence of HER2-positive tumors decreases with the patient age, some elderly patients do develop HER2-positive tumors. In contrast to younger patients in whom HER2-positive tumors are associated with ER-negative status, HER2-positive tumors in elderly patients were paradoxically ER-positive (Poltinnikov et al. 2006).

HER2, EGFR, and the biomarker combination EGFR/HER2 co-positivity significantly predicts for poor survival, HER2, and/or EGFR-positive tumor being more frequent in the population of poorly differentiated and large size tumors. In the subgroup of elderly patients, Poltinnikov et al. (Poltinnikov et al. 2006) reported no association between HER2 amplification and histology, vascular invasion, age, ER status, presence of DCIS and comedo-necrosis or second primaries including breast second primaries. However, HER2 positivity was associated with high-grade, T2 stage and positive nodal status. Therefore, in elderly patients, HER2 predicts the development of combined nodal and distant failure, and negatively influences the cause-specific survival in elderly patients (Poltinnikov et al. 2006).

Therefore, similarly to the trend in younger patients, HER2 positivity may be used to consider more aggressive treatment strategies in elderly patients. Moreover, in the absence of cardiac contraindications, adjuvant trastuzumab should be offered to older patients with HER2-positive breast cancer when chemotherapy is indicated, but cardiac monitoring is essential.

2.8   Proliferation and Genetic Instability

Contrary to the expectation that age-associated epithelial cancers arise due to time-dependent accumulation of genomic mutations, several studies reported that genetic instability biomarkers such as high nuclear grade, aneuploidy, HER2 amplification, and p53 mutation demonstrate a strong inverse correlation with ageing. These results are in agreement with the fact that ER is inversely correlated with abnormal p53. All indices of tumor growth and cellular turnover are also substantially under-expressed in these tumors; S phase fraction, mitotic index, and Ki-67/MIB1 declining more rapidly after age 60 (Durbecq et al. 2008; Molino et al. 2006).

Nevertheless, the pattern of genetic alteration (absence of steroid receptor, tumor aneuploidy, p53 overexpression, and weak or absent bcl2 expression) associated with a rapid proliferation is maintained in some elderly patients. Thus, despite the overall decrease of tumor proliferation in the elderly population, we were able to identify a nonnegligible proportion of high-grade and highly proliferating tumors in the subgroup of patient older than 70 (Durbecq et al. 2008). These results are in agreement with several studies that reported that tumors from elderly women were not always well-differentiated and are more likely to have nodal invasion.

Biological aggressiveness could then be defined on the basis of such features even for tumors from elderly women. Less than 30% of elderly patients presented at diagnosis four or more factors for which an unfavorable prognosis is well recognized (tumor size >2 cm, ER-, high proliferation) or putatively recognized (p53 overexpression or absent/weak bcl-2 expression) compared to about 50% of patients 34 years old or younger, and 40% of patients 35–64 years. The fact that elderly patients appeared to have a better prognosis compared to younger ones is only relative to the higher proportion of low-risk cancer among these patients. Therefore, therapies targeting tumor cell proliferation, either with cytotoxic agents, ionizing radiation, or targeted therapies toward growth factor signaling pathways should not be less efficient in tumors growing in older patients. These results are corroborated by the fact that adjuvant chemotherapy improves overall survival in elderly patients with ER-negative tumors and that the benefit was similar for women above and below the age of 70 years.

2.9 Apoptosis

A number of studies have shown a reduced apoptotic response to DNA damage with increasing age in rodents, suggesting that the mammary epithelium may be less capable of eliminating aberrant cells with age (Rose-Hellekant et al. 2006). The finding of a statistically significant reduction of the apoptotic response with age in humans supports the hypothesis that such reduction may play a significant role in the age-related increase of cancer. A significant reduction in mean apoptotic response was reported with increasing age in breast cancer patients lacking P53 mutations as well as normal controls. Moreover, after adjusting for age, cancer patients showed a significantly reduced apoptotic response compared to normal controls (Camplejohn et al. 2003).

P53, the guardian of the genome also acts on apoptosis through the induction of bax and the repression of bcl-2. P53 positivity/mutation and bcl2 expression were respectively inversely and directly associated with patient's age; P53 positivity and apoptotic index decreasing faster after age 50. Aging was also associated with a lower sensitivity of the potent anti-apoptotic gene, bcl-2 to pro-apoptotic stimuli (Warner and Hodes 1997).

2.10 Angiogenesis

Angiogenesis, the development of new vessels from preexisting vasculature, is reduced with aging and has been suggested to constitute a possible mechanism of the reduced tumor progression rate in older patients; the degree of tumor progression correlating with the extent of angiogenesis. In postmenopausal patients with breast cancer, angiogenesis in tumors decreases with advanced age. It has been suggested that decreased concentrations of growth factors that enhance angiogenesis as well as increased concentrations of angiogenesis inhibitors arise as a protective response against the increase incidence of tumors with ageing (Kudravi and Reed 2000; Nickoloff et al. 2004).

Alterations in angiogenesis noted in several animal models include endothelial cell dysfunction, reduced expression of the growth factor VEGF, TGF-β [beta] 1 and FGF expression, and increased expression of the modulator of the angiogenic response (TSP-1 and 2) in the aged animal compared to young control (Sadoun and Reed 2003). A defective inflammatory response in aged mice and humans has also been reported to slow angiogenesis during cutaneous wound healing via both direct (lack of angiogenic chemokines) and indirect (deficient induction of angiogenic growth factors by inflammatory mediators) mechanisms. The change in immune response was associated with delayed infiltration of monocytes/macrophages and lymphocytes as well as deficient expression of endothelial cell adhesion molecules (Swift et al. 2001).

These results demonstrate that delayed angiogenesis in aged tissues does not merely reflect a slower model of angiogenesis in young tissues, but is due to the fact that multiple pathways are affected. These data were relying on the fact that an anti-angiogenic drug was found to be more efficient against tumors of old animals (Kaptzan et al. 2006).

2.11   Immune Regulation

As we age, the efficiency of our immune system declines especially after about age 65, reducing the effectiveness of therapies that rely on provoking immune system responses. Moreover, it has been suggested that age-acquired immune deficiency is related to the increased incidence of cancer in older patients.

A decrease in the number of naive T cells at older age is considered to play a role in the age-related decline in T cell responses, responsible for the well-described decline in vaccine responsiveness in elderly patients. A significant decrease of the percentage of CD4+ T lymphocytes was observed in the lymph nodes of aged mice as well as in the peripheral blood of BALB/c and C57B6 mice as a function of age. Dominguez et al. (Dominguez and Lustgarten 2008) demonstrated that T regulatory (T-reg) cells accumulate in the aging immune system and that there is a direct correlation between T-reg accumulation and immune system decline. New data also indicate that other molecules important to immune system regulation are disrupted in the elderly. Conversely, Gravekamp et al. (Gravekamp et al. 2004) reported that CD8 cells were attracted by the tumors in old mice.

Thus, some adjuvants with the potential to stimulate the immune system in young patients may not necessarily be effective in the older patients.

2.12   Inflammatory Pathway

Chronic inflammation, as age-related, low-grade systemic inflammation, may promote carcinogenesis and predispose an individual to cancer (Vasto et al. 2009; Balkwill et al. 2005; Schwertfeger et al. 2006). Free radicals released at the site of inflammation are involved in carcinogenesis, not only damaging DNA but also modifying cancer-related proteins and regulating transcription. The microenvironment is characterized by the presence of smoldering inflammation, fuelled primarily by stromal leukocytes and by hypoxic conditions. Associated macrophages are a major player in the inflammatory response and produce a multitude of growth factors for epithelial and endothelial cells as well as inflammatory cytokines and chemokines that affect angiogenesis and may enhance cell proliferation, promotion, and eventually progression of cancer cells. In addition, immunosuppressive mediators released by local inflammatory or tumor cells extinguish host-mediated, anti-tumor responses and facilitate tumor progression (Mantovani et al. 2008; Sica et al. 2008).

Increased levels of inflammatory markers (IL6, CRP, TNFalpha) are associated with increased risk of cancer and linked to the presence of metastases (Il'Yasova et al. 2005). In particular, elevated levels of CRP and IL6 are associated with poor prognosis in metastatic breast cancer (Zhang and Adachi 1999). Moreover, PAI and uPA, two markers of poor prognosis for breast cancer and whose activation is regulated by inflammation, are highly expressed by fibroblasts and myofibroblasts with ageing (Dublin et al. 2000; Offersen et al. 2003). uPA/PAI-1 deregulation may therefore influence intra-tumoral signaling and alter the tumor microenvironment leading us to speculate that the microenvironment is more permissive to tumors in elderly patients.

2.13   Micro-environment

While both inflammation and wound healing are causally involved in cancer, senescent fibroblasts may also favor disease development by altering tumor microenvironment. Senescent human fibroblasts can enhance proliferation in vitro and tumorigenic potential in vivo of premalignant and malignant mammary epithelial cells, whilst normal mammary cells are not affected. This mechanism appears to be due to both soluble and insoluble factors (cytokines, epithelial growth factors, matrix metalloproteinases) secreted by senescent fibroblasts (Fig. 2.1). Parrinello et al. (Parrinello et al. 2005) demonstrated that premalignant mammary epithelial cells exposed to senescent human fibroblasts in mice irreversibly lose differentiated properties, become invasive, and undergo full malignant transformation. As no variation was observed in angiogenesis, invasive or proteolytic markers, they speculated that the senescent fibroblast may not alter the biological profile of the malignant epithelium.

All these results lead us to hypothesize that in young women the tissue microenvironment (senescent fibroblast, inflammation) as well as the immune system are poorly permissive to the development of breast cancer, thus influencing the development of high-grade ER-negative cells. This assumption is corroborated by the fact that an association was noted between high-grade tumors and the degree of lympho-plasmacytic reaction, considered to be an expression of host defense reaction. On the contrary, in older women the tissue microenvironment might be more permissive allowing less aggressive ER-positive cells to establish. We may also speculate that the tumor microenvironment influences tumor proliferation as all

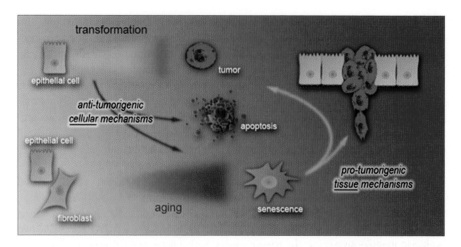

Fig. 2.1 Microenvironment and tumor: the impact of ageing. Through accumulated genetic mutations cell division can transform cells, leading to tumors. Nature stops this tumorigenesis process through apoptosis or senescence. However, as organisms age, the accumulation of senescent cells can create a pro-tumorigenic tissue environment. Courtesy of Judith Campisi

tumors developed by young women were more proliferating than the ones developed by older women, whatever the subtype considered (Durbecq et al. 2008).

2.14 Genetic Profiling

Genomic and transcriptome changes associated with aging were identified using DNA and RNA prospectively collected from stage- and grade-matched ER-positive breast cancer from younger (age ≤45) and older women (age ≥70) (Yau et al. 2007). Array CGH confirmed that ER-positive breast cancers were composed of two basic genotypes: a subtype characterized by few genomic copy number changes and a mixed amplifier subtype characterized by recurrent amplifications but no genomic subtypes showed any particular age bias. Direct comparison of the two age cohorts revealed also no significant differences in the fraction of genome altered.

In contrast, microarray profiling showed an average of 65-fold range in ER transcript levels across the entire collection of ER-positive breast cancer, with the older cohort showing significantly higher ER levels as compared with the younger cohort. Reported gene signatures representing luminal, proliferation, and MAPK markers were tested for their enrichment in the age-stratified cohorts and only the proliferation gene signature showed any significant age bias being more highly expressed in the younger cohort (Yau et al. 2007).

Of the 75 genes differentially expressed between younger and older cohorts, 75% would appear to be independent of menopausal status and therefore potentially informative of age-related differences in ER-positive breast cancer biology. A comprehensive database search confirmed that at least 40% of these genes have been reported to have a direct link with malignancy. Enrichment of cell-cycle-associated genes was observed in the younger patients whereas older patients showed differential expression of negative cell-cycle regulators and developmentally essential homeobox genes. HOXB7, in particular, known to be dependant on stromal signaling is transcriptionally upregulated in breast cancer metastatic to bone, and is thought to play a role in promoting angiogenesis, growth factor-independent proliferation and DNA double-strand break repair conferring breast cancer resistance to the genome destabilizing effects of DNA damage (Rubin et al. 2007). This result highlights the implication of the microenvironment on breast cancer development in elderly patients.

Recently, our group identified a tumor "genomic grade index" signature (GGI) reflecting differentiation and tumor progression and which was effectively associated with disease outcome in breast cancer far beyond the currently used clinico-pathological parameters (Sotiriou et al. 2006; Loi et al. 2007). This genomic grade is able to identify two clinically distinct ER-positive molecular subgroups (Loi et al. 2007): the "luminal A" subgroup of lower GGI levels and of good prognosis and the "luminal B" subgroup of worse clinical outcome and of higher GGI levels.

On the basis of this article and according to their biological characteristics evaluated by IHC, we were able to assign 1,666 breast tumors to a molecular subtype: the "HER-2+," the "ER & HER2 negative" or one of the two "luminal-like" subtypes divided according to their histological grade ("A" [HER-2-/ER+/low grade] and "B" [HER-2-/ER+/high grade]). We observed that age is highly influencing the incidence of breast cancer molecular subtypes. Patients younger than 40 develop a statistically higher rate of high-grade proliferating "HER-2" (27%) and "ER & HER2 negative" (31%) breast cancer whereas patients older than 50 develop mostly less aggressive hormone-dependant "luminal-A" breast cancer (>67%). Nevertheless, a significant proportion of patients older than 70 develop "luminal-B" (19%) tumors associated with high proliferation, high grade, large size, and nodal invasion (Durbecq et al. 2008).

These analyses corroborate clearly the assumption that elderly patients appeared to have a better prognosis compared to younger ones as a result of a higher proportion of low-risk "luminal A" tumors among these patients. Nevertheless, elderly patients may develop a nonnegligible proportion of highly aggressive "luminal B" tumors.

2.15 Interaction between Aging Process and Breast Cancer Development

Recent studies have indicated that both "convergent" and "divergent" mechanisms may relate cancer and ageing to each other: (1) either molecular pathways which simultaneously provide protection against cancer and ageing resistance by acting on the generation and accumulation of cellular damage or (2) process which protect from cancer but promote ageing as the shortening of telomeres and the de-repression of the CDKN2A locus (which play an important role in the p53 pathway) (Beausejour and Campisi 2006). It is also interesting to note that some genetic characteristics (i.e., some SNPs) could be associated with a decreased risk at younger ages but increased risk at older ages (Ralph et al. 2007).

Breast cancer incidence rises sharply to a high constant rate at a genetically determined age. Normal human ageing has been linked to increased genomic instability, global and promoter-specific epigenetic changes, and to altered expression of genes involved in cell division and extracellular matrix remodeling (Geigl et al. 2004). Therefore, the cancer-prone phenotype of older individual results from the combined effects of cumulative mutational load, increased epigenetic gene silencing, telomere dysfunction and altered extracellular matrix, and secreted products of senescent fibroblasts.

Finkel et al. (2007) view cancer and ageing as a pure stem cell disease, with cancer representing the effect of additional growth promoting mutations within a given stem cell and ageing representing the natural exhaustion and depletion of the stem and progenitor pool (Fig. 2.2).

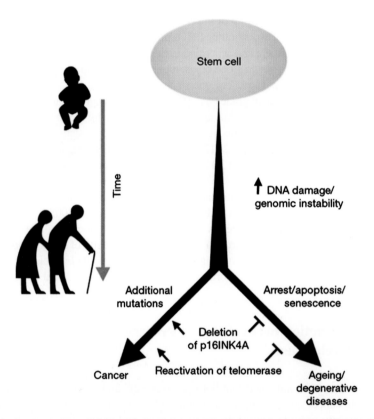

Fig. 2.2 Ageing and cancer from the perspective of alterations within the stem and progenitor cell pool. Cancer and ageing result primarily from accumulating damage to the stem and progenitor cell compartment. Mutations that allow stem cells to continue to proliferate in the setting of normal growth arrest signals such as DNA damage (i.e., loss of p16INK4a or reactivation of telomerase) would temporarily expand the stem cell pool and hence delay age-related pathologies. Over the long term, these mutations would also increase the likelihood of cancer. From Finkel et al. (2007)

2.16 Summary and Overall Impact on Prognosis

A strict similarity was observed on the clinical role of biological markers whatever the age of the patients at diagnosis. The 7-year probability of relapse was higher for patients with tumors having higher proliferative rates, higher frequency of p53 accumulation, weak or no bc12 expression, no ER and ≥4 positive nodes. Moreover the metastatic potential of breast cancer in the elderly patients does not differ significantly from the metastatic potential in younger women.

Therefore, even though older women mostly develop tumors with more favorable biological characteristics, specific subsets of elderly patients with tumors of high risk can be identified. In the subset of ER-positive tumors, cell proliferation, p53 accumulation, bc12 expression, and lymph node involvement provide significant and independent information for relapse and, in association, identified two subgroups of patients with relapse probability of 20 and 90%, the so-called luminal-A and luminal-B cancers respectively. It is important to understand that the most aggressive subtype of cancer may arise in elderly patients although less commonly than in younger women. This fact further stresses the importance of a biological characterization of all tumors, even in elderly patients.

Consequently, the difference in therapeutic approach can be explained by greater treatment toxicity in older patients, with significant co-morbid conditions but we have to exclude the indolent nature of breast tumors in such patients. Available trials suggest that breast cancer treatments are not significantly altered by age and that older breast cancer patients have a disease-specific survival similar to that of young patients when they are similarly treated.

2.17 Future Studies

Limited data on elderly cancer patients enrolled in clinical trials suggest that age itself, in the absence of severe concomitant illnesses or psychological, cognitive, or functional impairment, is not an independent risk factor for either increased toxicity or lack of treatment efficacy. Nevertheless, clinical trials specifically designed for elderly patient subpopulations with breast cancer are critically needed as underrepresentation of the elderly in clinical trials leads to inadequate information on the effect of age with regard to new anticancer treatments. Performance status—which takes into account level of activity, ambulation, and ability to care for oneself—and the presence of co-morbid conditions that may be exacerbated by the treatment are more reliable criteria for clinical trial eligibility than age. However, while age alone should never make a patient ineligible for a trial or other treatment, the effects of aging on bodily functions and physiology cannot be ignored when making treatment and referral decisions. Pharmacokinetic processes such as the absorption, metabolism, and excretion of drugs appear to be different in older patients, and in general, a person's physiologic tolerance or reserve diminishes with increasing age.

Finally, for early stage breast cancer management, the use of microarray technology which was able to identify a markedly increased number of patients at low risk who can be spared adjuvant chemotherapy, is of great interest especially in elderly patients who more frequently have co-morbidities and/or impaired organ functions (Veer LJ et al. 2002).

References

Balkwill F, Charles KA, Mantovani A (2005) Smoldering and polarized inflammation in the initiation and promotion of malignant disease. Cancer Cell 7:211–7

Beausejour CM, Campisi J (2006) Balancing regeneration and cancer. Nature 443:404–405

Camplejohn RS, Gilchrist R, Easton D et al (2003) Apoptosis, ageing and cancer susceptibility. British Journal of Cancer 88:487–490

Caywood J, Gray RJ, Hentz J et al (2005) Older age independently predicts a lower risk of sentinel lymph node metastasis in breast cancer. Annals Surg Oncol 12:1061–1065

Creighton C, Cordero K, Larios J et al (2006) Genes regulated by estrogen in breast tumor cells in vitro are similarly regulated in vivo in tumor xenografts and human breast tumors. Genome Biol 7:R28

Dominguez AL, Lustgarten J (2008) Implications of aging and self-tolerance on the generation of immune and antitumor immune responses. Cancer Res 68:5423–31

Dublin E, Hanby A, Pastel NK et al (2000) Immunohistochemical expression of uPA, uPAR, and PAI-1 in breast carcinoma. Fibroblastic expression has strong associations with tumor pathology. Am J Pathol 157:1219–1227

Durbecq V, Ameye L, Veys I et al (2008) A significant proportion of elderly patients develop hormone dependant "luminal-B" tumors associated with aggressive characteristics. Crit Rev Oncol Hematol 67:80–92

Evron E, Goldberg H, Kuzmin A et al (2006) Breast cancer in octogenarians. Cancer 106:1664–1668

Finkel T, Serrano M, Blasco MA (2007) The common biology of cancer and ageing. Nature 448:767–774

Geigl JB, Langer S, Barwisch S et al (2004) Analysis of gene expression patterns and chromosomal changes associated with aging. Cancer Res 64:8550–8557

Gravekamp C, Sypniewska R, Gauntt S et al (2004) Behavior of metastatic and non metastatic breast tumors in old mice. Exp Biol med 229:665–675

Il'Yasova D, Colbert LH, Harris TB et al (2005) Circulating levels of inflammatory markers and cancer risk in the health aging and body composition cohort. Cancer Epidemiol Biomarkers Prev 14:2413–2418

Kaptzan T, Skutelsky E, Itzhaki O et al (2006) Efficacy of anti-angiogenic treatment of tumors in old versus young mice. Mech Ageing Dev 127:398–409

Kudravi SA, Reed MJ (2000) Aging, cancer, and wound healing. In vivo 14:83–92

Loi S, Haibe-Kains B, Desmedt C et al (2007) Definition of clinically distinct molecular subtypes in estrogen receptor-positive breast carcinomas through genomic grade. J Clin Oncol 25:1239–1246

Mantovani A, Romero P, Palucka AK, Marincola FM (2008) Tumor immunity: effector response to tumor and role of the microenvironmant. Lancet 371:771–783

Molino A, Giovannini M, Auriemma A et al (2006) Pathological, biological and clinical characteristics, and surgical management, of elderly women with breast cancer. Crit Rev Oncol Hematol 59:226–233

Nickoloff BJ, Lingen MW, Chang BD et al (2004) Tumor suppressor maspin is upregulated during keratinocyte senescence, exerting a paracrine antiangiogenetic activity. Cancer Res 64:2956–2961

Offersen BV, Nielsen BS, Hoyer-Hansen G et al (2003) The myofibroblast is the predominant plasminogen activator inhibitor-1-expressing cell type in human breast carcinomas. Am J Pathol 163:1887–1899

Parrinello S, Coppe JP, Krtolica A et al (2005) Stromal-epithelial interactions in aging and cancer: senescent fibroblasts alter epithelial cell differentiation. J Cell Sci 118:485–496

Poltinnikov IM, Rudoler SB, Tymofyeyev Y et al (2006) Impact of Her2 Neu overexpression on outcome of elderly women treated with wide local excision and breast irradiation for early stage breast cancer. Am J Clin Oncol 29:71–79

Ralph DA, Zhao LP, Aston CE et al (2007) Age-specific association of steroid hormone pathway gene polymorphisms with breast cancer risk. Cancer 109:1940–1948

Resnick B, McLeskey SW (2008) Cancer screening across the aging continuum. AJMC 14:267–276

Rose-Hellekant TA, Wentworth KM, Nikolai S et al (2006) Mammary carcinogenesis is preceded by altered epithelial cell turnover in transforming growth factor factor alpha and c-myc transgenic mice. Am J Pathol 169:1821–1832

Rubin E, Wu X, Zhu T et al (2007) A role for the HoxB7 homeodomain protein in DNA repair. Cancer Res 67:1527–1535

Sadoun E, Reed MJ (2003) Impaired angiogenesis in aging is associated with alterations in vessel density, matrix composition, inflammatory response and growth factor expression. J Histochem Cytochem 51:1119–1130

Schwertfeger KL, Xian W, Kaplan AM et al (2006) A critical role for the inflammatory response in a mouse model of preneoplastic progression. Cancer Res 66:5676–5685

Sica A, Allavena P, Mantovani A, 2 (2008) Cancer related inflammation: the macrophage connection. Cancer Lett 267:204–215

Smigal C, Jemal A, Ward E et al (2006) Trends in breast cancer by race and ethnicity: update 2006. CA Cancer J Clin 56:168–183

Sotiriou C, Wirapati P, Loi S et al (2006) Gene expression profiling in breast cancer: understanding the molecular basis of histologic grade to improve prognosis. J Natl Cancer Inst 98:262–272

Swift ME, Burns AL, Gray KL, DiPietro LA (2001) Age-related alterations in the inflammatory response to dermal injury. J Invest Dermatol 117:1027–1035

Van Zee KJ, Manasseh DM, Bevilacqua JL et al (2003) A nomogram for predicting the likelihood of additional nodal metastases in breast cancer patients with a positive sentinel node biopsy. Ann Surg Oncol 10:1140–1151

Vasto S, Carruba G, Lio D et al (2009) Inflammation, ageing and cancer. Mech Ageing Dev 130(1-2):40–45

Veer LJ van 't, Dai H, van de Vijver MJ et al (2002) Gene expression profiling predicts clinical outcome of breast cancer. Nature 415:530–536

Warner HR, Hodes RJ (1997) Pocinki; What does cell death have to do with aging? Am J Geriatr Soc 45:1140–6

Yau C, Fedele V, Roydasgupta R, 5 et al (2007) Aging impacts transcriptomes but not genomes of hormone-dependent breast cancers. Breast Cancer Res 9:R59

Zhang GJ, Adachi I (1999) Serum interleukin-6 levels correlate to tumor progression and prognosis in metastatic breast carcinoma. Anticancer Res 19:1427–1432

Chapter 3
Clinical Epidemiology and the Impact of Co-Morbidity on Survival

Adri C. Voogd, Marieke J. Louwman, and Jan Willem W. Coebergh

3.1 Breast Cancer in the Elderly: A Changing Picture

Breast cancer will increasingly affect the lives of older women, especially in developed countries. In the last three decades, women of all age groups have experienced the benefits of a lowering mortality rate though earlier diagnosis and effective treatment. These benefits have been counteracted by the rising incidence, resulting from higher levels of exposure to risk factors and possibly also from the increased detection of occult, non lethal invasive breast cancers. At the same time, demographics are characterized by a large increase in the elderly population, which will become even more pronounced during the next decades. The most remarkable increase in the absolute number of newly diagnosed breast cancer patients and long-term survivors (at risk for recurrent disease or second breast cancers) will thus exhibit among the higher age groups, the prevalence doubling from 3.5% in 2000 to 7% in 2015 in the Netherlands (Poll-Franse et al. 2004). Being confronted with these rising numbers of patients or anticipating them, many doctors and clinical researchers have taken a special interest in the study of breast cancer in older women (Bouchardy et al. 2007), as is reflected by the increasing number of papers with a special focus on this group.

As part of a recent review of the literature on the clinical epidemiology of breast cancer in the elderly, 22 population-based studies were identified in PubMed, describing age-related differences in detection, staging, treatment, and prognosis of breast cancer (Louwman et al. 2007). The main conclusions of this review with respect to older breast cancer patients were as follows:

- A relatively large proportion of (7–16%) remained unstaged.
- The proportion with advanced disease (stage III & IV) was clearly higher among elderly patients compared to younger ones.
- The treatment was generally less aggressive than for younger patients.

A.C. Voogd (✉)
Department of Epidemiology, Maastricht University Medical Centre,
P.O. Box 616, 6200 MD Maastricht, The Netherlands
e-mail: adri.voogd@epid.unimaas.nl

M.W. Reed and R.A. Audisio (eds.), *Management of Breast Cancer in Older Women*,
DOI 10.1007/978-1-84800-265-4_3, © Springer-Verlag London Limited 2011

- Although more patients have received chemotherapy since the early 1990s, its use is still very moderate among the elderly.
- Older patients were less likely to receive radiotherapy than younger patients, illustrating the preference for mastectomy without radiotherapy, instead of breast-conserving treatment (consisting of lumpectomy with axillary dissection (AD) and radiotherapy).
- Disease-specific (or relative) survival was generally lower compared to younger patients.
- Co-morbidity was present more often and was also related to (sub-optimal) treatment.

This chapter expands on the findings of this review by presenting the most recent trends in incidence, treatment, and prognosis of breast cancer in older women based on a variety of registries and provides explanations for these trends. These trends will be illustrated in depth by the data of the Eindhoven Cancer Registry, because of its unique clinical data on co-morbidity, and by European data. Population-based data show actual variations in patterns of detection, staging, and treatment by age and thus offer a scope for improvement of care and for feeding guidelines and future, randomized clinical trials. However, because of the limitations to perform randomized studies in the elderly, other research strategies also need to be explored for information synthesis, as will be done in this chapter.

3.2   Recent Trends in Epidemiology and Treatment of Breast Cancer in the Elderly

3.2.1   Diagnosis

Already in the 1970s and early 1980s there was a clear tendency toward earlier diagnosis of breast cancer, especially in the younger age groups, as illustrated by the Eindhoven Cancer Registry data (Coebergh et al. 1990). The percentage of tumors measuring ≤2 cm rose from more than 20% to almost 45%. The steadily increasing use of early detection and screening strategies since the mid-1970s, in combination with the rising public awareness of breast cancer, are the most likely explanations for this favorable trend. However, since the mid-eighties no further improvement has been observed in the stage distribution for patients aged <50 years. For patients aged 50–69 years, the stage distribution continued to improve as a result of the introduction of mass mammographic screening, with particularly high attendance rates (85%) (Annual Report 2005). A similar improvement was observed for women aged 70–79 years, following the extension of the upper age limit of the screening program to 75 years in 1998. Recent data show that the stage distribution of patients aged 70–79 years is now almost similar to younger age groups (Fig. 3.1). Women of 80 years and older, however, remained at a higher risk of being diagnosed with more advanced disease.

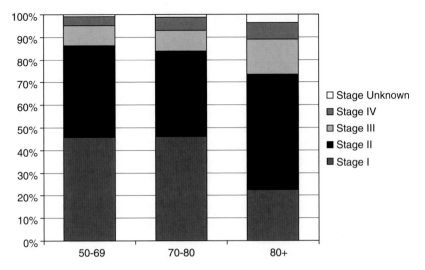

Fig. 3.1 Stage distribution among patients with invasive breast cancer aged 50 years or older, according to age group. Period of diagnosis 2000–2005. (Source: Eindhoven Cancer Registry)

The detection of small nonpalpable lesions by screening has boosted the development and introduction of less invasive staging procedures, such as large core needle biopsy, and localization procedures (Duijm et al. 2007). Although not invited for the screening program, women aged 75+ years will certainly have benefited from these developments as well.

3.2.2 Prognosis

Relative survival is the preferred way to describe the prognosis of older (breast) cancer patients, because it takes into account the risk of dying from other causes than the disease of interest. An alternative method is to calculate disease-specific survival. However, obtaining reliable information on the cause of death carries the risk of misclassification, especially when the patient has more than one tumor. Getting an adequate diagnosis or retrieving the cause of death especially may be more difficult for older patients, especially in the presence of comorbidity. Fourteen percent of the newly diagnosed patients at age 70–79 and 22% older than age 80 suffered from ≥2 concomitant serious conditions. Such patients are more likely to be admitted to nursing homes and thus disappear from the view of the treating physician or general practitioner. International comparisons of cancer survival estimates, such as in the EUROCARE studies, may also be complicated by the proportion of cases registered purely from death certificate information (DCO cases). A recent analysis of the impact of incomplete ascertainment of cancer cases and the presence of DCO cases concluded that these phenomena should be taken into account when comparing survival estimates between different populations (Robinson et al. 2007) especially for older patients, as incompleteness and DCO registration is associated with increasing age (Pollock and Vickers 1995).

Relative survival of breast cancer patients of patients aged 40–75 years is largely similar, as is indicated by recent data of the Eindhoven Cancer Registry (Fig. 3.2). A somewhat lower relative survival rate was observed for patients of 75 years or older. These results are confirmed by data from EUROCARE, including data from more than 400,000 patients diagnosed in 20 European countries during 1995–1999. According to these European data, 5-year relative survival percentages were 82, 85, 83, 79, and 71%, respectively, for patients aged 15–44, 45–54, 55–64, 65–74, and 75 years or older. The slightly worse relative survival of older patients could be explained by their poorer stage distribution, under-treatment or by a combination of both factors. However, when looking at the tumor characteristics, there also appears to be an association between increasing age at diagnosis and the presence of more favorable biologic characteristics of the tumor.

In spite of the larger tumor size, older patients have tumors showing a higher expression of steroid receptors, a lower proliferation rate, more diploid cells, more normal p53, and less frequent expression of the HER2/neu receptor (Diab et al. 2000;

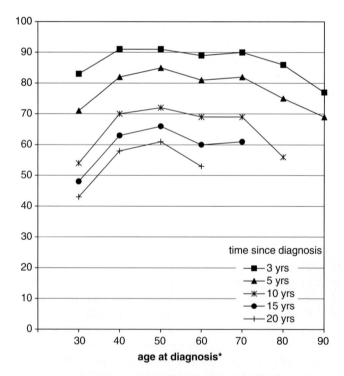

Fig. 3.2 Relative survival of breast cancer patients diagnosed between 1990 and 2002 in southeastern Netherlands, according to age at diagnosis (*midpoint of 10-year age interval) and time since diagnosis

Molino et al. 2006). The prognostic impact of the poorer stage distribution among older women thus seems to be counterbalanced by more favorable tumor biology. Moreover, slower growing tumors can remain undetected for long. Just like for the other age groups, there probably is much variability in aggressiveness of disease in older women, stressing the need for a better understanding of the tumor biology to improve prognostication and choice of therapy (Mandelblatt 2006). Large-scale genome analysis may help to define the prognostic profile of a tumor and identify molecular subtypes as a basis for potential therapeutic targets, specifically for the elderly (Anders et al. 2008).

3.2.3 Treatment

Like their younger counterparts, older breast cancer patients have benefited from the development and introduction of less invasive staging and treatment procedures, and new drugs. Still, age continues to play an important role in the use of these and other procedures, which are considered standard care for younger women. For example, data from the Netherlands Cancer Registry indicate that there was not much difference between patients younger than 70 and those aged 70–79 years with respect to the use of breast-conserving surgery (BCS) and radiotherapy following BCS (Siesling et al. 2007). However, the picture was completely different for women of 80 years and older, who constituted 8% of the total patient group. In the Eindhoven Cancer Registry age appeared to be a stronger predictor for the use surgery or the administration of radiotherapy following BCS than co-morbidity (Vulto et al. 2006) (Fig. 3.3). In fact, after BCS, patients aged 80 years or older

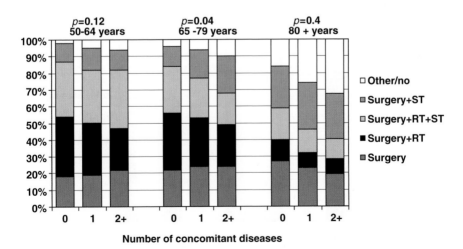

Fig. 3.3 Primary treatment of patients with invasive breast cancer from 1995 to 2002, according to age and concomitant disease. RT: radiotherapy (Source: Eindhoven Cancer Registry)

were 10 times less likely to receive radiotherapy than those of 50–64 years of age (OR 0.1; 95% CI 0.1–0.2). Factors, such as the distance to radiotherapy facilities, and the protracted radiotherapy course, frailty, limited social support, and psychological and economic factors and patients' or family's preference are mentioned as explanatory factors in this respect.

The same age-related pattern was observed with respect to axillary lymph node staging. In 1997, just before the introduction of sentinel node biopsy (SNB) in the southeast Netherlands, 23% of the women of 70–80 years did not undergo an axillary staging procedure (i.e., AD), compared to 42% of the patients of 80 years or more (Fig. 3.4). Considering the limited morbidity associated with SNB and the valuable prognostic information resulting from it, one would expect the introduction of this procedure to lead to a substantial decrease in the proportion of elderly patients not undergoing axillary staging. This was only true for women of 70–79 years, where this proportion decreased to 13%. In 2005, only 33% of patients 80 years and older underwent a sentinel node procedure and 41% still did not undergo axillary staging.

Age also plays an important role in the decision to use chemotherapy. Like data from many other studies, data from the Eindhoven Cancer registry showed that in 2006 the use of chemotherapy, alone or in combination with hormonal therapy, decreased with increasing age. Of the patients aged 50–69 years with positive axillary lymph nodes, almost 60% received chemotherapy, whereas of the patients 70 years and older, less than 2% received chemotherapy (Fig. 3.5) (Sukel et al. 2008). Much higher proportions have been observed in other countries such as Italy, where a recent multicenter observational cohort study, covering the period 2000–2002 reported the use of chemotherapy in 45% of all patients aged 70–75 years and

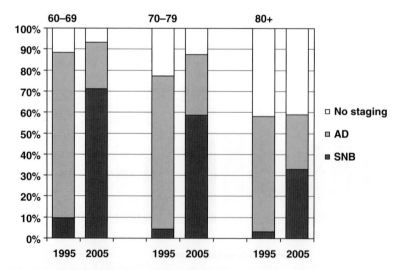

Fig. 3.4 The proportion of patients undergoing axillary dissection (AD), sentinel node biopsy (SNB), or no axillary staging procedure in 1995 and 2005, according to age group (Source: Eindhoven Cancer Registry)

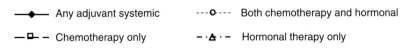

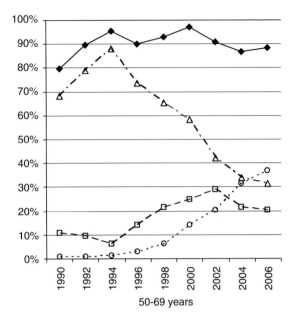

50-69 years

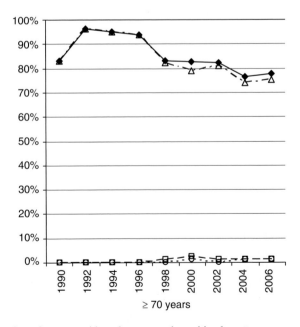

≥ 70 years

Fig. 3.5 Proportion of women with early stage node-positive breast cancer receiving adjuvant systemic treatment, by age and year of diagnosis

17% for those older than 75 years (Mustacchi et al. 2007). This international variation is almost certainly the consequence of a different interpretation of the available evidence for the benefit of chemotherapy for older patients.

The previous data illustrate that special efforts should be put in studying the
safety of less aggravating treatment plans, such as intra-operative radiotherapy and
cytotoxic drugs with a more favorable toxicity profile, as well as the implementation
of such alternatives in daily practice. In effect, omitting axillary staging, limited use
of breast-conserving surgery and omitting postoperative radiotherapy have remained
rather common practices among elderly patients, especially in those of 80 years and
older; these differences are only partly explained by the presence of concurrent
diseases in these patients, but rather seem to imply that older age tends to be confused
with chronic illness. Similar deviations from practice guidelines in the elderly have
been observed in other studies (Hebert-Croteau et al. 1999; Giordano et al. 2005),
but still little is known about the possible reasons.

3.3   Current Dilemmas and Directions for Future Research

Clinical trials are credited for a large proportion of the improvements in cancer
therapy. The major thread for the implementation and reproducibility of trial results
is the selective uptake of older patients in randomized controlled trials because of
co-morbidity, lack of understanding of the consent procedure, and deficient social
support. If still desirable, trials testing less aggressive and less arduous treatment
strategies and aiming at the majority of the elderly will be much more likely to
succeed in entering a sufficient number of patients and providing widely applicable
results than trials designed exclusively for patients without functional limitations
(Siu 2007).

There is evidence that selection of patients may explain differences in outcome
between randomized patients and patients not entering a trial (Bijker et al. 2002).
However, little evidence exists for effective strategies for trial enrolment among
elderly cancer patients (Eaker et al. 2006; Kimmick et al. 2005). To enable valid
generalization of trial results, a thorough administration of the total number of eligible patients in each participating center is needed, as well as the reasons why
patients were not entered into the trial.

In modern trials, comparing loco-regional or systemic treatments, explicit age
limits are no longer in use. However, many of the elderly are not considered eligible
because of co-morbidity or other factors which hamper time-consuming informed
consent procedures, intensive treatment, and follow-up prescribed by the trial
protocol. In some cases, overall results of trials show a beneficial effect for the total
group, but the effect appears to increase or decrease with age. Although 96% of
recent breast cancer randomized clinical trials report age, only 28% present evaluation of outcomes by age. However, subgroup analyses often do not solve the
problem, as most of the trials are not powered for analyses according to age
group, leading to small numbers in the different age strata, especially for the elderly.

This explains why difficulties remain when applying results from important trials but even meta-analyses to older patients. Examples are the use of chemotherapy, especially anthracycline-containing regimens, for estrogen-receptor-negative breast cancer (Clarke et al. 2008), the use of a radiotherapy boost following breast-conserving treatment of invasive breast cancer (Bartelink et al. 2007) and the use of radio-therapy following lumpectomy for ductal carcinoma in situ (Holmberg et al. 2008). These issues may be solved by trials with a primary focus on the elderly. To guarantee sufficient uptake in such trials, broad inclusion criteria are needed, allowing patients with different levels of disease severity and a wide range of coexisting illnesses to be randomized. Such trials are also desirable to study interventions with a more acceptable toxicity profile and a smaller burden on patients' daily life, such as intra-operative radiotherapy.

In the absence of evidence-based guidelines and/or while waiting for the results from randomized clinical trials to come, decision-making should be guided by risk–benefit analysis for each individual patient, taking into account tumor charac-teristics as well as patient-related factors. Nowadays, physicians have a host of validated and standardized instruments at their disposal to determine individual heterogeneity at the tumor level, ranging from the TNM classification system to the measurement of tumor grade, steroid receptor status, HER2/neu receptor, and different proliferation markers. Currently, this arsenal is being extended by genetic assays, which allow the distinction between high- and low-risk tumors at the molecular level. In contrast to younger patients, individual variation among older patients is not mainly a question of differences in disease characteristics, but is also considerable at other levels. Substantial interindividual variation exists with respect to physical and mental health, social network, and patients' expectations. In the elderly, these factors are at least of equal importance as the disease characteristics in providing tailored treatment, and therefore more effort should be put into the development and validation of instruments to measure them.

The difficulty of developing and performing randomized controlled trials for the elderly and the uncertainties about the applicability of the results to general practice leave ample room for descriptive studies (Hillner and Mandelblatt 2006) based on data of cancer registries or hospital-based registries (Table 3.1). Collecting standard data on tumor stage, disease characteristics (i.e., grade, steroid receptor status), and staging procedures and treatment (i.e., surgery, radiotherapy and adjuvant systemic treatment) will be sufficient to monitor adherence to guidelines or the implementation of new guidelines. It should be noted here that large staging and treatment variations between hospitals should not always be interpreted as a proof of inade-quate care, but may also point at absence of guidelines, lack of precision in the indications for treatment, or lack of consensus because of insufficient evidence for the recommendations given in the guidelines.

Adding co-morbid conditions to a population- or hospital-based cancer registry will help to find explanations for noncompliance with guidelines. Moreover, such cancer registries could be of help by collecting follow-up data to give an impression of treatment outcome. Loco-regional control of disease may be such a parameter, but also the assessment of quality of life, treatment-related complications, and

Table 3.1 Research Strategies to Understand and Improve Care for Elderly Cancer Patients

Strategy	Strengths	Limitations
Randomized controlled trials	Controlled conditions of the trial provide strong conclusive evidence of cause-and-effect relationships. With good preparation and involvement large and quick recruitment should be feasible.	Implementation and reproducibility because of selective uptake of older patients (related to co-morbidity, lack of understanding of the consent procedure, and deficient social support)
Descriptive studies (cancer registry or hospital-based registry)	Collecting standard data on tumor stage, disease characteristics, and treatment will be sufficient to monitor adherence to guidelines or the implementation of new guidelines.	Documentation of data for the very elderly patients is as good as practice delivers and that is likely to be variable.
	Adding co-morbid conditions to the database will help to find explanations for noncompliance with guidelines. Collection of follow-up data will give an impression of outcome (such as loco-regional control, treatment-related complications, and healthcare utilization) Sampling frame for quality-of-life studies.	Completeness and quality of the data are dependent on the continuous accuracy and discipline of (many) doctors to document information in their clinical files. These limitations with respect to completeness and quality of the data might hamper comparability across institutions and over time.
Qualitatively oriented (identification and accurate documentation of the critical steps preceding diagnosis and treatment for each individual patient)	Patterns in the structure or organization of breast cancer care, underlying suboptimal diagnosis and treatment and unfavorable treatment outcomes, can be recognized, which would otherwise have remained undetected. Enables evaluation of new concepts, such as the role of shared decision-making and assessment of patient and doctor preferences.	Documentation for a considerable period of time is needed. Completeness and quality of the data are dependent on the willingness and discipline of (many) doctors and other healthcare workers to provide extra information on their way of working.

healthcare utilization at certain points during follow-up in a random sample of the patients should be relatively easy to organize by a cancer registry.

The following examples illustrate how such data may be used to fill the gaps in knowledge and provide us the evidence to improve the decision-making process.

- A recent prospective study by Marinello et al. shows how observational studies can help to define a subgroup of elderly patients in which chemotherapy is well-tolerated by using information on co-morbidity and performance status (Marinello et al. 2008): Of 110 consecutive patients older than 70 years of age with lung, colon, or breast cancer, only one-third were found to have completed the scheduled chemotherapy regimen and 66% experienced adverse events as early death ($n=14$) and grade III and IV toxicity ($n=40$). Several predictors of treatment failure were identified, such as advanced stage of disease, toxicity of treatment, co-morbidity score, and Karnofsky performance status.
- A study by Smith et al. shows how data on life expectancy and a co-morbidity score may be used to calculate the number of patients needing radiotherapy to prevent second breast cancer events (Table 3.2) (Smith et al. 2006). This "number needed to treat (NNT)" is a useful tool to weigh the benefits of a breast-cancer-specific intervention against the (short-term) harms and competing risk of dying from other causes in each individual patient (Gorin et al. 2006).
- Doyle et al. used tumor data from the Surveillance, Epidemiology and End-Results (SEER) program and linked them with Medicare files to estimate the risk of cardiomyopathy, congestive heart failure, and heart disease following the use of chemotherapy among women aged 65 years or older, taking into account the presence of heart disease at baseline (Doyle et al. 2007). Their conclusion was that chemotherapy, especially with anthracyclines, is associated with a substantially increased risk of cardiomyopathy.

But cancer-registry-based studies also have their limitations (Table 3.1). Documentation of data for the very elderly patients is as good as practice delivers and that is likely to be variable. Completeness and quality of the data is dependent on the accuracy and discipline of doctors to document information in their clinical files. Electronic patient records with predefined data fields may increase the completeness of the data and may be used by the cancer registry to link with other relevant clinical data and follow-up data. But even these extra efforts to increase the

Table 3.2   Number Needed to Irradiate (Nnt) to Prevent One Second Breast Cancer Event[a](Smith et al. 2006)

Age group (years)	Co-morbidity score	No. in study	8-year survival (%) (95% CI)	Adjusted NNT(95% CI)
70–74	0	2188	84 (83–89)	21 (16–31)
	1	540	72 (68–76)	24 (18–36)
	2–9	226	47 (40–55)	37 (28–55)
80–84	0	1096	51 (57–64)	29 (22–43)
	1	388	47 (40–53)	38 (28–56)
	2–9	218	29 (21–36)	61 (46–90)

[a]combined outcome of second ipsilateral breast cancer reported and/or subsequent mastectomy

accuracy and the completeness of the data might be insufficient to visualize and analyze the complexity of the decision-making process.

A more qualitatively oriented strategy would be to analyze the decision-making process in each individual patient by an accurate documentation of the steps preceding diagnosis and treatment (Table 3.1). For example, which clinical information was available when a medical decision was made and what information was taken into account? Which disciplines were involved in the decision-making process? In combination with a structured evaluation and discussion of the data, this method may result in recognizing patterns in the structure or organization of breast cancer care underlying suboptimal care and unfavorable treatment outcomes and which would otherwise have remained undetected. Such a strategy may also be useful to evaluate the potential contribution of comprehensive geriatric assessment (Extermann et al. 2005) and of new concepts such as shared decision-making (Mandelblatt 2006) with assessment of patients' and doctor preferences (Jansen et al. 2004; Duric and Stockler 2001; Mandelblatt et al. 2006) to the improvement of quality of care in older patients.

References

Annual report 2005 in Dutch. 's (2006) Hertogenbosch: Stichting Bevolkingsonderzoek Borstkanker Zuid

Anders CK, Hsu DS, Broadwater G, Acharya CR, Foekens JA, Zhang Y et al (2008) Young age at diagnosis correlates with worse prognosis and defines a subset of breast cancers with shared patterns of gene expression. J Clin Oncol 26(20):3324–3330

Bartelink H, Horiot JC, Poortmans PM, Struikmans H, Van den Bogaert W, Fourquet A et al (2007) Impact of a higher radiation dose on local control and survival in breast-conserving therapy of early breast cancer: 10-year results of the randomized boost versus no boost EORTC 22881–10882 trial. J Clin Oncol 25(22):3259–3265

Bijker N, Peterse JL, Fentiman IS, Julien JP, Hart AA, Avril A et al (2002) Effects of patient selection on the applicability of results from a randomised clinical trial (EORTC 10853) investigating breast-conserving therapy for DCIS. Br J Cancer 87(6):615–620

Bouchardy C, Rapiti E, Blagojevic S, Vlastos AT, Vlastos G (2007) Older female cancer patients: importance, causes, and consequences of undertreatment. J Clin Oncol 25(14):1858–1869

Clarke M, Coates AS, Darby SC, Davies C, Gelber RD, Godwin J et al (2008) Adjuvant chemotherapy in oestrogen-receptor-poor breast cancer: patient-level meta-analysis of randomised trials. Lancet 371(9606):29–40

Coebergh JW, Crommelin MA, Kluck HM, van Beek M, van der Horst F, Verhagen-Teulings MT (1990) Breast cancer in southeast North Brabant and in North Limburg; trends in incidence and earlier diagnosis in an unscreened female population, 1975–1986. Ned Tijdschr Geneeskd 134(15):760–765

Diab SG, Elledge RM, Clark GM (2000) Tumor characteristics and clinical outcome of elderly women with breast cancer. J Natl Cancer Inst 92(7):550–556

Doyle JJ, Neugut AI, Jacobson JS, Wang J, McBride R, Grann A et al (2007) Radiation therapy, cardiac risk factors, and cardiac toxicity in early-stage breast cancer patients. Int J Radiat Oncol Biol Phys 68(1):82–93

Duijm LE, Groenewoud JH, Roumen RM, de Koning HJ, Plaisier ML, Fracheboud J (2007) A decade of breast cancer screening in The Netherlands: trends in the preoperative diagnosis of breast cancer. Breast Cancer Res Treat 106:113–119

Duric V, Stockler M (2001) Patients' preferences for adjuvant chemotherapy in early breast cancer: a review of what makes it worthwhile. Lancet Oncol 2(11):691–697

Eaker S, Dickman PW, Bergkvist L, Holmberg L (2006) Differences in management of older women influence breast cancer survival: results from a population-based database in Sweden. PLoS Med 3(3):e25

Extermann M, Aapro M, Bernabei R, Cohen HJ, Droz JP, Lichtman S et al (2005) Use of comprehensive geriatric assessment in older cancer patients: recommendations from the task force on CGA of the International Society of Geriatric Oncology (SIOG). Crit Rev Oncol Hematol 55(3):241–252

Giordano SH, Hortobagyi GN, Kau SW, Theriault RL, Bondy ML (2005) Breast cancer treatment guidelines in older women. J Clin Oncol 23(4):783–791

Gorin SS, Heck JE, Cheng B, Smith SJ (2006) Delays in breast cancer diagnosis and treatment by racial/ethnic group. Arch Intern Med 166(20):2244–2252

Hebert-Croteau N, Brisson J, Latreille J, Blanchette C, Deschenes L (1999) Compliance with consensus recommendations for the treatment of early stage breast carcinoma in elderly women. Cancer 85(5):1104–1113

Hillner BE, Mandelblatt J (2006) Caring for older women with breast cancer: can observational research fill the clinical trial gap? J Natl Cancer Inst 98(10):660–661

Holmberg L, Garmo H, Granstrand B, Ringberg A, Arnesson LG, Sandelin K et al (2008) Absolute risk reductions for local recurrence after postoperative radiotherapy after sector resection for ductal carcinoma in situ of the breast. J Clin Oncol 26(8):1247–1252

Jansen SJ, Otten W, Stiggelbout AM (2004) Review of determinants of patients' preferences for adjuvant therapy in cancer. J Clin Oncol 22(15):3181–3190

Kimmick GG, Peterson BL, Kornblith AB, Mandelblatt J, Johnson JL, Wheeler J et al (2005) Improving accrual of older persons to cancer treatment trials: a randomized trial comparing an educational intervention with standard information: CALGB 360001. J Clin Oncol 23(10):2201–2207

Louwman WJ, Vulto JC, Verhoeven RH, Nieuwenhuijzen GA, Coebergh JW, Voogd AC (2007) Clinical epidemiology of breast cancer in the elderly. Eur J Cancer 43(15):2242–2252

Mandelblatt J (2006) Treating breast cancer: the age old dilemma of old age. J Clin Oncol 24(27):4369–4370

Mandelblatt J, Kreling B, Figeuriedo M, Feng S (2006) What is the impact of shared decision making on treatment and outcomes for older women with breast cancer? J Clin Oncol 24(30):4908–4913

Marinello R, Marenco D, Roglia D, Stasi MF, Ferrando A, Ceccarelli M et al (2008) Predictors of treatment failures during chemotherapy: A prospective study on 110 older cancer patients. Arch Gerontol Geriat 48(2):222–226

Molino A, Giovannini M, Auriemma A, Fiorio E, Mercanti A, Mandara M et al (2006) Pathological, biological and clinical characteristics, and surgical management, of elderly women with breast cancer. Crit Rev Oncol Hematol 59(3):226–233

Mustacchi G, Cazzaniga ME, Pronzato P, De Matteis A, Di Costanzo F, Floriani I (2007) Breast cancer in elderly women: a different reality? Results from the NORA study. Ann Oncol 18(6):991–996

Poll-Franse, L.V. van de, Coebergh, J.W., Houterman, S., Mols, F., Alers, J.C., Berg, F.A. van den, Haes,, Koning,, Leeuwen,, Schornagel,, Oost,, Soerjomataram,, Voogd,, & Vries (2004) SignaleringscommissieKanker. Kanker in Nederland. Trends, prognoses en implicaties voor zorgvraag. KWF Kankerbestrijding, Amsterdam

Pollock AM, Vickers N (1995) Why are a quarter of all cancer deaths in south-east England registered by death certificate only? Factors related to death certificate only registrations in the Thames Cancer Registry between 1987 and 1989. Br J Cancer 71(3):637–641

Robinson D, Sankila R, Hakulinen T, Moller H (2007) Interpreting international comparisons of cancer survival: the effects of incomplete registration and the presence of death certificate only cases on survival estimates. Eur J Cancer 43(5):909–913

Siesling S, van de Poll-Franse LV, Jobsen JJ, van Driel OJ Repelaer, Voogd AC (2007) Explanatory factors for variation in the use of breast conserving surgery and radiotherapy in the Netherlands, 1990–2001. Breast 16(6):606–614

Siu LL (2007) Clinical trials in the elderly—a concept comes of age. N Engl J Med 356(15): 1575–1576

Smith BD, Gross CP, Smith GL, Galusha DH, Bekelman JE, Haffty BG (2006) Effectiveness of radiation therapy for older women with early breast cancer. J Natl Cancer Inst 98(10):681–690

Sukel MP, van de Poll-Franse LV, Nieuwenhuijzen GA, Vreugdenhil G, Herings RM, Coebergh JW et al (2008) Substantial increase in the use of adjuvant systemic treatment for early stage breast cancer reflects changes in guidelines in the period 1990–2006 in the southeastern Netherlands. Eur J Cancer 44(13):1846–54

Vulto AJ, Lemmens VE, Louwman MW, Janssen-Heijnen ML, Poortmans PH, Lybeert ML et al (2006) The influence of age and co-morbidity on receiving radiotherapy as part of primary treatment for cancer in South Netherlands, 1995 to 2002. Cancer 106(12):2734–42

Part II
Special Considerations in the Managemant
of Older Women

Chapter 4
Comprehensive Geriatric Assessment

Margot A. Gosney

4.1 Why do we need to assess older patients with cancer?

Epidemiological studies show us that the aging population, which is well known to clinicians and healthcare planners, will continue to increase in number. With increasing age, the development of cancer becomes more likely, and many older individuals will be diagnosed with a malignancy in later life or may survive from a younger age with such a diagnosis. As individuals become older, there is little doubt that comorbidity becomes a major issue in the presence or absence of cancer. Although clinicians may view older people as being a minor part of their day-to-day workload, there are few specialties with the obvious exceptions of obstetrics and pediatrics who do not deal with older people on a daily basis. Within the last 10– 20 years, there has been an increasing awareness of geriatric oncology as a specialty in its own right, and many have attempted to measure comorbidity to improve the management of patients with cancer. The giants of geriatric medicine as described by Bernard Isaacs (incontinence, instability and falls, impaired hearing and vision, and intellectual decline) are all more prevalent with increasing age. Other conditions particularly related to environmental exposure are also frequently present. Comorbidities are highly relevant to the prognosis of cancer patients. This is not only due to the effect on prognosis of the additional comorbidities, but also their influence on the treatment of such patients.

When observing elderly women with breast cancer, it becomes abundantly clear that biological and chronological age are not identical. Despite similar genetic makeup and environmental factors, one 80-year-old woman may be physically and mentally robust and another may exhibit the frailty syndrome.

There are three occasions when the clinical assessment of an older person with breast cancer is important. Initially, prior to the decision to undertake therapy, a patient's suitability for surgery and/or adjuvant therapy must be determined. Without attention to comorbidity, patient selection may not be ideal, therapy may

M.A. Gosney
Clinical Health Sciences, University of Reading, Reading, RG1 5AQ, Berkshire, UK
e-mail: m.a.gosney@reading.ac.uk

M.W. Reed and R.A. Audisio (eds.), *Management of Breast Cancer in Older Women*,   53
DOI 10.1007/978-1-84800-265-4_4, © Springer-Verlag London Limited 2011

not be evidence based, and untreated comorbidity will not be identified and actively managed. Second, during treatment, it is vital that response to therapy is monitored and this must include the continued assessment of existing conditions and an active search for the development of new conditions, which may or may not be related to therapy. Third, and perhaps more important for service planning, is the assessment of disease free survival, as well as overall survival. To many older people, the argument of quantity versus quality may result in patient derived decisions being made which are different from clinicians.

4.2 What assessment methodologies have been used in the past?

Extermann in her 1999 review identified four commonly used measures of comorbidity and reported not only a systematic review of these methodologies, but also an expert opinion on each of the indices. She studied the Charlson Comorbidity Index, the Cumulative Illness Rating Scale (CIRS), the Index of Coexistent Disease (ICED), and the Kaplan-Feinstein Index (Extermann 2000).

4.2.1 The Charlson Comorbidity Index

The Charlson Comorbidity Index was designed in 1987 and was initially used in general internal medicine patients to analyze mortality at 1-year, as a result of different comorbidities. While it was not developed for use in patients with malignant disease, it was validated in a cohort of breast cancer patients using 10-year mortality as the end point. It has been used to predict mortality, outcomes of postoperative complications, length of hospital stay, and discharge to a nursing home. Its validation in the older cancer patient has resulted in its wide use. While the Charlson has good interrater and test-retest reliability, it does have some problems. It ignores certain comorbidities, including hematopoietic disorders and moderate renal dysfunction, both of which may be critical in patients who may have impaired renal function as a consequence of aging, or hematological problems due to bone marrow infiltration or chemotherapy. It must also be remembered that four of the Charlson items relate to cancer, and therefore, the use of this scale in patients with a primary diagnosis of breast cancer may result in skewed results.

4.2.2 The Cumulative Illness Rating Scale (CIRS)

This assessment scale was first designed in 1968 and assesses comorbidities according to the organ system affected and the severity of the affect. The items use a 0–4 scale (i.e. none, mild, moderate, severe, extremely severe/life threatening).

Although the CIRS score does correlate with hospitalization rates, hospital readmission, medication usage, functional disability, and mortality, it has been less used in elderly patients within oncology. It correlates well with the Charlson when studying prognosis, though unfortunately unless the observer is using the CIRS regularly, the assessment of disease severity often includes errors.

4.2.3   The Index of Coexistent Disease (ICED)

This scale was developed in 1987 and addresses both physical and functional ability. It assesses the presence and severity of fourteen different categories of conditions. It has been validated in patients with breast cancer and correlates with both the intensity of treatment, as well as the use of axillary node dissection in breast cancer. Unfortunately, the ICED like the CIRS requires a considerable amount of medical knowledge to ensure that the severity of diseases is accurately determined, and therefore, a relatively senior clinician is required to complete; thus, limiting its usefulness in everyday practice.

4.2.4   The Kaplan-Feinstein Index

This index, which was developed in 1974, has a narrower rating of severity (0–3) of a number of conditions that are considered to impair a patient's long-term survival. It has been used in patients with breast cancer, where it has been found to correlate with mortality (Newschaffer et al. 1997).

4.3   Surgical Assessment Scales

There are a number of surgical assessment scales that may be more appropriate to the preoperative assessment of elderly women with breast cancer. They include both APACHE and POSSUM.

4.3.1   The Acute Physiology and Chronic Health Evaluation (APACHE) Index

The APACHE was first published in 1981 and then replaced in 1985 by APACHE II. It includes twelve physiological parameters, usually measured during the first 24 h after admission to an intensive care unit. Headley and colleagues found that patients with breast cancer admitted to the intensive care unit had their mortality accurately predicted using the APACHE II score (Headley et al. 1992).

4.3.2 Physiological and Operative Severity Score in Enumeration of Mortality and Morbidity (POSSUM)

This scale, developed by Copeland and colleagues in the North West in 1991, was initially used as a scoring system for hospital audit. It predicts morbidity and postoperative mortality in general surgery. Its usefulness has been assessed as part of the initial validation of PACE (Preoperative Assessment of Cancer in the Elderly), but has no other formal evaluation in older people with breast cancer (Copeland et al. 1991).

There are few papers that have compared APACHE II, POSSUM, and ASA (American Society of Anesthesiologists) scoring systems. Much of the comparison has been undertaken in patients with head and neck tumors which clearly influence maintenance of airway, respiratory complications, and the issues of local tumor dissection (de Cassia Braga Ribeiro and Kowalski 2003). Little evidence exists in breast cancer patients.

4.3.3 Adult Comorbidity Evaluation-27 (ACE-27)

The ACE-27 was initially derived from the Kaplan-Feinstein Index (Paleri and Wight 2002). Its usefulness in older patients with tumors related to alcohol and cigarette smoking is well documented, but data in breast cancer patients are lacking (Gosney 2005).

4.4 Comprehensive Geriatric Assessment

The Comprehensive Geriatric Assessment (CGA) evaluates a number of aspects of normal aging. This enables patients to be thoroughly assessed in a holistic fashion, to ensure that their pretreatment comorbidities are treated and the overall outcome of any specific cancer treatment is optimized. It is essential that the CGA includes measures of functional status, comorbidity, nutritional status, drug therapy, socio-economic issues, and the presence of geriatric syndromes. The CGA will ensure that all patients at the time of treatment selection receive appropriate therapy and even the frailest benefit from palliative treatment (Balducci 2003).

There is little doubt that many of the frailest individuals with breast cancer will benefit from active intervention. It is known that outside oncology, the CGA is very effective when planning the management of frail, older individuals with complex medical needs. The CGA is superior to usual care in the management of older patients with common conditions such as hip fracture and congestive cardiac failure. A number of randomized controlled trials have tested the effectiveness of CGA in the care of older patients in a variety of settings (Ferrucci et al. 2003).

While it might be considered that comorbidities are different in patients with and without cancer, when one compares the 10 most prevalent comorbid conditions in age matched groups; arthritis, hypertension, digestive, cardiac, and vascular diseases constitute the top five in both cancer and noncancer elderly patients (Repetto and Comandini 2000).

CGA has been used frequently in a variety of cancer and noncancer studies. Even in the early 1990s, a systematic review identified 28 trials that had employed comprehensive assessments. Unfortunately, the majority of these trials were studying a variety of geriatric medicine services such as day hospitals and hospital at home, as well as looking at chronic care management models (Stuck et al. 1993).

The CGA can be used in both relatively fit and the most frail. In a US review by Wieland and Hirth, the use of CGA in the most frail and oldest old cancer patients ensured that the care was cost effective. This also provides evidence for the use of CGA in elderly patients from outside Europe, thereby providing more evidence for a standardized form of assessment (Wieland and Hirth 2003).

It is vital that frailty is identified and quantified. A frailty index CGA (FI-CGA) has been used to identify different levels of frailty (i.e. mild, moderate, and severe), and not surprisingly, has found that greater frailty is associated with worse functional and mental status. In a Canadian study, the FI-CGA allowed identification of those most at risk for both decompensation of clinical status and mortality. They found that higher levels of frailty were associated with an increase in risk of an adverse outcome of death or institutionalization and the risk was highest for those with the most severe frailty. Although they found limited benefit in the intervention group (multidisciplinary input), the population was so frail with a number of irreversible geriatric syndromes that this finding may not be entirely surprising (Jones et al. 2004).

4.4.1 How does CGA compare with other Assessment Scales?

In an Italian study of cancer patients aged up to 94 years, CGA was assessed by its comparison with performance status, using both Activities of Daily Living (ADL) and Instrumental Activities of Daily Living (IADL). This prospective study allowed early identification of the frailest patients and, therefore, ensured provision of individualized cancer management. They found that up to a third of individuals required help with transportation and 13% required some form of assistance, to enable them to take their prescribed medication. Although many of these issues were identified by the ADL and the IADL, the authors were keen to stress that these individual scoring systems were merely part of the CGA (Serraino et al. 2001).

There has been speculation about the role of the CGA in various subgroups of elderly patients with cancer. The CGA may add information to some groups, but not others. In a study of over 360 elderly cancer patients, the CGA was compared with performance status and comorbidity and assessed by logistic regression (Repetto et al. 1998). The majority of the patients were independent in ADL and this is not a consistent finding in all cancer patients. Repetto and colleagues found a strong association between CGA and performance status, particularly in those elderly patients who had a good performance status at baseline. They, in keeping with others, found arthritis to be the most common comorbid condition, but somewhat surprisingly found only a prevalence of 5.2% for urinary incontinence and that 0.3% of their patients had dementia. This does, therefore, cause concern as to whether their selected patients were truly representative of those seen in everyday geriatric medicine practice.

The use of the CGA in older patients with cancer not only detects the geriatric syndromes/problems, but also adds prognostic value to each of the variables that are measured if there is a therapeutic impact of the CGA.

Extermann suggests that the performance status of patients undergoing therapy for cancer has deteriorated since the 1990s (Extermann 2003). She suggests that in many series, almost half of the cancer patients have two or more comorbidities, with the result that health problems in the older cancer patients are high.

4.4.2   Survival

A systematic review undertaken by Kuo and colleagues in 2004 identified nine studies providing survival data on patients in whom a CGA had been undertaken (Kuo et al. 2004). Their study, which incorporated all papers published on Medline from 1966 to March 2003, included papers where there was a randomized trial of outpatient CGA versus usual care. The majority of the studies were in primary care, with only three in a hospital consultation setting. They found that outpatient CGA had no demonstrable benefit for the survival of frail, older patients when compared to usual care. While statistically convincing, there are notable deficiencies in this systematic review. It did expand the earlier meta-analysis of CGA, performed by Stuck and colleagues in 1993, but included only studies from the U.S. It did not include either in-patient or home usage of CGA and was poorly powered. Such findings should not discourage clinicians from using the CGA in the in-patient setting and in frail patients with cancer.

4.4.3   Who should have a CGA performed?

There remains some doubt as to which patients are ideal candidates for the CGA (Bernabei et al. 2000). There is little doubt that it is not necessary in younger, fit cancer patients, but some suggest that even fit older cancer patients should undergo the CGA. What is quite clear is its positive role in the very frail individuals when making decisions about treatment and prognosis. However, there are a number of older individuals with cancer in whom the CGA may potentially pick up early-stage disability and geriatric syndromes, which are treatable. It is essential that the CGA is evaluated in prospective clinical trials to ensure that the oncology profession continues to use it. In patients with breast cancer, those receiving a CGA have a better prognosis than in non-CGA patients, though numbers studied are small.

Despite oncologists and geriatricians working together, there is often some doubt as to whether a patient can tolerate aggressive, life-prolonging treatment following a diagnosis of cancer. Treatment has a variety of effects on a patient and a number of issues are present that may have been previously undetected. The CGA may, therefore, help in the management of older individuals by detecting frailty, ensuring that there is treatment for previously unsuspected conditions, and that all social barriers to treatment are removed to ensure that no ageist attitudes occur (Balducci and Beghe 2000).

4.4.4 What is the evidence in breast cancer?

In a pilot study, 15 patients with early breast cancer, with a mean age of 79 years, were assessed every 3 months by a multidisciplinary team for a total of 6 months. They found that from this small sample, comorbidities as measured by the CIRS-G ranged between 3 and 9 (median 5). Two-thirds of patients were at pharmacological risk, a third at psychosocial risk, and just over half at nutritional risk. While initially each patient had, on average, six problems, a further three problems developed during follow-up (Extermann et al. 2004). This study highlighted that even when there were a limited number of comorbidities, patients were at risk from a variety of other problems and each required, on average, 17 recommendations or actions. Of the 184 interventions undertaken, 48 were multidisciplinary and 50 were pharmacy-led. More importantly, the patients did appear to benefit as determined by both the researcher's assessment and patient self-reported questionnaires. The authors concluded that a full CGA being performed every 3 months was too cumbersome, and indeed, one of the issues during follow-up was patients being outside the geographical area at times of re-review. They suggested that telephone follow-up by a nurse practitioner, followed by targeted interventions by particular specialists, may be a way forward in the future, but studies need to be undertaken.

In the U.S. study of older patients with early breast cancer, a CGA performed every 3 months with monthly telephone follow-up detected, on average, six unaddressed or under-addressed problems at the initial examination and a further three new problems over the following 6 months. With this in mind, tailoring the therapy according to identified issues appears to be both pragmatic and well validated. Areas such as cognition and social support interact to affect decision-making, drug compliance, and functional dependence. Extermann has highlighted that a multidisciplinary team may use the CGA in a constructive fashion. The team includes a nurse, a nurse practitioner who then administers the core geriatric assessment, a dietician, a social worker, and a pharmacist. The team meets weekly, thereby enabling the patient to access support in the areas required. The full CGA is only undertaken if the primary nurse identifies patients at risk from a short screening protocol, which may suggest that her case mix is different from others where all individuals required the CGA (Extermann 2003).

Wedding and Höffken in 2003 advocated the use of CGA in breast cancer patients (Wedding and Höffken 2003). They found that in a 2003 PUBMED search combining the search terms "breast cancer" and "geriatric assessment" resulted in 27 items. Unfortunately, since then there has been little substantial change in the situation, and while a further 16 papers are now identified, the only papers with original data are confined to small prospective studies (Extermann et al. 2004; Hurria et al. 2005), though other authors have used the CGA in patients with breast cancer to identify the number with no comorbidity (26.4%) (Koroukian et al. 2006).

Some of the later validation of CGA in breast cancer patients has been through its inclusion in PACE (Preoperative Assessment of Cancer in the Elderly). While PACE includes CGA, it also has a measure of fatigue and performance status. It is not, however, within PACE being used to assess the selection of patients prior to surgery, but simply to document the presence of comorbidity (Pope et al. 2006).

4.4.5   Does the CGA correlate with laboratory measures?

While CGA has been compared to a number of measures of physical, emotional, and social functioning, there are little data about the correlation between serum pro-inflammatory cytokines, including IL-6 and CGA. IL-6 plays a major role in acute inflammatory response and high levels of IL-6 and TNF-α have been found in both humans and animals with cancer. There has been particular interest in IL-6 due to its association with the development of cancer cachexia, which is common in older cancer humans. In a study of 84 elderly patients with advanced cancer, a number of clinical characteristics, as well as measures of serum levels of pro-inflammatory cytokines, were undertaken. Mantovani and colleagues found that IL-6 and C-reactive protein (CRP) were significantly higher in elderly (65–96 years) cancer patients than adult cancer patients (<65 years). They found a significant association between serum levels of IL-6 and CGA variables in the elderly cancer patients; IL-6 also correlated well with CGA variables, with a statistically significant Spearman's Rank correlation coefficient between measures of functional status using the Katz Activities of Daily Living (Katz ADL), ADL, IADL, and nutritional status. While the authors suggested that IL-6 may be a reliable marker as disease outcome, it is interesting to speculate whether the now clear association between CGA variables and IL-6 merely confirms that CGA is a good indicator of outcome and IL-6 may be useful in the prospective follow-up of cancer patients (Mantovani et al. 2004).

4.5   Application of Comprehensive Geriatric Assessment in clinical practice

There is little doubt that many authors advocate the use of geriatric assessment in the elderly cancer patient in an effort to avoid impairment of activities and performance, recognize the need for supporting independence, and delay or avoid the need for care and the resulting dependence (Harlacher and Fusgen 2000).

It is also important that the patient be enabled to remain at home in a familiar environment. A number of social issues, including income, availability of transportation, and home support, will undoubtedly influence the tolerance of different cancer treatments (Monfardini and Balducci 1999). While CGA has been advocated by a number of authors, taskforces, and as a result of courses on the management of older people with cancer, some clinicians find it long and cumbersome (Hurria et al. 2006; Audisio et al. 2004; Extermann et al. 2005; Bruce et al. 2004). In these cases the abbreviated comprehensive geriatric assessment (a-CGA) may be more appropriate. The a-CGA was developed by selection of various instruments that make up the CGA. Fifteen items were chosen and the a-CGA was validated in over 500 patients with cancer, of whom 43% had a primary diagnosis of breast cancer (Overcash et al. 2005). Unfortunately, there was no assessment of the time taken for the a-CGA to be administered, as it was part of a larger battery of tests. The authors, however, have suggested that it may take as little as 5 min when compared with the 30 min to administer the CGA. The full use of the a-CGA in identifying patients who require more intensive assessment has been recommended (Overcash et al. 2006).

While there is little doubt by individual clinicians, taskforce groups, or organizations of oncologists and geriatricians that there is a role for assessment of older people with cancer, there is still a lack of published data. The taskforce on CGA from the International Society of Geriatric Oncology (SIOG) was quite clear in its 2005 recommendations that there was evidence to support the use of CGA in elderly cancer patients (Extermann et al. 2005). They found that although CGA was well used within geriatric medicine, its relevance in oncology was difficult to determine, as most of the data were from patients who may incidentally have cancer rather than from a primary group of elderly individuals with cancer. There is very little doubt that the CGA when used in the oncology clinic does identify unrecognized geriatric problems. However, the data does not determine whether these problems would have been identified by the involvement of a geriatrician or a clinician skilled in geriatric medicine. Thus it may be that the CGA simply identifies deficiencies in training and further supports the increased collaboration of geriatricians with oncologists. Of particular concern is the under-recognition of cognitive impairment and depression, and while the former should have been identified in the community prior to the presentation of the individual with cancer, the latter may be simply related to the new diagnosis rather than to a preexisting condition.

If the CGA improves survival in only those individuals with advanced stage disease and not early stage cancer, it must be considered as to whether the CGA has been used to identify coexisting conditions that were more likely to result in death, than as a result of the tumor itself. There are little data that tell us whether the CGA alone has influenced the treatment that oncologists and surgeons offer to their patients with breast cancer. Although PACE may turn out to be an alternative to CGA, the need for a short screening test which the a-CGA provides may target the use of PACE in the future. In future research, it must be quite clear as to the primary outcomes of any study, using a-CGA or CGA prior to the treatment of an older person with cancer. This will unfortunately be a difficult study to undertake. The ethics of identifying coexisting comorbidity and not treating it is clearly difficult.

It must, therefore, rest with individual clinicians when designing research studies, to ensure that primary and secondary outcomes are clear, that patient quality of life has as high a priority as quantity, (i.e. survival) and that individual patients help determine outcome measures that are important to them.

While geriatricians and oncologists continue to work together and there is a large body of evidence that has developed from the International SIOG, there is still a gap between research data and application of clinical practice. Undoubtedly, the CGA has much to offer in the early assessment and ongoing monitoring of elderly patients with breast cancer, though data are still at times anecdotal or the result of retrospective analysis.

With improving therapies, more frail patients will require assessment and the CGA will be of particular benefit.

References

Audisio RA, Bozzetti F, Gennari R et al (2004) The surgical management of elderly cancer patients; recommendations of the SIOG surgical task force. Eur J Cancer 40(7):926–938

Balducci L (2003) New paradigms for treating elderly patients with cancer: the comprehensive geriatric assessment and guidelines for supportive care. J Support Oncol 1(4 Suppl 2):30–37

Balducci L, Beghe C (2000) The application of the principles of geriatrics to the management of the older person with cancer. Crit Rev Oncol Hematol 35(3):147–154

Bernabei R, Venturiero V, Tarsitani P, Gambassi G (2000) The comprehensive geriatric assessment: when, where, how. Crit Rev Oncol Hematol 33(1):45–56

Bruce C, Osman N, Audisio RA, Aapro MS (2004) European School of Oncology Advanced Course on Cancer in the Elderly Liverpool, 29–30 April 2004. Surg Oncol 13(4):159–167

Copeland GP, Jones D, Walters M (1991) POSSUM: a scoring system for surgical audit. Br J Surg 78(3):355–360

de Cassia Braga Ribeiro K, Kowalski LP (2003) APACHE II, POSSUM, and ASA scores and the risk of perioperative complications in patients with oral or oropharyngeal cancer. Arch Otolaryngol Head Neck Surg 129(7):739–745

Extermann M (2000) Measuring comorbidity in older cancer patients. Eur J Cancer 36(4):453–471

Extermann M (2003) Studies of comprehensive geriatric assessment in patients with cancer. Cancer Control 10(6):463–468

Extermann M, Meyer J, McGinnis M, Crocker TT, Corcoran MB, Yoder J et al (2004) A comprehensive geriatric intervention detects multiple problems in older breast cancer patients. Crit Rev Oncol Hematol 49(1):69–75

Extermann M, Aapro M, Bernabei R et al (2005) Use of comprehensive geriatric assessment in older cancer patients: recommendations from the task force on CGA of the International Society of Geriatric Oncology (SIOG). Crit Rev Oncol Hematol 55(3):241–252

Ferrucci L, Guralnik JM, Cavazzini C et al (2003) The frailty syndrome: a critical issue in geriatric oncology. Crit Rev Oncol Hemat 46(2):127–137

Gosney MA (2005) Clinical assessment of elderly people with cancer. Lancet Oncol 6:790–797

Harlacher R, Fusgen I (2000) Geriatric assessment in the elderly cancer patient. J Cancer Res Clin Oncol 126(7):369–374

Headley J, Theriault R, Smith TL (1992) Independent validation of APACHE II severity of illness score for predicting mortality in patients with breast cancer admitted to the intensive care unit. Cancer 70(2):497–503

Hurria A, Gupta S, Zauderer M et al (2005) Developing a cancer-specific geriatric assessment. Cancer 104(9):1998–2005

Hurria A, Lachs MS, Cohen HJ, Muss HB, Kornblith AB (2006) Geriatric assessment for oncologists: rationale and future directions. Crit Rev Oncol Hematol 59(3):211–217

Jones DM, Song X, Rockwood K (2004) Operationalizing a frailty index from a standardized comprehensive geriatric assessment. J Am Geriatr Soc 52(11):1929–1933

Koroukian SM, Murray P, Madigan E (2006) Comorbidity, disability, and geriatric syndromes in elderly cancer patients receiving home health care. J Clin Oncol 24(15):2304–2310

Kuo HK, Scandrett KG, Dave J, Mitchell SL (2004) The influence of outpatient comprehensive geriatric assessment on survival: a meta-analysis. Arch Gerontol Geriatr 39(3):245–254

Mantovani G, Madeddu C, Gramignano G et al (2004) Association of serum IL-6 levels with comprehensive geriatric assessment variables in a population of elderly cancer patients. Oncol Rep 11(1):197–206

Monfardini S, Balducci L (1999) A comprehensive geriatric assessment (CGA) is necessary for the study and the management of cancer in the elderly. Eur J Cancer 35(13):1771–1772

Newschaffer CJ, Bush TL, Penbarthy LT (1997) Comorbidity measurement in elderly female breast cancer patients with administrative and medical records data. J Clin Epidemiol 50(6):725–733

Overcash JA, Beckstead J, Extermann M, Cobb S (2005) The abbreviated comprehensive geriatric assessment (aCGA): a retrospective analysis. Crit Rev Oncol Hematol 54(2):129–136

Overcash JA, Beckstead J, Moody L, Extermann M, Cobb S (2006) The abbreviated comprehensive geriatric assessment (aCGA) for use in the older cancer patient as a prescreen: scoring and interpretation. Crit Rev Oncol Hematol 59(3):205–210

Paleri V, Wight RG (2002) Applicability of the adult comorbidity evaluation—27 and the Charlson indexes to assess comorbidity by notes extraction in a cohort of United Kingdom patients with head and neck cancer: a retrospective study. J Laryngol Otol 116(3):200–205

Pope D, Ramesh H, Gennari R, Corsini G, Maffezzini M, Hoekstra HJ et al (2006) Pre-operative assessment of cancer in the elderly (PACE): a comprehensive assessment of underlying characteristics of elderly cancer patients prior to elective surgery. Surg Oncol 15(4):189–197

Repetto L, Comandini D (2000) Cancer in the elderly: assessing patients for fitness. Crit Rev Oncol Hematol 35(3):155–160

Repetto L, Venturino A, Vercelli M, Gianni W, Biancardi V, Casella C et al (1998) Performance status and comorbidity in elderly cancer patients compared with young patients with neoplasia and elderly patients without neoplastic conditions. Cancer 82(4):760–765

Serraino D, Fratino L, Zagonel V (2001) Prevalence of functional disability among elderly patients with cancer. Crit Rev Oncol Hematol 39(3):269–273

Stuck AE, Siu AL, Wieland GD, Adams J, Rubenstein LZ (1993) Comprehensive geriatric assessment: a meta-analysis of controlled trials. Lancet 342(8878):1032–1036

Wedding U, Höffken K (2003) Care of breast cancer in the elderly woman—what does comprehensive geriatric assessment (CGA) help? Support Care Cancer 11(12):769–774

Wieland D, Hirth V (2003) Comprehensive geriatric assessment. Cancer Control 10(6):454–462

Chapter 5
A Practical Mini-Guide to Comprehensive Geriatric Assessment

Siri Rostoft Kristjansson

The Comprehensive Geriatric Assessment (CGA) is a practical tool used by geriatricians in their daily work. Unfortunately, there is no such thing as an internationally standardized CGA, but we will present some of the tools that are most frequently used in the field of geriatric oncology.

5.1 Functional Measurements

These measurement tools help define patients' functional capabilities.

5.1.1 Eastern Cooperative Oncology Group Performance Status

The Eastern Cooperative Oncology Group Performance Status (ECOG PS) (Table 5.1) is widely used in oncology settings and is a well-established prognostic factor for most cancers. However, medical doctors outside the oncology setting, such as internal medicine specialists and surgeons, are not always familiar with ECOG PS.

5.1.2 Katz Index of Independence in Basic Activities of Daily Living

This index measures basic (or personal) activities of daily living including toileting, feeding, transferring, grooming, continence, and bathing (Table 5.2). Dependency in any of these activities will usually require help from a caregiver on a daily basis. In Europe, the Barthel index is more widely used.

S.R. Kristjansson (✉)
Department of Geriatric Medicine, Oslo University Hospital Ullevål, Oslo, N-0407, Norway
e-mail: sirikristjansson@gmail.com

M.W. Reed and R.A. Audisio (eds.), *Management of Breast Cancer in Older Women*,
DOI 10.1007/978-1-84800-265-4_5, © Springer-Verlag London Limited 2011

Table 5.1 Eastern cooperative oncology group performance status (Oken et al. 1982)

Grade	ECOG
0	Fully active, able to carry on all predisease performance without restriction
1	Restricted in physically strenuous activity, but ambulatory and able to carry out work of a light or sedentary nature, e.g., light house work, office work
2	Ambulatory and capable of all self-care, but unable to carry out any work activities. Up and about more than 50% of waking hours
3	Capable of only limited self-care, confined to bed or chair more than 50% of waking hours
4	Completely disabled. Cannot carry on any self-care. Totally confined to bed or chair
5	Dead

The ECOG Performance Status is in the public domain and, therefore, available for public use. The Eastern Cooperative Oncology Group, Robert Comis M.D., Group Chair

Table 5.2 Katz index of independence in activities of daily living

ActivitiesPoints (1 or 0)	Independence (1 Point) No supervision, direction, or personal assistance	Dependence (0 Points) With supervision, direction, personal assistance, or total care
Bathing Points: _____	Bathes self completely or needs help in bathing only a single part of the body such as the back, genital area or disabled extremity	Need help with bathing more than one part of the body, getting in or out of the tub or shower. Requires total bathing
Dressing Points: _____	Get clothes from closets and drawers and puts on clothes and outer garments complete with fasteners. May have help tying shoes.	Needs help with dressing self or needs to be completely dressed.
Toileting Points: _____	Goes to toilet, gets on and off, arranges clothes, cleans genital area without help.	Needs help transferring to the toilet, cleaning self or uses bedpan or commode.
Transferring Points: _____	Moves in and out of bed or chair unassisted. Mechanical transfer aids are acceptable	Needs help in moving from bed to chair or requires a complete transfer.
Continence Points: _____	Exercises complete self control over urination and defecation.	Is partially or totally incontinent of bowel or bladder
Feeding Points: _____	Gets food from plate into mouth without help. Preparation of food may be done by another person.	Needs partial or total help with feeding or requires parenteral feeding.
Total Points: _____		

Score of 6 = High, Patient is independent.
Score of 0 = Low, patient is very dependent.
Adapted from (Katz et al. 1970), © The Gerontological Society of America. Reproduced by permission of the publisher

5.1.3   The Lawton Instrumental Activities of Daily Living Scale

Instrumental activities of daily living (IADL) include more specialized activities such as abilities to manage money, to shop, to use transportation, housekeeping, and food preparation (Table 5.3). Dependency in IADL will require help from a caregiver, but not necessarily on a daily basis.

Table 5.3   The Lawton instrumental activities of daily living scale

Ability to use telephone	
Operates telephone on own initiative; looks up and dials numbers	1
Dials a few well-known numbers	1
Answers telephone, but does not dial	1
Does not use telephone at all	0
Shopping	
Takes care of all shopping needs independently	1
Shops independently for small purchases	0
Needs to be accompanied on any shopping trip	0
Completely unable to shop	0
Food preparation	
Plans, prepares, and serves adequate meals independently	1
Prepares adequate meals if supplied with ingredients	0
Heats and serves prepared meals or prepares meals, but does not maintain adequate diet	0
Needs to have meals prepared and served	0
Housekeeping	
Maintains house alone with occasional assistance (heavy work)	1
Performs light daily tasks such as dishwashing, bed making	1
Performs light daily tasks, but cannot maintain acceptable level of cleanliness	1
Needs help with all home maintenance tasks	1
Does not participate in any housekeeping tasks	0
Laundry	
Does personal laundry completely	1
Launders small items, rinses socks, stockings, etc.	1
All laundry must be done by others	0
Mode of transportation	
Travels independently on public transportation or drives own car	1
Arranges own travel via taxi, but does not otherwise use public transportation	1
Travels on public transportation when assisted or accompanied by another	1
Travel limited to taxi or automobile with assistance of another	0
Does not travel at all	0
Responsibility for own medications	
Is responsible for taking medication in correct dosages at correct time	1
Takes responsibility if medication is prepared in advance in separate dosages	0
Is not capable of dispensing own medication	0

(continued)

Table 5.3 (continued)

Ability to handle finances	
Manages financial matters independently (budgets, writes checks, pays rent and bills, goes to bank); collects and keeps track of income	1
Manages day-to-day purchases, but needs help with banking, major purchases, etc.	1
Incapable of handling money	0

Scoring: For each category, circle the item description that most closely resembles the client's highest functional level (either 0 or 1).

From (Lawton and Brody 1969) Copyright The Gerontological Society of America. Used with permission of the publisher

5.2 Comorbidity

Comorbidity can be assessed using a numbered scale, such as Cumulative Illness Rating Scale (CIRS) or Charlson Comorbidity Index.

The manual for scoring the CIRS is published as an appendix in "A Manual of Guidelines to Score the Modified CIRS and Its Validation in Acute Hospitalized Elderly Patients". (Salvi et al. 2008)

The Charlson Comorbidity Index was published in 1987. (Charlson et al. 1987) An example of the scoring sheet is shown in Table 5.4.

Satariano et al. (Satariano and Ragland 1994) found that breast cancer patients who had three or more of seven selected comorbid conditions had a 20-fold higher rate of mortality from causes other than breast cancer and a 4-fold higher rate of all-cause mortality when compared with patients who had no comorbid conditions. The seven comorbidities found to be independently associated with breast cancer were as follows:

- Myocardial infarction
- Other types of heart disease
- Diabetes
- Other forms of cancer
- Respiratory conditions
- Gallbladder conditions
- Liver conditions

5.3 Nutritional Status

A well-validated tool in the geriatric population is the Mini Nutritional Assessment (MNA) (Fig. 5.1).

Table 5.4 Charlson comorbidity index

Comorbidity	Present	Points
Myocardial infarct		1
Congestive heart failure		1
Peripheral vascular disease		1
Cerebrovascular disease (except hemiplegia)		1
Dementia		1
Chronic pulmonary disease		1
Connective tissue disease		1
Ulcer disease		1
Mild liver disease		1
Diabetes (without complications)		1
Diabetes with end organ damage		2
Hemiplegia		2
Moderate or severe renal disease		2
2nd solid tumor (nonmetastatic)		2
Leukemia		2
Lymphoma, MM…		2
Moderate or severe liver disease		3
Second metastatic solid tumor		6
AIDS		6

Reprinted from (Charlson et al. 1987) With permission from Elsevier

5.4 Cognitive Function

The most widely used screening instrument for cognitive dysfunction is the Mini Mental State Examination (MMSE). A sample of the MMSE is shown in Table 5.5.

5.5 Depression

Depression is common among elderly patients, and a screening instrument for depression is often included in the CGA. The Geriatric Depression Scale is validated in an elderly population (Table 5.6). Although differing sensitivities and specificities have been obtained across studies, for clinical purposes, a score > 5points is suggestive of depression and should warrant a follow-up interview. Scores >10 points are almost always depression.

Mini Nutritional Assessment
MNA®

Last name:		First name:	Sex:	Date:
Age:	Weight, kg:	Height, cm:	I.D. Number:	

Complete the screen by filling in the boxes with the appropriate numbers.
Add the numbers for the screen. If score is 11 or less, continue with the assessment to gain a Malnutrition Indicator Score.

Screening

A Has food intake declined over the past 3 months due to loss of appetite, digestive problems, chewing or swallowing difficulties?
0 = severe loss of appetite
1 = moderate loss of appetite
2 = no loss of appetite ☐

B Weight loss during the last 3 months
0 = weight loss greater than 3 kg (6.6 lbs)
1 = does not know
2 = weight loss between 1 and 3 kg (2.2 and 6.6 lbs)
3 = no weight loss ☐

C Mobility
0 = bed or chair bound
1 = able to get out of bed/chair but does not go out
2 = goes out ☐

D Has suffered psychological stress or acute disease in the past 3 months
0 = yes   2 = no ☐

E Neuropsychological problems
0 = severe dementia or depression
1 = mild dementia
2 = no psychological problems ☐

F Body Mass Index (BMI) (weight in kg) / (height in m²)
0 = BMI less than 19
1 = BMI 19 to less than 21
2 = BMI 21 to less than 23
3 = BMI 23 or greater ☐

Screening score (subtotal max. 14 points) ☐☐
12 points or greater   Normal – not at risk – no need to complete assessment
11 points or below   Possible malnutrition – continue assessment

Assessment

G Lives independently (not in a nursing home or hospital)
0 = no   1 = yes ☐

H Takes more than 3 prescription drugs per day
0 = yes   1 = no ☐

I Pressure sores or skin ulcers
0 = yes   1 = no ☐

Ref. Vellas B, Villars H, Abellan G, et al. Overview of the MNA® - Its History and Challenges. J Nut Health Aging 2006;10:456-465.
Rubenstein LZ, Harker JO, Salva A, Guigoz Y, Vellas B. Screening for Undernutrition in Geriatric Practice: Developing the Short-Form Mini Nutritional Assessment (MNA-SF). J. Geront 2001;56A: M366-377.
Guigoz Y. The Mini-Nutritional Assessment (MNA®) Review of the Literature - What does it tell us? J Nutr Health Aging 2006; 10:466-487.

© Nestlé, 1994, Revision 2006. N67200 12/99 10M
For more information : www.mna-elderly.com

J How many full meals does the patient eat daily?
0 = 1 meal
1 = 2 meals
2 = 3 meals ☐

K Selected consumption markers for protein intake
• At least one serving of dairy products (milk, cheese, yogurt) per day   yes ☐   no ☐
• Two or more servings of legumes or eggs per week   yes ☐   no ☐
• Meat, fish or poultry every day   yes ☐   no ☐
0.0 = if 0 or 1 yes
0.5 = if 2 yes
1.0 = if 3 yes ☐.☐

L Consumes two or more servings of fruits or vegetables per day?
0 = no   1 = yes ☐

M How much fluid (water, juice, coffee, tea, milk...)is consumed per day?
0.0 = less than 3 cups
0.5 = 3 to 5 cups
1.0 = more than 5 cups ☐.☐

N Mode of feeding
0 = unable to eat without assistance
1 = self-fed with some difficulty
2 = self-fed without any problem ☐

O Self view of nutritional status
0 = views self as being malnourished
1 = is uncertain of nutritional state
2 = views self as having no nutritional problem ☐

P In comparison with other people of the same age, how does the patient consider his/her health status?
0.0 = not as good
0.5 = does not know
1.0 = as good
2.0 = better ☐.☐

Q Mid-arm circumference (MAC) in cm
0.0 = MAC less than 21
0.5 = MAC 21 to 22
1.0 = MAC 22 or greater ☐.☐

R Calf circumference (CC) in cm
0 = CC less than 31   1 = CC 31 or greater ☐

Assessment (max. 16 points) ☐☐.☐

Screening score ☐☐

Total Assessment (max. 30 points) ☐☐.☐

Malnutrition Indicator Score
17 to 23.5 points   at risk of malnutrition ☐
Less than 17 points   malnourished ☐

Fig. 1 Mini Mutational Assessment (MNA)

Table 5.5   Sample from the mini mental state examination (MMSE)

Orientation to time	"What is the date?"
Registration	"Listen carefully. I am going to say three words. You say them back after I stop. Ready? Here they are…APPLE (pause), PENNY (pause), TABLE (pause). Now repeat those words back to me." [Repeat up to five times, but score only the first trial.]
Naming	"What is this?" [Point to a pencil or pen.]
Reading	"Please read this and do what it says." [Show examinee the words on the stimulus form.] Close your eyes

Reproduced by special permission of the publisher, Psychological Assessment Resources, Inc., 16204 North Florida Avenue, Lutz, Florida 33549, from the Mini Mental State Examination, by Marshal Folstein and Susan Folstein, © 1975, 1998, 2001 by Mini Mental LLC, Inc. Published 2001 by Psychological Assessment Resources, Inc. Further reproduction is prohibited without permission of PAR, Inc. The MMSE can be purchased from PAR, Inc. by calling (813) 968–3003

Table 5.6   Geriatric depression scale: (Short form – Gds-15)

Choose the best answer for how you have felt over the past week:
1. Are you basically satisfied with your life? YES/**NO**
2. Have you dropped many of your activities and interests? **YES**/NO
3. Do you feel that your life is empty? **YES**/NO
4. Do you often get bored? **YES**/NO
5. Are you in good spirits most of the time? YES/**NO**
6. Are you afraid that something bad is going to happen to you? **YES**/NO
7. Do you feel happy most of the time? YES/**NO**
8. Do you often feel helpless? **YES**/NO
9. Do you prefer to stay at home, rather than going out and doing new things? **YES**/NO
10. Do you feel you have more problems with memory than most? **YES**/NO
11. Do you think it is wonderful to be alive now? YES/**NO**
12. Do you feel pretty worthless the way you are now? **YES**/NO
13. Do you feel full of energy? YES/**NO**
14. Do you feel that your situation is hopeless? **YES**/NO
15. Do you think that most people are better off than you are? **YES**/NO

Answers in bold indicate depression. Although differing sensitivities and specificities have been obtained across studies, for clinical purposes a score >5 points is suggestive of depression and should warrant a follow-up interview. Scores >10 are almost always depression. Yesavage JA, Brink TL, Rose TL, Lum O, Huang V, Adey MB, Leirer VO: Development and validation of a geriatric depression screening scale: A preliminary report. Journal of Psychiatric Research 17: 37–49, 1983

5.6   Screening Tools

The need for shorter screening tools to identify patients who need a full CGA has been advocated. The Vulnerable Elders Survey (VES-13) (Table 5.7) and the Groningen Frailty Indicator (Table 5.8) are two examples of such tools. The role of screening tools in geriatric oncology needs further validation.

Table 5.7 *Vulnerable elders survey (VES-13)*

Vulnerable elders survey (VES-13)

1. Age_____ (One point for age 75-84, 3 points for age 85 or greater)
2. In general, compared to other people your age, would you say that your health is:
   A. Poor, * (1 Point)
   B. Fair,* (1 Point)
   C. Good
   D. Very Good, or
   E. Excellent
3. How much difficulty, on average, do you have with the following physical activities: (SCORE 1 POINT FOR EACH * RESPONSE, MAXIMUM OF 2 POINTS)

	No difficulty	A little difficulty	Some difficulty*	A lot of difficulty*	Unable to do*
Stooping, crouching or kneeling					
Lifting, or carrying objects as heavy as 10 pounds					
Reaching or extending arms above shoulder level					
Writing, or handling and grasping small objects					
Walking a quarter of a mile					
Heavy housework such as scrubbing floors or washing windows					

4. Because of your health or a physical condition, do you have any difficulty: (SCORE 4 POINTS FOR ONE OR MORE * YES RESPONSES IN THIS SECTION)
   A. Shopping for personal items (like toilet items or medicine)?
   o   YES>> Do you get help with shopping?   YES*   NO
   o   NO
   o   DON"T DO>> Is that because of your health   YES*   NO

   B. Managing money (like keeping track of expenses or paying bills)?
   o   YES>> Do you get help with managing money?   YES*   NO
   o   NO
   o   DON'T DO>> Is it because of your health?   YES*   NO

   C. Walking across the room? USE OF CANE OR WALKER IS OKAY
   o   YES>> Do you get help with walking   YES*   NO
   o   NO
   o   DON"T DO>> Is that because of your health?   YES*   NO

   D. Doing light housework (like washing dishes, straightening up, or light cleaning?
   o   YES>> Do you get help with light housework?   YES*   NO
   o   NO
   o   DON'T DO>> Is that because of your health?   YES*   NO

   E. Bathing or showering?
   o   YES>> Do you get help with bathing or showering?   YES*   NO
   o   NO
   o   DON"T DO>> Is that because of your health?   YES*   NO

Scoring 3 or greater identifies an individual that has 4.2 times the risk of death or functional decline over the next two years.

From: The Vulnerable Elders Survey (VES-13): A Tool for Identifying Vulnerable Elders in the Community – 2001. Saliba, S, Elliott M, Rubenstein LA, Solomon DH, et al. Journal of the American Geriatric Society 2001;49:1691-9.

Table 5.8 Groningen frailty indicator

	YES	NO
Mobility		
Can the patient perform the following tasks without assistance from another person (walking aids such as a cane or wheelchair are allowed)		
Grocery shopping	0	1
Walking outside house (around house or to neighbors)	0	1
Getting (un)dressed	0	1
Visiting restroom	0	1
Vision	1	0
Does the patient encounter problems in daily life because of impaired vision?		
Hearing		
Does the patient encounter problems in daily life because of impaired hearing?	1	0
Nutrition		
Has the patient unintentionally lost a lot of weight in the past 6 months (6 kg in 6 months or 3 kg in a month)	1	0
Comorbidity		
Does the patient use 4 or more different types of medication?		

	YES	NO	SOMETIMES
Cognition	1	0	0
Does the patient have any complaints about his/her memory (or diagnosed with dementia)			
Psychosocial	1	0	1
Does the patient ever experience emptiness around him?			
Does the patient ever miss the presence of other people around him?	1	0	1
Does the patient ever feel alone?	1	0	1
Has the patient been feeling down or depressed lately?	1	0	1
Has the patient felt nervous or anxious lately?	1	0	1
Physical fitness	1	0	
How would the patient rate his/her own physical fitness? (0–10, 0 is very bad, 10 is very good)			
Total score GFI			

Circle the appropriate answers and add scores\
Reprinted [adapted] from (Slaets 2006), with permission from Elsevier

5.7   Physical Performance Assessment

The ability to perform certain physical tests can predict mortality and physical dependence. Objective physical measurements of gait speed and grip strength are included in the definition of the phenotypic frailty syndrome (Fried et al. 2001).

A widely used example of a physical test is the "Timed Up-and-Go" (TUG): A person sits on an armchair is asked to walk 3 m, turn around, then walk back, and sit down on the chair. The time used to complete this task is recorded. A cut-off of 19 s approximately identifies the slowest quintile in a sample of noninstitutionalized elderly individuals (Rockwood et al. 2007).

References

Charlson ME, Pompei P, Ales KL, McKenzie CR (1987) A new method of classifying prognostic comorbidity in longitudinal studies: development and validation. J Chron Dis 40(5):373–383

Fried LP, Tangen CM, Walston J, Newman AB, Hirsch C, Gottdiener J et al (2001) Frailty in Older Adults - Evidence for a Phenotype. J Gerontol A BiolMed Sci 56(3):146–157

Katz S, Down TD, Cash HR et al (1970) Progress in the development of the index of ADL. Gerontologist 10:20–30

Lawton MP, Brody EM (1969) Assessment of older people: self-maintaining and instrumental activities of daily living. Gerontologist 9(3):179–186

Oken MM, Creech RH, Tormey DC, Horton J, Davis TE, McFadden ET, Carbone PP (1982) Toxicity And Response Criteria Of The Eastern Cooperative Oncology Group. Am J Clin Oncol 5:649–655

Rockwood K, Andrew M, Mitnitski A (2007) A comparison of two approaches to measuring frailty in elderly people. J Gerontol A Biol Sci Med Sci 62(7):738–743

Saliba S, Elliott M, Rubenstein LA, Solomon DH et al (2001) The Vulnerable Elders Survey: A Tool for Identifying Vulnerable Older People in the Community. J Am Geriatric Soc 49:1691–1699

Salvi F et al (2008) A Manual of Guidelines to Score the Modified Cumulative Illness Rating Scale and Its Validation in Acute Hospitalized Elderly Patients. J Am Geriatr Soc 56(10):1926–1931

Satariano WA, Ragland DR (1994) The Effect of Comorbidity on 3-Year Survival of Women with Primary Breast Cancer. Ann Intern Med 120:104–110

Slaets JPJ (2006) Vulnerability in the elderly: frailty. Med Clin N Am 90(4):593–601

Chapter 6
Impact of the Physiological Effects of Aging on the Pharmacokinetics and Pharmacodynamics of Systemic Breast Cancer Treatment

Paul Hamberg, Maja J.A. de Jonge, and Caroline M. Seynaeve

6.1 Introduction

The physiological changes in the process of aging are the sum of multiple factors affecting each individual to a different extent. The result of these changes and the impact on pharmacokinetics (PKs) and pharmacodynamics (PDs) of systemic anti-cancer treatment are linked mechanistically to altered drug handling and altered physiological reserve. The risk of death does increase with chronological age, which is consistent with a progressive and independently evolving aging process; yet aging is better reflected by the biological age than the calendar age. Determining the biological age or the functional status of an elder is one of the challenges facing those involved in the treatment of the elderly as no universal instrument or test is available to estimate the individual biological age (as discussed in Chap. 4). No treatment should commence, especially concerning cytotoxic anticancer therapy, before careful evaluation of the physiological reserve of an older individual has been assessed, while during treatment an ongoing routine must assure that in case of preceding under- or overestimation of the assumed biological age of a patient, it is recognized in an early phase and treatment is adjusted accordingly.

In this chapter, we will focus on the physiological effects of aging on the PK and PD properties of systemic breast cancer therapies. Efficacy data of the different therapies are not addressed, as these are extensively discussed in other chapters in this book.

6.1.1 Changes in the Elderly

Changes of importance of PK and PD properties of anticancer treatment in the healthy older population are not merely limited to purely physical factors. In general,

P. Hamberg (✉)
Department of Medical Oncology, Erasmus University Medical Center–Daniel den Hoed Cancer Center, Rotterdam, The Netherlands
e-mail: p.hamberg@mchaaglanden.nl

M.W. Reed and R.A. Audisio (eds.), *Management of Breast Cancer in Older Women*,
DOI 10.1007/978-1-84800-265-4_6, © Springer-Verlag London Limited 2011

Table 6.1 Types of changes in older women relevant to pharmacokinetics and pharmacodynamics

Type of change	Examples of changing aspects
Lifestyle changes	Social interactions/activities
	Diet habits
Physiological changes	Altered body composition
	Decreased drug absorption from the gastrointestinal tract
	Decreased glomerular filtration rate,
	Altered hepatic metabolism
	Lower bone marrow cellularity
	Changes in cardiac capacity
	Decline in neurological performances
Pathophysiological changes	Comorbidity
	Poly-pharmacy

three groups of factors might have an impact on PK and PD properties of drugs in older women as compared to their younger counterpart (Table 6.1), including changes in lifestyle and habits, physiological changes occurring as a function of age, and pathophysiological alterations.

In patients reaching older age, changes in diet habits as well as in social interactions occur that are unrelated to health issues, and resulting in an altered pastime. Elderly seek food activities as a means for companionship brought on by the social context, and once in that social context, generally eat what is served. (Koehler and Leonhaeuser 2008) As changes in pharmacokinetics of oral drugs due to food intake in general are variable depending on the specific drug taken, physicians should be aware of these nonmedical changes affecting their prescribed treatment. For this purpose, attention at intake and start of breast cancer therapy is warranted in order to specifically address relevant issues.

Pathophysiological changes are of crucial importance in the elderly as compared to younger women: the incidence of diseases rises during the age timeline, resulting in a higher frequency of comorbidity and related medication use. Comorbidity, with a reported incidence of 50–80% in the age group between 65–101 years (Aapro et al. 2005; Janssen-Heijnen et al. 2005), is affecting anticancer treatment at several levels. For instance: comorbidity with an impact on organ function will directly generate alterations in the PKs, and subsequently this change in PKs as well as the diminished organ function/reserve itself will result in an altered PD profile. Medication prescribed in relation to the comorbidity will put the elderly at risk for drug-drug interactions. Further, the risk for drug-drug interaction(s) increases with the number of drugs taken, with a likelihood of interaction of almost 50% while taking five different drugs, increasing to nearly 100% when using eight drugs concomitantly (Blower et al. 2005). Given the fact that in an oncology ward, the median number of drugs prescribed per patient was eight, everyone caring for oncology patients should be aware of likely interactions and their sequelae. The relevance of comorbidity (Chap. 3) as well as drug-drug interactions (Chap. 20) in the management of the elderly with breast cancer is discussed extensively elsewhere in this book.

6.2 Physiological Changes Occurring as a Function of Increasing Age

Most prominent physiological changes in otherwise healthy older subjects can be classified into two main categories:

- PK changes, including the influence of altered body composition, decreased drug absorption from the gastro-intestinal (GI) tract, decreased glomerular filtration rate, and altered hepatic metabolism; and
- Factors resulting in a changed PD profile like lower bone marrow cellularity, changes in cardiac capacity, and decline in neurological and cognitive performances (Table 6.1).

The most relevant body composition changes associated with increasing age constitute of a decrease of lean body mass and total body water, accompanied by an increased proportion of body fat (Elmadfa and Meyer 2008). The part of total body weight that is accounted for by fat increases by about 50% during aging, whereas the loss of total body water is estimated at 6 L between the ages of 20 and 80 years (Elmadfa and Meyer 2008). These changes give rise to a different volume of distribution for both lipophilic and hydrophilic drugs with a reduction or rise in peak plasma levels, respectively. Also, the volume of distribution of drugs is affected by the decrease in albumin that is consistently shown in the older population (Salive et al. 1992), resulting in a larger unbound fraction of drugs in serum known to be responsible for both efficacy and toxicity of a therapeutic agent. Especially for drugs with a narrow therapeutic window, such as cytotoxic drugs, this might result in increased toxicity.

During healthy aging, the autonomic nervous system of the GI tract is deteriorating in a neuropathic way, contributing to the declining function of the GI tract (Phillips and Powley 2007). A delay in gastric emptying as well as a slowing down of peristalsis will alter the pharmacokinetics of drugs, usually by a delay in time to maximal concentration, and sometimes, due to a longer exposure time to the intestinal surface in an increased absorption (McLean and Le Couteur 2004). On the other hand, the increased absorption rate due to longer exposure time can be counterbalanced by the well-known decline in splanchnic blood flow, resulting in a decrease in absorption rate. For a long time it has been assumed that gastric acidity declines as a function of age; however, more recent reports have shown that the majority of patients maintain gastric acid secretion for their entire life. At the moment, one assumes that the very frequent use of concomitant medication like H_2-receptor antagonists and proton pump inhibitors in the older patient groups is causing the observed diminished gastric acidity (McLean and Le Couteur 2004). The ultimate effect of these changes on absorption of a drug in the individual remains unpredictable.

Furthermore, healthy aging is coupled with a decline in kidney function due to an increased degree in fibrosis of renal tissue and a lack of regenerative ability, causing a decreased glomerular filtration rate (Percy et al. 2008). It is obvious that this physiological event may have a major impact on the clearance of a substantial part of drugs used in breast cancer therapy, becoming even more relevant in case comedication is taken.

As with the kidney, the liver also suffers due to the aging process, as hepatic blood flow, liver volume, and metabolic capacities decrease resulting in a considerable decrease in physiological hepatic clearance of drugs in the older population (Zeeh and Platt 2002; Durnas et al. 1990). This may result in a higher exposure to drugs that are cleared by the liver, but may also have an effect on the extent of the formation of (active) metabolites. Given the fact that both comedication and breast cancer therapies may be cleared by the liver, as well as the reality that a considerable part of breast cancer patients suffers from liver metastases (potentially further limiting liver function), this should carefully be evaluated, especially in older breast cancer patients.

6.3 Physiological Effects of Aging on Pharmacokinetics and Pharmacodynamics of Hormonal Treatment

Hormonal therapy for breast cancer is typically administered orally (except for fulvestrant, being intramuscularly given), resulting in all previously mentioned factors potentially influencing the PK-PD profile of hormonal treatment in older patients, in contrast to, for example, cytotoxic drugs that usually are administered by intravenous injection, bypassing potential limitations in absorption from the intestinal tract. The mechanism of action of hormonal therapy for breast cancer is aiming to reduce estrogen levels or block signaling through the inhibition of estrogen receptors. Available drugs are classified according to the mechanism of action, and consist of selective estrogen receptor modulators (SERMs), aromatase inhibitors (AIs), and progestins or selective estrogen receptor down regulators (SERDs). Below, the available data evaluating the impact of age on PK-PD properties of hormonal agents in patients with breast cancer are reviewed (Tables 6.2 and 6.3).

6.3.1 SERMs

Bioavailability of the two SERMs currently approved for the treatment of breast cancer, tamoxifen, and toremifene (a chlorinated derivative of tamoxifen), is close to 100%. Protein binding (>95%) and hepatic metabolization are also similar in both agents.

The PKs of tamoxifen, the most widely used SERM in breast cancer, is unmistakenly altered during aging. The concentrations of tamoxifen as well as of its main metabolites (N-desmethyltamoxifen, N-desdimethyltamoxifen, primary alcohol, and 4-hydroxytamoxifen) are consistently increasing over age cohorts; concentrations being 2–3 times higher in women in the older cohorts as compared to the group of women under 40 years of age (Peyrade et al. 1996; Sheth et al. 2003). A remarkable finding is that the concentration of tamoxifen as well as of every single metabolite

Drug	Pharmacokinetic changes due to aging	Reference
Hormonal therapy		
Tamoxifen	Plasma concentrations of tamoxifen as well as its metabolites are 2–3 times higher in elderly	(Peyrade et al. 1996; Sheth et al. 2003)
Letrozole	No effect	(Buzdar et al. 2002)
Anastrozole	No data	
Exemestane	No data	
Megestrol acetate	No data	
Fulvestrant	No data	
Cytotoxic therapy		
Doxorubicin	No effect	(Dobbs et al. 1995; Rudek et al. 2004)
Pegylated doxorubicin	No data	
Epirubicin	No data	
Epirubicin in multiagent regimens	Decreased clearance	(Wade et al. 1992)
Idarubicin	No effect	(Toffoli et al. 2000)
Mitoxantrone	No effect	(Repetto et al. 1999)
Docetaxel	No effect	(Dobbs et al. 1995; Ten Tije et al. 2005; Hurria et al. 2006)
	Lower Lawton score (meaning more dependent in instrumental activities) and higher score on Geriatric Depression scale correlated with longer terminal T ½.	(Hurria et al. 2006)
Paclitaxel	Decreased clearance and volume of distribution	(Smorenburg et al. 2003; Joerger et al. 2006)
Vinorelbin	Conflicting results:	
	No effect vs.	(Sorio et al. 1997; Wong et al. 2006; Vogel et al. 1999)
	Decreased clearance	(Gauvin et al. 2000)
Continuous 5-FU	Decreased clearance	(Etienne et al. 1998)
Capecitabine	No effect	(Cassidy et al. 1999)
UFT	No data	
Doxifluridine	No data	
CMF	Modest increase in 5-FU clearance	(Gelman and Taylor 1984)
	No effect on methotrexate or cyclophosphamide	
AC	No effect	(Crivellari et al. 2000)
Biologicals		
Trastuzumab	No data	
Bevacizumab	No data	

5-FU 5-fluorouracil; *UFT* tegafur-uracil; *CMF* cyclophosphamide, methotrexate and 5-FU; *AC* doxorubicin and cyclophosphamide
Combination regimens are only mentioned in the table if PK data are available

Table 6.3 Impact of age assessed by direct comparison or modeling on the pharmacodynamics of therapy directed at breast cancer

Drug	Pharmacodynamic changes due to aging	Reference
Hormonal therapy		
Tamoxifen	No data	
Letrozole	No effect with regard to the level of estrogen suppression	(Pfister et al. 2001)
Anastrozole	No data	
Exemestane	No data	
Megestrol acetate	No data	
Fulvestrant	No data	
Cytotoxic therapy		
Doxorubicin	Increased incidence of cardiotoxicity	(Pinder et al. 2007)
Pegylated doxorubicin	Dose-dependent:	(O'Brien et al. 2004)
	60 mg/m^2 every 6 weeks: higher incidence of hematological toxicity, asthenia, stomatitis	
	50 mg/m^2 every 4 weeks: No effect	
Epirubicin	Increased incidence of cardiotoxicity	(Ryberg et al. 2008)
Idarubicin	No data	
Mitoxantrone	No data	
Docetaxel (weekly)	Higher incidence of neutropenia	(Ten Tije et al. 2005)
Docetaxel (3-weekly)	No data	
Paclitaxel (weekly)	No effect	(Perez et al. 2002)
Paclitaxel (3-weekly)	Higher incidence of grade 3 neutropenia	(Lichtman et al. 2006)
Vinorelbin	No data	
Continuous 5-FU	No data	
Capecitabine	No data	
UFT	No data	
Doxifluridine	No data	
Doxorubicin-based	No effect on hematological toxicity	(Ibrahim et al. 1996)
	No effect on infectious complications	
FEC	No effect	(Cascinu et al. 1996)
Epirubicin/paclitaxel followed by CMF (all cycles dose dense with growth factor support)	Higher incidence of neutropenia	(Kümmel et al. 2006)
Epirubicin/cyclophosphamide followed by CMF	Higher incidence of neutropenia	(Kümmel et al. 2006)
Biologicals		
Trastuzumab	No data	
Bevacizumab	No data	

5-FU 5-fluorouracil *UFT* tegafur-uracil
CMF cyclophosphamide, methotrexate and 5-FU
FEC 5-FU, 4-epidoxorubicin and cyclophosphamide

does increase to the same extent, resulting in an unchanged relative proportion of tamoxifen and its metabolites at aging (Peyrade et al. 1996). Theoretically, this phenomenon might be explained by an increased bioavailability, a better compliance, a decreased elimination of tamoxifen and metabolites, or an increased enterohepatic circulation, though a decreased elimination is less likely as all the elimination routes do have to be affected to the same extent.

The toxicity profile of SERMs, in general, is relatively mild, with vasomotor complaints and ocular toxicity being the most frequently occurring side effects, while thromboembolic and endometrial carcinoma are the most clinically relevant.

Currently, there are no clues pointing toward a correlation between serum levels of tamoxifen and/or its metabolites and the presence of adverse events. On the contrary, one PK study performed in 316 patients reported an incidence of all grades of side effects of tamoxifen to be 8.9%, whereby no correlation between serum levels and toxicity profile was found (Peyrade et al. 1996).

Interpretation of the data on toremifene and its metabolites is hampered by the lack of sufficient data, partly due to the fact that this drug is not frequently used anymore. A single pharmacokinetic study has been comparing PKs and toxicity of toremifene, given as a single dose of 120 mg, in 10 elderly women (65–74) and 20 young men (19–33 years), introducing two variables in a small study. No age-dependent change was seen with regard to toremifene absorption, while the volume of distribution increased in the elderly, giving rise to a prolonged half-life (4.2 vs. 7.2 days) as clearance was unaltered (Sotaniemi and Anttila 1997). There were no data on steady state exposure (Sotaniemi and Anttila 1997).

Renal impairment does not affect the PKs of both SERMs, in contrast to hepatic impairment that leads to raised serum-levels of both agents (Anttila et al. 1995; DeGregorio et al. 1989). Regarding the latter, it has been advised to adjust the toremifene dose in patients with impaired hepatic function (Anttila et al. 1995).

6.3.2 Aromatase Inhibitors

Currently, three third-generation AIs are relevant in the treatment of breast cancer: anastrozole, letrozole, and exemestane. Anastrozole and letrozole are nonsteroidal, competitive (reversible) inhibitors of the aromatase enzyme, while exemestane is a steroidal, noncompetitive (irreversible) aromatase inhibitor. The clinical relevance of the differences in mechanism of action(s) remains to be established, as all three agents are acting by inhibiting the aromatase enzyme, resulting in an effective reduction of estrogen levels ranging from 81 to 98%. (Buzdar 2003; Buzdar et al. 2002; Lonning 2003) Data regarding oral bioavailability of AIs are limited to letrozole and found to be close to 100% without influence of food ingestion (Lonning 2003). Half-lives are 24, 48, and 40–50 h for exemestane, letrozole, and anastrozole, respectively (Buzdar 2003; Buzdar et al. 2002; Lonning 2003), whereas for letrozole, it was noticed that with chronic dosing, as compared to a single dose, a larger increase in half-life (42%) than in the area under the curve (AUC) (28%) was found, which was consistent with saturation of metabolizing enzymes (Pfister et al. 2001).

Of the AIs, letrozole has been sufficiently studied with respect to the impact of age on PKs and PDs. These data are lacking for anastrozole and exemestane. In a single- and multiple-dose study evaluating the impact of age on PKs, no significant differences were found in the exposure of the drug and half-life of letrozole at steady state between the different age groups. Furthermore, no relevant differences in suppression of estrogen levels between the age groups were evident (Pfister et al. 2001).

Several large trials on adjuvant hormonal therapy in postmenopausal breast cancer patients have been published: ATAC (anastrozole vs. tamoxifen vs. the combination) (The Arimidex, Tamoxifen, Alone or in Combination Trialists' Group et al. 2006); ABCSG-8, ARNO-95, and ITA (all three: 5 years tamoxifen vs. switch strategy tamoxifen 2–3 years followed by anastrozole for 3–2 years) (Jonat et al. 2006); IES (tamoxifen vs. switch strategy tamoxifen/exemestane, period of therapy 5 years) (Coombes et al. 2007); BIG 1–98 (tamoxifen vs. letrozole vs. sequential therapies tamoxifen/letrozole and letrozole/tamoxifen) (Crivellari et al. 2008); and MA.17 (after 5 years of tamoxifen randomization between placebo and letrozole for another 5 years) (Muss et al. 2008). Only two of these studies, however, are providing data on toxicity in the older subgroup (Crivellari et al. 2008; Muss et al. 2008).

The large ($n=5,169$) NCIC CTG Intergroup MA.17 trial is the only trial generating placebo-controlled data on toxicity regarding older patients treated with an AI. It was shown that in the age group 60–70 years, a higher incidence of hot flushes, insomnia, arthralgias, and alopecia occurred in the letrozole group, while in women who were 70 years of age or older, there was no significant difference in toxicity in the letrozole group as compared to the placebo group (Muss et al. 2008). However, women 70 years of age or older treated with letrozole, as compared to placebo, had a significantly worse quality of life at 6 months in several domains (vitality score, bodily pain, physical scale, and vasomotor domain), still being present but limited to the vasomotor domain at 24 months, while there was no difference at 36 months (Muss et al. 2008).

Furthermore, letrozole has been compared to tamoxifen in a subgroup analysis of the BIG 1–98 trial ($n=4,922$) by using the following age-cohorts in postmenopausal women: ≤64 years, 65–74 years, and ≥75 years. In patients aged 75 years and older, a higher discontinuation rate was found (38%) as compared to patients younger than 75 years of age (23%); however, no difference existed in this respect between the two treatment groups (Crivellari et al. 2008). No convincing overall patterns of differences were observed in thromboembolic or cardiac events in the group 75 years or older, but in the age group 65–74 years of age, thromboembolic events appeared more commonly during tamoxifen treatment and cardiac events during letrozole treatment (Crivellari et al. 2008). This pattern of an increased incidence in ischemic cardiac events and a decreased rate of thromboembolic events during treatment with an AI as compared with tamoxifen is consistent with the findings in the general group, regardless of age (Pritchard and Abramson 2006).

An adverse event of special concern in older patients treated with AIs for a prolonged period of time (like the patients treated with 5 years of adjuvant aromatase inhibition) is osteoporosis as AIs promote accelerated bone loss (Lester and Coleman 2005). In the aging population a progressive decrease in bone mineral density is seen. A large study ($n = 1,70,000$ women) showed a median T-score −0.37 in women between 50 and 59 years of age, while this rapidly decreased to −0.82, −1.34, −1.85 in the subsequent age cohorts, (60–69, 70–79, 80–99) (Siris et al. 2006). The impact of a decrease in bone mineral density is reflected by an increase in fracture risk across the age-cohorts (Siris et al. 2006). Next to an increase in fracture risk, there is also an earlier occurrence of fractures in elderly patients treated with letrozole as compared with tamoxifen (Crivellari et al. 2008). As AIs promote acceleration of bone loss, this treatment will put patients at risk for an even further increase in fracture risk. Attention to osteoporotic risk factors in this patient group, therefore, is warranted, and in the cases with additional risk factors, monitoring of bone mineral density is indicated (if treatment with bisphosphonates is not given yet).

6.3.3 Progestins and SERD

There are no data on the impact of age on the use of megestrol acetate (progestin) and fulvestrant. Megestrol acetate is a synthetically constructed progestin with a good oral bioavailability. After hepatic metabolization, it is excreted mainly by urine and to a lesser extent by feces.

Fulvestrant is administered as a monthly intramuscular injection and, due to a long half-life (40–60 days), steady state concentration is reached after about 6 monthly injections, though the major part of the 2/3 fold accumulation occurs during the first 3 months. Fulvestrant is metabolized in the liver and mainly excreted by the fecal route (Robertson et al. 2004; Robertson and Harrison 2004).

6.4 Physiological Effects of Aging on Pharmacokinetics and Pharmacodynamics of Cytotoxic Therapy

As the toxicity profile of cytotoxic drugs for breast cancer treatment is substantially less favorable as compared to that of hormonal therapy and the therapeutic window is small, the context in which the therapy is given becomes more important. The indication of treatment (adjuvant or advanced disease), the extent of disease load, and prior treatment does definitely influence the PD profile, and in some cases, the PK-profile as well. Although still limited data are available (Table 6.2 and Table 6.3), more studies evaluated the influence of age on the PK-PD profile of cytotoxic agents, as compared to hormonal agents. Below, we address the available data hereon, primarily obtained from studies in patients with breast cancer and in view of the emphasis on elderly supplemented by relevant data derived from elderly patients with other malignancies.

6.4.1   General Considerations of Adjuvant Cytotoxic Therapy in the Elderly

It has been reported that the risk of toxicity of adjuvant chemotherapy for breast cancer patients over the age of 65 years mainly depends on the type of administered treatment—CMF (cyclophosphamide, methotrexate, and 5-fluoro-uracil [5-FU]), anthracyclines, or taxanes—rather than on the chronological age or comorbidity of the patient. It should be taken into account, however, that these data are derived from a retrospective cohort analysis, being open to selection bias as oncologists may have been reluctant to initiate adjuvant chemotherapy in those patients thought to be too vulnerable on the basis of, for example, comorbidity (Hurria et al. 2005). In general, there is an increase in the incidence of neutropenia in elderly compared to younger patients (Kümmel et al. 2006; Dees et al. 2000), which is even more pronounced with dose-dense chemotherapy, most likely due to a more limited bone marrow reserve (Kümmel et al. 2006). In addition, nonhematological toxicity of adjuvant chemotherapy in older breast cancer patients seems to be either quite similar (Hurria et al. 2005; Kümmel et al. 2006; Dees et al. 2000; Muss et al. 2005; Ibrahim et al. 2000) or increased (Crivellari et al. 2000), while in contrast, elderly patients tend to experience less nausea and/or vomiting (DeMaio et al. 2005; Gelman and Taylor 1984). Despite possible changes in the toxicity pattern, the quality of life of older women receiving adjuvant chemotherapy was not found to be worse than that of younger women (Dees et al. 2000; Crivellari et al. 2000).

It has been reported, however, that in women >70 years of age treated with adjuvant CMF, a significantly higher frequency of treatment interruption (25.9 vs. 4.7%, respectively), mostly due to toxicity and patient refusal, is occurring (Brunello et al. 2005). Further, treatment-related mortality seems to increase linearly with increasing age, and therefore, is higher in older breast cancer patients treated with adjuvant cytotoxic therapy, as the observed incidence was 0.2% ($\leq$50 years), 0.7% (51–64 years), and 1.5% ($\geq$65 years) (Muss et al. 2005).

6.4.2   General Considerations of Cytotoxic Therapy for Metastatic Breast Cancer in the Elderly

A considerable part of the evidence on combination regimens for metastatic breast cancer (MBC) in the elderly is based on retrospective studies and subset-analysis. In a retrospective analysis of five trials studying multidrug regimens for MBC (five doxorubicin-based schedules, and one schedule consisting of CMF in combination with vincristine and prednisone), 70 women $\geq$70 years were compared to randomly selected patients being under 50, and between 50–69 years of age. Although the performance score (PS) in the elderly was worse (PS 2: 11%, 16%, 23%; PS 3: 7%, 2%, 14% in the age groups: <50 years, 50–69 years, $\geq$70 years, respectively), there was no significant difference in administered dose-intensity and observed toxicity between the different age groups. However, apart from the obvious limitations associated with retrospective analyses, a true comparison is hampered because in three of the five protocols the given dose of a specific regimen was already reduced by 25% upfront for patients ≥65 years of age, not being the case for the younger cohort (Christman et al. 1992). As this is a reflection of the attitude of physicians regarding the utilization of chemotherapeutic treatment in elderly, the data from every retrospective study have to be carefully weighted with respect to the obvious limitations as often a geriatric assessment was not incorporated and usually the elderly fit patients were enrolled.

6.4.3   Anthracycline- and Anthracenedione-Based Cytotoxic Therapy

The clearance of doxorubicin as part of combination cytotoxic regimens, as studied in two trials ($n=27$ and 110 patients) in patients with a solid malignancy, was found to be unaffected by increasing age (Dobbs et al. 1995; Rudek et al. 2004), though unfortunately doxorubicin PKs administered as single agent have not been investigated separately in older patients with breast cancer. This may be important as anthracyclines are among the most effective drugs to treat breast cancer, and it has been observed that in patients with breast cancer the clearance of doxorubicin is significantly lower than in patients with other tumors (Dobbs et al. 1995). Pharmacokinetic analyses in breast cancer patients treated with adjuvant doxorubicin in combination with cyclophosphamide showed no age-related changes in clearance or distribution of either of these drugs (Crivellari et al. 2000), though in other studies performed in cancer patients with different tumor types, it has been observed that the coadministration of cyclophosphamide is reducing the clearance of doxorubicin by approximately 30% (Rudek et al. 2004). The absence of an age-related effect on the PK properties of doxorubicin was confirmed as age is not considered a relevant factor in the population PK-PD model (Joerger et al. 2007).

Data on age-related differences in the PK-profile of pegylated doxorubicin are not available at the moment. The clearance of epirubicin, administered as part of multiagent regimens, was found to be decreased in elderly women (Wade et al. 1992), though this could not be confirmed while modeling the PKs of patients treated with FEC (5-FU, 4-epidoxorubicin, and cyclophosphamide) (Sandstrom et al. 2006). The PKs of two infrequently used anthracyclines in breast cancer, idarubicin and mitoxantrone, are unaltered by the healthy aging process (Crivellari et al. 2006; Repetto et al. 1999).

As cardiotoxicity is one of the classic and most burdensome toxicities of anthracyclines, this is especially of concern in elderly patients. Both age and anthracycline-based chemotherapy are associated with an increased rate of heart disease (Doyle et al. 2005; Ibrahim et al. 1999; Ryberg et al. 2008), and cardiotoxic therapy with anthracyclines resulted in an even higher incidence of congestive heart failure in patients aged 66–70 years compared to a younger age group (hazard rate [HR] 1.3) (Pinder et al. 2007). Data from a retrospective study in a large population of non-Hodgkin lymphoma patients ($n=3{,}164$) treated with doxorubicin-based chemotherapy confirmed this finding, and also revealed a synergistic effect of doxorubicin treatment and hypertension on the occurrence of congestive heart failure (HR 1.8) (Hershman et al. 2008). In general, the pegylated liposomal formulation of doxorubicin is less cardiotoxic than doxorubicin (O'Brien et al. 2004), and this also appears to apply to the elderly (Biganzoli et al. 2007). The incidence of cardiotoxicity due to pegylated liposomal doxorubicin in patients ≥70 years of age with MBC (6%, $n=62$) was comparable to the cardiotoxicity observed in younger patients with MBC (Biganzoli et al. 2007). The incidence of clinically relevant cardiac events associated with epirubicin treatment, studied in the only randomized phase III study performed in a true cohort of elderly patients (≥60 years, $n=397$) with metastatic BC, was 24% (vs. 17% in the comparative group receiving gemcitabine, not being considered as a cardiotoxic agent), while a decline in left ventricular ejection fraction of ≥10% was observed in 27% of the patients in the epirubicin group (Feher et al. 2005). Of note is that epirubicin was administered in a weekly schedule (35 mg/m^2, days 1, 8, and 15 of 4-weekly cycle), which is not a very commonly used regimen. Also, we have to keep in mind that patients enrolled in randomized trials fulfill the inclusion criteria, including those with respect to an adequate cardiac condition. Recently, new insights became available based on retrospective collection of data on 1,097 anthracycline-naïve epirubicin-treated patients with MBC (Ryberg et al. 2008). Age was a clear risk factor for cardiotoxicity with a HR of 1.28 for every additional ten years of age at the start of epirubicin. So, the recommended maximum epirubicin dose has been adjusted downwards for the elderly. As the current model incorporates other risk factors as well (previous hormonal therapy, previous CMF therapy, previous mediastinal irradiation, predisposition to heart disease, number of metastatic sites), the range of recommended maximum epirubicin dose for women of 70 years of age is 303–820 mg/m^2 (Ryberg et al. 2008). Currently, there are no clear recommendations whether the maximal cumulative dose of the other anthracyclines should be lower in the elderly as compared to younger patients.

Further, a large retrospective subset analysis from 18 studies ($n=1,011$, 244 patients ≥65 years; treatment period 1973–1984), using doxorubicin-based combination chemotherapy for metastatic breast cancer, showed comparable hematological toxicity and infectious complications in patients ≥65 years and patients between 50–64 years of age. After a full dose being administered in the first cycle in all patients, the dose intensity achieved from cycle two and onwards was lower in the elderly (80 vs. 91%). The specific reason for this difference is not yet clear, whether they be toxic effects or a lower threshold to arbitrary dose reductions in the elderly compared with the younger patient (Ibrahim et al. 1996).

A higher incidence of hematological toxicity, anorexia, asthenia, and stomatitis was observed in older as compared to younger patients with MBC when a 6-week schedule of pegylated doxorubicin at a dose of 60 mg/m^2 was administered. No difference in toxicity profile between the two groups was found at a dose of 50 mg/m^2, repeated every 4 weeks (Biganzoli et al. 2007). The combination of pegylated doxorubicin (40 mg/m^2) with cyclophosphamide (500 mg/m^2), both given on day 1 every 4 weeks as first line chemotherapy in 35 MBC patients older than 65 years of age, resulted in 31% grade 3–4 neutropenia and 11% grade 3 mucositis.

There were no episodes of neutropenic fever or treatment-related deaths reported (Kurtz et al. 2007). Based on the incidence of toxicity (mucositis and myelotoxicity), the authors concluded that this schedule of pegylated doxorubicin and cyclophosphamide cannot be recommended in routine practice in this population (Kurtz et al. 2007). Another phase II trial evaluated the combination of pegylated doxorubicin (40 mg/m^2 day 1) with vinorelbine (25 mg/m^2 intravenously day 1, and 40 mg/m^2 by oral route on day 15) in a 4-weekly schedule as first-line chemotherapy for MBC in 34 women of 65 years of age or older (Addeo et al. 2008). During a median of five cycles that have been administered, grade 3–4 neutropenia occurred in 26% of patients, while febrile neutropenia was reported in 9% of patients, all episodes occurring after the sixth cycle. Among nonhematological toxicity, gastrointestinal side effects were the most frequent (grade 3–4 nausea, 6%; vomiting, 12%) (Addeo et al. 2008).

Currently, the recommendation with regard to the use of pegylated doxorubicin in elderly is as single agent at a dose of 45–50 mg/m^2, repeated every 4 weeks.

Only randomized phase III trial in a true cohort of elderly MBC patients (≥65 years) toxicity data from the epirubicin group (35 mg/m^2, days 1,8,15 of a 28-day cycle) are available from 192 patients as compared to toxicity data of the gemcitabine group (1,200 mg/m^2 dL,8,15 of a 28-day cycle) from 190 patients (Feher et al. 2005). Epirubicin resulted in less hematological toxicity, as compared to gemcitabine (grade 3–4 neutropenia, 17.9 vs. 25.3%; grade 3–4 thrombocytopenia 1.5 vs. 9%). With increasing age, shifts in toxicities were seen with increasing incidence of leukopenia (but not neutropenia), mucositis (both in the epirubicin arm), and pulmonary toxicity (in the gemcitabine arm). Serious adverse events leading to therapy discontinuation occurred in both groups, being 8.5 vs. 6.1% ($p=0.44$) for epirubicin and gemcitabine, respectively. Of the 28 deaths, three were considered related to chemotherapy treatment, all three occurring in the gemcitabine group in patients ≥70 years of age (Feher et al. 2005).

The toxicity profile of the FEC combination (600 mg/m^2 day 1 and 8, 75 mg/m^2 day 1, 600 mg/m^2 day 1 every 28 days), reported as part of a greater retrospective analysis in patients with several types of advanced cancer, was not different in patients being younger vs. older than 70 years of age (Cascinu et al. 1996).

The impact of age (range: 60–71 years of age) regarding the feasibility of a dose-dense regimen was evaluated in a subset ($n=52$) analysis of a dose-dense trial comparing a 2-weekly regimen consisting of four cycles epirubicin/paclitaxel (90 mg/m^2; 175 mg/m^2) followed by three cycles of intravenous CMF (600 mg/m^2; 40 mg/m^2; 600 mg/m^2) with growth factor support (=dose–dense regimen) vs. a 3-weekly schedule consisting of four courses epirubicin/cyclophosphamide (90 mg/m^2; 600 mg/m^2) followed by three cycles CMF (600 mg/m^2; 40 mg/m^2; 600 mg/m^2) (Kümmel et al. 2006). Delays of chemotherapy administration were more common in the older patients than in younger patients (13 vs. 7%), being even more frequent in the elderly treated with the dose-dense as compared to the 3-weekly schedule (17 vs. 11%). Delayed hematological recovery more frequently was the reason for delays in chemotherapy administration among older women than among young ones. Nonhematologic toxicity did occur at similar rates in both age groups (Kümmel et al. 2006).

The tolerance of dose-dense chemotherapy regimes in elderly has also retrospectively been evaluated by reviewing the charts of all breast cancer patients 60 years or older ($n=2600$) treated at the Memorial Sloan Kettering Cancer Center between 2002 and 2005 and selecting all patients treated with dose-dense adjuvant chemotherapy consisting of four cycles of doxorubicin 60 mg/m^2 and cyclophosphamide 600 mg/m^2, given every 2 weeks, followed by four cycles of paclitaxel 175 mg/m^2 every 2 weeks, with standard white blood cell growth factor support (Zauderer et al. 2008). In the 160 identified female breast cancer patients (median age 65 years; range: 60–76 years), next to one toxic death, grade 3–4 toxicity occurred in 41% of the patients, mainly consisting of neutropenia (12%), infection (9%), neutropenic fever (5%), and fatigue (6%). Toxicity and patient preference resulted in early discontinuation in 22% of the patients. A noteworthy finding is that 50% of the patients were treated with erythrocyte growth factor support. A further subdivision in the age-categories <70 years of age and 70 years or older did show that advanced age was not associated with a higher probability of grade 3–4 toxicity (Zauderer et al. 2008). In the total cohort of older women, the presence of comorbidity was predictive for the occurrence of grade 3–4 toxicity (odds ratio 2.15) (Zauderer et al. 2008).

Although the oral administration of chemotherapy is more convenient and attractive to patients, idarubicin, an orally administered anthracycline, is hardly used anymore in breast cancer. In older women with MBC ($n=26$), a dose dependent, severe toxicity pattern (including toxic deaths) was observed (Crivellari et al. 2006; Chevallier et al. 1990; Freyer et al. 2004). In the elderly experiencing grade 3–4 neutropenia in comparison to patients experiencing ≤grade 2 neutropenia, significantly higher levels of idarubicin and its principal metabolite, idarubicinol, were found (Toffoli et al. 2000). Mitoxantrone in elderly, despite relevant antitumor activity (Repetto et al. 1999; Repetto et al. 1995), is limited in its use due to frequently occurring neutropenia, a general decrease in bone marrow cellularity, a persisting decrease in red cell colony forming units, as well as a persisting decrease in circulating hematopoietic progenitor cells (Repetto et al. 1999). The duration of neutropenia or thrombocytopenia could not be explained by changes in peak plasma levels or AUC (Repetto et al. 1999).

In summary, the anthracyclines (pegylated) doxorubicin and epirubicin are tolerable treatment options in the fit elderly breast cancer patient, though a tendency of more pronounced toxicity, especially myelosuppression, is observed being unrelated to available PK parameters. Oncologists, however, should be aware of the higher likelihood of congestive heart failure, especially in case of a history of cardiac events. Therefore, monitoring of the cardiac function during anthracycline therapy remains indicated for this patient group.

6.4.4   Taxanes

Next to anthracyclines, taxanes are an important class of active agents in the treatment of BC. In elderly patients, both taxanes, docetaxel and paclitaxel, mainly have been studied using a weekly schedule (Perez et al. 2002; ten Tije et al. 2004; Del Mastro et al. 2005; Smorenburg et al. 2003; Repetto et al. 2004; D'hondt et al. 2004; Hainsworth et al. 2001; Maisano et al. 2005).

Age itself does not seem to alter the clearance of docetaxel irrespective of the administration in a weekly or a 3-weekly schedule (Rudek et al. 2004; Ten Tije et al. 2005; Hurria et al. 2006). Patients aged ≥65 years appeared to be more sensitive to docetaxel-induced neutropenia. In this respect, it is noteworthy that in a small study ($n=51$) in patients with different types of cancer, 3 out of 20 elderly patients suffered from an episode of febrile neutropenia, all three patients having an AUC-value in the upper quartile, while none of the patients in the age group below 65 years of age had an episode of febrile neutropenia (Ten Tije et al. 2005). In a more recent PK study ($n=20$, 10 patients with MBC) using weekly docetaxel (35 mg/m^2 for three subsequent weeks, followed by 1-week break) in patients aged 66–84 years, the absence of an effect of age on the pharmacokinetics of docetaxel was confirmed. However, based on grade ≥3 hematological toxicity in 19% and grade ≥3 nonhematological toxicity in 53% of the patients, the authors advocated to initially start with a dose of 26 mg/m^2 docetaxel and escalate the dose if no toxicity has been observed (Hurria et al. 2006). Interestingly, PK variables were evaluated for their correlations with baseline geriatric assessment variables. A lower score on the Lawton Instrumental Activities of Daily Living scale (indicating increased need for assistance in completing instrumental activities of daily living) and a higher score at the Geriatric Depression Scale were correlated with a longer half-life of bound docetaxel (Hurria et al. 2006). These data underscore that further data hereon are warranted, and may be helpful regarding a more optimal assessment of which older patients to treat with chemotherapy.

Furthermore, the most invalidating, consistently observed side-effect of a weekly regimen of docetaxel in the elderly was fatigue/asthenia, sometimes being the reason to discontinue the chemotherapy (Rudek et al. 2004; Ten Tije et al. 2005; Massacesi et al. 2005; Nuzzo et al. 2008).

In the randomized ELDA-trial (elderly breast cancer-docetaxel adjuvant), breast cancer patients aged between 65–79 years who are candidates for adjuvant systemic therapy are randomized between docetaxel (35 mg/m^2, days 1, 8, 15, repeated every 4 weeks) and intravenous CMF (600 mg/m^2; 40 mg/m^2; 600 mg/m^2, given on days 1 and 8 every 4 weeks). Safety and toxicity data have recently been reported for 103 patients, having received a median of four cycles of chemotherapy (Nuzzo et al. 2008). The docetaxel therapy had a more favorable toxicity profile than the CMF regimen, whereby especially a lower incidence and severity of hematological toxicity was observed (grade 3–4 neutropenia in 8.3 vs. 66.0% and grade 3–4 thrombocytopenia 0 vs. 7.6%) (Nuzzo et al. 2008). Grade 3–4 nonhematological toxicity was observed in 31.2 and 22.6% of the docetaxel and CMF treated patients, respectively. Constipation, mucositis, nausea, and vomiting were significantly more common in patients treated with CMF, while fatigue, diarrhea, abdominal pain, dysgeusia, neuropathy, and liver toxicity were more common in those treated with weekly docetaxel (Nuzzo et al. 2008). Of patients assigned to chemotherapy, 15%

did not receive the preplanned doses of docetaxel and 19% did not receive the preplanned dose of CMF.

Data on 3-weekly docetaxel (dose range 75–100 mg/m^2) administered to older women with BC are only available from abstracts and show contradictory and nonconclusive results (Rossi et al. 2005; Aapro et al. 2003). In older patients and other patients having a poor performance ($n=111$; median age 75 years; range 46–86 years) with advanced nonsmall cell lung cancer (NSCLC), docetaxel has been studied in a 3-weekly and a weekly regimen (at a dose of 75 mg/m^2 3-weekly, and 30 mg/m^2 on days 1, 8 and 15 every 28 days, respectively) as first-line therapy. This study observed a higher incidence of neutropenia during the 3-weekly regimen, though the incidence of severe infectious complications (sepsis, febrile neutropenia) did not seem to be significantly different between the two treatment regimens (Lilenbaum et al. 2007).

Pharmacokinetic data of docetaxel, administered in a 3-weekly regimen, in an older cohort of patients were derived from a small study in patients with stage III/IV NSCLC. Fifteen of the 35 screened patients met the inclusion criteria, and only 12 patients treated with 60 mg/m^2 (the approved dose in Japan) were evaluable for PK analysis. The data of these patients (median age 78 years; range 76–87 years) were compared with data of a historic group of younger patients treated with the same dose of docetaxel, at another infusion-rate, resulting in slight changes in AUC and half-life (Takigawa et al. 2004).

The other taxane used in standard regimens for breast cancer treatment is paclitaxel. The clearance of unbound paclitaxel was significantly diminished (Smorenburg et al. 2003; Joerger et al. 2006) as was the volume of distribution at steady state in MBC patients of ≥70 years of age (Smorenburg et al. 2003). A weekly dose of 100 mg/m^2 of paclitaxel in younger cancer patients with different tumor types ($n=15$) and of 80 mg/m^2 in older patients with MBC (≥70 years), given on days 1, 8, 15 every 28 days, resulted in comparable hematological pharmacodynamics, with a similar decrease in white blood cell counts (Smorenburg et al. 2003). No impact of age on toxicity of weekly administered paclitaxel (80 mg/m^2, days 1, 8, 15, repeated on day 29) was found in a trial evaluating patients with MBC ($n=212$; 73 patients being ≥65 years of age) (Perez et al. 2002). In another pharmacokinetic/ pharmacodynamic study ($n=153$, 39 patients with MBC, 23 (59%) of the MBC patients >65 years) in which patients were treated with 3-weekly paclitaxel (175 mg/m^2), a decreased clearance of paclitaxel and increased AUC of paclitaxel in relation to age were found, as well as a significant increase in the incidence of grade 3 neutropenia (not grade 4 neutropenia) in older patients. These findings, however, were not translated in a different risk of hospitalization for toxicity or receiving intravenous antibiotics (Lichtman et al. 2006). Furthermore, no significant correlation between the increased paclitaxel exposure and the lower neutrophil nadir was found (Lichtman et al. 2006). In contrast with the findings obtained for docetaxel, scores on geriatric assessment scales (Charlson score, and Instrumental Activities of Daily Life scale) assessed in patients with MBC were not predictive for toxicity of paclitaxel (Del Mastro et al. 2005).

In summary, the findings with regard to a weekly regimen of docetaxel do not show an altered PK profile in the elderly, except for the findings indicative of a correlation with the outcome of geriatric assessment. In general, fatigue is consistently seen as invalidating event and myelosuppression is more pronounced in older women with BC treated with weekly docetaxel as compared to younger patients. It is very likely that the further increase in myelosuppression by using a 3-weekly schedule of docetaxel, instead of a weekly schedule, as is seen in patients with NSCLC, is also and even more applicable to the BC population, though full data of confirmatory studies are lacking.

For paclitaxel, there are no PK or PD data relevant to the elderly, to deviate from the schedule currently considered as standard of care in all breast cancer patients with metastatic disease, being a weekly dose of 80 mg/m^2 administered on days 1, 8, 15 every 4 weeks.

6.4.5   Fluoropyrimidine-Based Cytotoxic Therapy

The clearance of 5-FU, administered as a continuous intravenous schedule, is decreased due to aging (Etienne et al. 1998). Bolus infusion of 5-FU was unaltered in elderly as age did not have an impact on the PKs of any of the components of intravenously administered CMF (600 mg/m^2; 40 mg/m^2; 600 mg/m^2 on day 1 every 3 weeks) (Batey et al. 2002). As early as 1984, a modified schedule of the classical CMF regimen (100 mg/m^2 orally days 1–14; 40 mg/m^2; 5-FU 600 mg/m^2 the latter two on days 1 and 8, and repeated every 4 weeks) for elderly ($\geq$65 years of age) with locally advanced or metastatic BC was proposed, wherein the absolute doses of cyclophosphamide and methotrexate were calculated by means of the creatinin clearance (Gelman and Taylor 1984). A significantly lower incidence of nausea and vomiting was observed at increasing age (Gelman and Taylor 1984), while the occurrence of other toxicity was not significantly different between older and younger patients (Gelman and Taylor 1984; Beex et al. 1992).

The influence of age on the PKs of capecitabine, the oral pro-drug of 5-FU, was evaluated in 25 patients (median age 62 years; range 41–80 years) with heterogeneous types of solid tumors (Cassidy et al. 1999). No effect of age on AUC and peak-concentrations (Cmax) of 5-FU and its metabolites could be detected (Cassidy et al. 1999). Importantly, and in line with the PK findings, the activity of dihydropyrimidine dehydrogenase, the initial enzyme in the catabolism of 5FU, was not found affected by increasing age (Etienne et al. 1994).

Conflicting data are available on the tolerability of the labeled, standard dose of capecitabine. Bajetta et al reported that the dose of capecitabine considered standard in younger patients (2,500 mg/m^2 daily, days 1–14, repeated every 3 weeks) was not feasible in older patients with MBC ($n=30$, $\geq$65 years, capecitabine given as first or second line) because of an excess of toxicity consisting of 7% toxic deaths, 13% grade 3–4 diarrhea, 10% grade 3–4 dyspnea, and need for dose reductions in 30% of the patients (Bajetta et al. 2005). In this trial, a reduced dose of capecitabine (2,000 mg/m² per day) was well tolerated by elderly with MBC (*n*=43) and could be given without dose reductions in 95% of the cohort, notwithstanding an increase in the incidence of toxicity, especially diarrhea, in women over 70 years as compared to women being 65—70 years of age (grade 3–4 diarrhea 32 vs. 10%, respectively) (Bajetta et al. 2005). In another trial, however, capecitabine at a dose of 2,510 mg/m² per day (days 1–14, repeated every 3 weeks) did seem to be well tolerated in a randomized phase II trial in older patients (≥55 years) treated with first-line therapy for metastatic breast cancer (*n*=93) (O'Shaughnessy et al. 2001). This study was early terminated due to a superior clinical benefit rate of capecitabine over intravenous CMF, the comparative regimen. Capecitabine was associated with nonhematological toxicity mainly consisting of hand-foot syndrome (15%), gastrointestinal symptoms (8–12%), and fatigue (5%), whereas CMF primarily induced gastrointestinal toxicity (9%) (O'Shaughnessy et al. 2001). Of note, discussion on the optimal and/or tolerable dose of capecitabine is also an issue in the total group of breast cancer patients. In a retrospective cohort from the MD Anderson Cancer Center, the safety and toxicity of different doses of capecitabine (daily doses of 2,500, 2,250, and 2,000 mg/m², respectively) administered as second/third-line for MBC in 141 patients have been evaluated (Hennessy et al. 2005). Toxicity profiles were less pronounced in the lowest dose cohort, while dose reductions due to toxicity were mandated in 40, 63, and 28% in the respective dose cohorts. Efficacy was not significantly affected. The authors concluded that the lowest dose of capecitabine is resulting in a more favorable therapeutic index.

The combination of vinorelbine and capecitabine was studied in a dose finding study in patients ≥65 years with MBC stratifying for the presence or absence of bone metastasis. More grade 3–4 neutropenia was found in patients with bone involvement. The recommended dose level in patients ≥65 years with bone metastases was lower than in patients without skeletal disease (daily capecitabine dose 2,000 mg/m², instead of 2,500 mg/m² days 1–14) in both groups of patients combined with vinorelbine 20 mg/m² days 1 and 8 every 3 weeks (Hess et al. 2004).

Tegafur-uracil (UFT) and doxifluridine are infrequently used fluoropyrimidines, the more in breast cancer, and in elderly patients, no PK data are available. PD data are obtained from a single study on either drug. In a very small study (*n*=10) in patients with advanced breast cancer 65 years and older, oral UFT induced diarrhea in all patients, consisting of grade 3–4 in 40% of the patients. Twenty percent of the patients in this study discontinued treatment after the first cycle because of gastrointestinal toxicity (Gupta et al. 2005). Diarrhea was also the major adverse event (grade 3 in 11%) in elderly with MBC treated with doxifluridine, but age did not affect tolerability (Bajetta et al. 1998).

To sum up, CMF administered as an intravenous or classic schedule are well-known regimens in the treatment of patients with BC and are tolerable in the elderly. Furthermore, capecitabine is a reasonable and an effective option for older patients with MBC, whereby the recommended starting dose consists of 2,000 mg/m² per day, given for 14 days in a 3-weekly regimen, though even a dose of 2,500 mg/m² instead of 2,000 mg/m² might be tolerable.

6.4.6   Vinca-Alkaloid Based Cytotoxic Therapy

Vinorelbine, as the only member of this family of inhibitors of microtubule polymerization, has been evaluated in the elderly with MBC. Most of the available data are pointing toward unaltered pharmacokinetics of intravenously administered vinorelbine in the elderly (Sorio et al. 1997; Wong et al. 2006; Nguyen et al. 2002), though in one study in patients with heterogeneous tumor types, a reduced vinorelbine clearance was observed (Gauvin et al. 2000). A positive correlation between the exposure to vinorelbine and neutropenia has been detected (Wong et al. 2006; Nguyen et al. 2002). Neutropenia and constipation were found to be the most important toxicities of vinorelbine (Wong et al. 2006; Vogel et al. 1999; Rossi et al. 2003). Oral vinorelbine as a single agent has been tested in women ≥65 years with MBC as first- or second-line chemotherapy for metastatic disease, at an initial dose of 60 mg/m^2 given weekly (without a break) for the first four doses, and being increased to 70 mg/m^2 for the subsequent administrations if there was no grade 4 neutropenia or a recurrent grade 3 neutropenia (Baweja et al. 2006). This strategy resulted in a mild toxicity pattern in the 25 treated patients, grade 3–4 toxicity mainly being neutropenia (13%), fatigue (13%), and dizziness (8%). Yet this regimen had only little antitumor activity (Baweja et al. 2006).

Next to the combination of vinorelbine and pegylated doxorubicin (above) and of vinorelbine and capecitabine (above), vinorelbine has been evaluated in combination with gemcitabine (Dinota et al. 2005). In a strongly selected population (26% of the patients excluded based on frailty) of women ≥65 years of age with advanced/metastatic BC ($n = 34$), the combination of gemcitabine and vinorelbine resulted in a substantial percentage of grade 3–4 hematological and gastrointestinal toxicity (anemia 8–18%, constipation 15–17%, abdominal pain 8%). Although an improvement in quality of life (QoL) was suggested, data on QoL were only available for 56% of the patients (Dinota et al. 2005). Another trial using the combination of vinorelbine and gemcitabine in a small group of MBC patients ≥70 years of age ($n = 12$) was prematurely interrupted due to serious and unacceptable toxicity (25% grade 3 neutropenia; 17% grade 3 gastrointestinal toxicity, 8% grade 3 anemia) (Basso et al. 2007).

The limitations of these data do not allow a definite recommendation toward one of these single agent or combination regimens, though it underlines the necessity for a careful determination of the tolerable dose in the cohort of older women.

6.5   Physiological Effects of Aging on Pharmacokinetics and Pharmacodynamics of Biologicals

The administration of biologicals (molecular targeted agents) such as trastuzumab or bevacizumab have not yet specifically been studied in elderly patients with MBC. In a retrospective analysis, collecting data from 19 phase I/II studies on molecular targeted agents (total group 401 patients, of whom 130 patients older than 65 years of age), toxicity was not related to age (Townsley et al. 2006). In colorectal cancer patients, analysis of a safety registry database did not reveal age >65 years to be a risk factor for developing arterial thromboembolic events during treatment with bevacizumab (Sugrue et al. 2007). Elderly patients received the same dose intensity as their younger counterparts, and the frequency and intensity of (severe) adverse events were similar (Townsley et al. 2006).

As age itself is a risk factor for cardiac toxicity during cytotoxic treatment, as explained in the section on anthracyclines, special attention should also be given to cardiac evaluation with regard to the use of trastuzumab in older patients, given the fact that trastuzumab is also associated with cardiac toxicity especially when given in combination with chemotherapy. Further, it has to be kept in mind that older patients, especially in the case of relevant comorbidity, were not eligible for the performed studies on trastuzumab therapy.

6.6   Conclusions

Overall, still only limited data are available on the PK and PD profile of anticancer therapies in older women with BC, this absence being even more explicit in the subgroups of endocrine drugs and the so-called biologicals. A substantial part of the data are based on retrospectively collected information, which inevitably introduces some patient selection bias and does not reflect real clinical practice. Age does have an impact on the PKs of tamoxifen and paclitaxel, whereas an impact on PD is more common during cytotoxic therapy. While the therapeutic armamentarium of the medical oncologist is expanding, usually on the basis of trials including patients of all ages, it remains important to address relevant questions for the elderly in studies specifically designed for this subgroup, also incorporating PK and PD endpoints, in order to let the elderly benefit from recent progress in treatment options and to improve the outcome of breast cancer in this age group.

References

Aapro MS, Olsen SR, Alakl M, Murawsky M, Hurria A (2003) Safety profile of docetaxel in older patients with metastatic breast cancer. Breast Cancer Res Treat 82(1):532

Aapro MS, Köhne CH, Cohen HJ, Extermann M (2005) Never too old? Age should not be a barrier to enrolment in cancer clinical trials. Oncologist 10:198–204

Addeo R, Faiola V, Guarrasi R et al (2008) Liposomal pegylated doxorubicin plus vinorelbine combination as first-line chemotherapy for metastatic breast cancer in elderly women ≥65 years of age. Cancer Chemother Pharmacol 62:285–292

Anttila M, Laakso S, Nyländen P, Sotaniemi EA (1995) Pharmacokinetics of the novel antiestrogenic agent toremifene in subjects with altered liver and kidney function. Clin Pharmacol Ther 57:628–635

Bajetta E, Biganzoli L, Carnaghi C et al (1998) Oral doxifluridine plus levoleucovorin in elderly patients with advanced breast cancer. Cancer 83:1136–1141

Bajetta E, Procopio G, Celio L et al (2005) Safety and efficacy of two different doses of capecitabine in the treatment of advanced breast cancer in older women. J Clin Oncol 23:2155–2161

Basso U, Fratino L, Brunello A et al (2007) Which benefit from adding gemcitabine to vinorelbine in elderly (≥70 years) women with metastatic breast cancer? Early interruption of a phase II study. Ann Oncol 18:58–63

Batey MA, Wright JG, Azzabi A et al (2002) Population pharmacokinetics of adjuvant cyclophosphamide, methotrexate and 5-fluorourail (CMF). Eur J Cancer 38:1081–1089

Baweja M, Suman VJ, Fitch TR et al (2006) Phase II trial of oral vinorelbine for the treatment of metastatic breast cancer in patients ≥65 years of age: an NCCTG study. Ann Oncol 17:623–629

Beex LVAM, Hermus ARMM, Pieters GFFM, van Hoesel QGCH, Nooy MA, Mignolet F (1992) Dose intensity of chemotherapy with cyclophosphamide, methotrexate and 5-fluoorouracil in the elderly with advanced breast cancer. Eur J Cancer 28:686–690

Biganzoli L, Coleman R, Minisini A et al (2007) A joined analysis of two European Organization for the Research and Treatment of Cancer (EORTC) studies to evaluate the role of pegylated liposomal doxorubicin (Caelyx TM) in the treatment of elderly patients with metatstatic breast cancer. Crit Rev Oncol Hematol 61:84–89

Blower P, de Wit R, Goodin S, Aapro M (2005) Drug-drug interactions in oncology: why are they important and can they be minimized? Crit Rev Oncol Hematol 55:117–142

Brunello A, Basso U, Pogliani C et al (2005) Adjuvant chemotherapy for elderly patients (> or =70 years) with early high-risk breast cancer: a retrospective analysis of 260 patients. Ann Oncol 16:1276–1282

Buzdar AU (2003) Pharmacology and pharmacokinetics of the newer generation aromatase inhibitors. Clin Cancer Res 9:468s–472s

Buzdar AU, Robertson JF, Eiermann W, Nabholtz JM (2002) An overview of the pharmacology and pharmacokinetics of the newer generation aromatase inhibitors anastrozole, letrozole and exemestane. Cancer 95:2006–2016

Cascinu S, Del Ferro E, Catalano G (1996) Toxicity and therapeutic response to chemotherapy in patients aged 70 years or older with advanced cancer. Am J Clin Oncol 19:371–374

Cassidy J, Twelves C, Cameron D et al (1999) Bioequivalence of two tablet formulations of capecitabine and exploration of age, gender, body surface area, and creatinine clearance as factors influencing systemic exposure in cancer patients. Cancer Chemother Pharmacol 44:453–460

Chevallier B, Monnier A, Metz R et al (1990) Phase II study of oral idarubicin in elderly patients with advanced breast cancer. Am J Clin Oncol 13:436–439

Christman K, Muss HB, Case LD, Stanley V (1992) Chemotherapy of metastatic breast cancer in the elderly. The Piedmont Oncology Association experience. JAMA 268:57–62

Coombes RC, Kilburn LS, Snowdon CF (2007) urvival and safety of exemestane versus tamoxifen after 2–3 years' tamoxifen treatment (Intergroup Exemestane Study): a randomised controlled trial. Lancet 369:559–570

Crivellari D, Bonetti M, Castiglione-Gertsch M et al (2000) Burdens and benefits of adjuvant cyclophosphamide, methotrexate, and fluorouracil and tamoxifen for elderly patients with breast cancer: the international breast cancer study group trial VII. J Clin Oncol 18:1412–1422

Crivellari D, Lombardi D, Corona G et al (2006) Innovative schedule of idarubicin in elderly patients with metastatic breast cancer: comprehensive results of a phase II multi-institutional study with pharmacokinetic drug monitoring. Ann Oncol 17:807–812

Crivellari D, Sun Z, Coates AS et al (2008) Letrozole compared with tamoxifen for elderly patients with endocrine-responsive early breast cancer: the BIG 1–98 trial. J Clin Oncol 26:1972–1979

D'hondt R, Paridaens R, Wildiers H et al (2004) Safety and efficacy of weekly docetaxel in frail and/or elderly patients with metastatic breast cancer: a phase II study. Anticancer Drugs 15:341–346

Dees EC, O'Reilly S, Goodmann SN et al (2000) A prospective pharmacologic evaluation of age-related toxicity of adjuvant chemotherapy in women with breast cancer. Cancer Invest 18:521–529

DeGregorio MW, Wiebe VJ, Venook AP, Holleran WM (1989) Elevated plasma tamoxifen levels in a patient with liver obstruction. Cancer Chemother Pharmacol 23:194–195

Del Mastro L, Perrone F, Repetto L et al (2005) On behalf of the Gruppo Italiano di Oncologia Geriatria (GIOGer). Weekly paclitaxel as first-line chemotherapy in elderly advanced breast cancer patients: a phase II study of the Gruppo Italiano di Oncologia Geriatrica (GIOGer). Ann Oncol 16:253–258

DeMaio E, Gravina A, Pacilio C et al (2005) Compliance and toxicity of adjuvant CMF in elderly breast cancer patients: a single-center experience. BMC Cancer 5:30

Dinota A, Bilancia D, Romano R, Manzione L (2005) Biweekly administration of gemcitabine and vinorelbin as first line therapy in elderly advanced breast cancer. Breast Cancer Res Treat 89:1–3

Dobbs NA, Twelves CJ, Gillies H, James CA, Harper PG, Rubens RD (1995) Gender affects doxorubicin pharmacokinetics in patients with normal liver chemistry. Cancer Chemother Pharmacol 36:473–476

Doyle JJ, Neugut AI, Jacobson JS, Grann VR, Hershman DL (2005) Chemotherapy and cardio-toxicity in older breast cancer patients: a population-based study. J Clin Oncol 23:8597–8605

Durnas C, Loi M, Cusack BJ (1990) Hepatic drug metabolism and ageing. Clin Pharmacokinet 19:359–389

Elmadfa I, Meyer AL (2008) Body composition, changing physiological functions and nutrient requirements of the elderly. Ann Nutr Metab 52(11):2–5

Etienne MC, Lagrange JL, Dassonville O et al (1994) Population study of dihydropyrimidine dehydrogenase in cancer patients. J Clin Oncol 12:2248–2253

Etienne M-C, Chatelut E, Pivot X et al (1998) Co-variables influencing 5-fluorouracil clearance during continous venous infusion. A NONMEM analysis. Eur J Cancer 34:92–97

Feher O, Vodvarka P, Jassem J et al (2005) First-line gemcitabine versus epirubicin in postmeno-pausal women aged 60 or older with metastatic breast cancer: a multicenter, randomized, phase III study. Ann Oncol 16:899–908

Freyer G, Lortholary A, Delcambre C et al (2004) Unexpected toxicities in elderly patients with oral idarubicin in metastatic breast cancer: the GINECO experience. Clin Oncol (R Coll Radiol) 16:17–23

Gauvin A, Pinguet F, Culine S, Astre C, Gomeni R, Bresolle F (2000) Bayesian estimate of vinorelbine pharmacokinetic parameters in elderly patients with advanced metastatic cancer. Clin Cancer Res 6:2690–2695

Gelman RS, Taylor SG IV (1984) Cyclophosphamide, Methotrexate and 5-fluorouracil chemo-therapy in women more than 65 years old with advanced breast cancer: the elimination of age trends in toxicity by using doses based on creatinin clearance. J Clin Oncol 2:1404–1413

Gupta S, Mauer AM, Ryan CW, Taber DA, Samuels BL, Fleming GF (2005) A phase II trial of UFT and leucovorin in women 65 years and older with advanced breast cancer. Am J Clin Oncol 28:65–69

Hainsworth JD, Burris HA III, Yardley DA et al (2001) Weekly docetaxel in the treatment of elderly patients with advanced breast cancer: a Minnie Pearl cancer research network phase II trial. J Clin Oncol 19:3500–3505

Hennessy BT, Gauthier AM, Michaud LB, Hortobagyi G, Valero V (2005) Lower dose capecit-abine has a more favorable therapeutic index in metastatic breast cancer: retrospective analysis of patients treated at M. D. Anderson Cancer Center and a review of capecitabine toxicity in the literature. Ann Oncol 16:1289–1296

Hershman DL, McBride RB, Eisenberger A, Tsai WY, Grann VR, Jacobson JS (2008) Doxorubicin, cardiac risk factors, and cardiac toxicity in elderly patients with diffuse B-cell non-Hodgkin's lymphoma. J Clin Oncol 26:3159–3165

Hess D, Thürlimann B, Pagani O et al (2004) Capecitabine and vinorelbin in elderly patients (≥ 65 years) with metastatic breast cancer: a phase I trial (SAKK 25/99). Ann Oncol 15:1760–1765

Hurria A, Brogan K, Panageas S et al (2005) Patterns of toxicity in older patients with breast cancer receiving adjuvant chemotherapy. Breast Cancer Res Treat 92:151–156

Hurria A, Fleming MT, Baker SD et al (2006) Pharmacokinetics and toxicity of weekly docetaxel in older patients. Clin Cancer Res 12:6100–6105

Ibrahim NK, Frye DK, Buzdar AU, Walters RS, Hortobagyi GN (1996) Doxorubicin-based chemotherapy in elderly patients with metastatic breast cancer. Tolerance and outcome. Arch Intern Med 156:882–888

Ibrahim NK, Hortobagyi GN, Ewer M et al (1999) Doxorubicin-induced congestive heart failure in elderly patients with metastatic breast cancer, with long-term follow-up: the M.D.Andersen experience. Cancer Chemother Pharmacol 43:471–478

Ibrahim NK, Buzdar AU, Asmar L, Theriault RL, Hortobagyi GN (2000) Doxorubicin-based adjuvant chemotherapy in elderly breast cancer patients: the M.D.Anderson experience, with long term follow-up. Ann Oncol 11:1597–1601

Janssen-Heijnen ML, Houterman S, Lemmens VE, Louwman MW, Maas HA, Coebergh JW (2005) Prognostic impact of increasing age and co-morbidity in cancer patients: a population-based approach. Crit Rev Oncol Hematol 55:231–240

Joerger M, Huitema ADR, van den Bongard DHJG, Schellens JHM, Beijnen JH (2006) Quantative effect of gender, age, liver function and body size on the population pharmacokinetics of paclitaxel in patients with solid tumors. Clin Cancer Res 12:2150–2157

Joerger M, Huitema AD, Richel DJ et al (2007) Population pharmacokinetics and pharmacody-namics of doxorubicin and cyclophosphamide in breast cancer patients: a study by the EORTC-PAMM-NDDG. Clin Pharmacokinet 46:1051–1068

Jonat W, Gnant M, Boccardo F et al (2006) Effectiveness of switching from adjuvant tamoxifen to anastrozole in postmenopausal women with hormone-sensitive early-stage breast cancer: a meta-analysis. Lancet Oncol 7:991–996

Koehler J, Leonhaeuser IU (2008) Changes in food preferences during aging. Ann Nutr Metab 52(S1):15–19

Kümmel S, Krocker J, Kohls A et al (2006) Dose-dense adjuvant chemotherapy for node-positive breast cancer in women 60 years and older: Feasibility and tolerability in a subset of patients in a randomized trial. Crit Rev Oncol Hematol 58:166–175

Kurtz JE, Rousseau F, Meyer N et al (2007) Phase II trial of pegylated liposomal doxorubicin-cyclophosphamide combination as first-line chemotherapy in older metastatic breast cancer patients. Oncology 73:210–214

Lester J, Coleman R (2005) Bone loss and the aromatase inhibitors. Br J Cancer 93(1):S16–22

Lichtman SM, Hollis D, Miller AA et al (2006) Prospective evaluation of the relationship of patient age and paclitaxel clinical pharmacology: Cancer and Leukemia group B (CALGB 9762). J Clin Oncol 24:1846–1851

Lilenbaum R, Rubin M, Samuel J et al (2007) A randomized phase II trial of two schedules od docetaxel in elderly or poor performance status patients with advanced non-small cell lung cancer. J Thorac Oncol 2:306–311

Lonning P (2003) Clinical pharmacokinetics of aromatase inhibitors and inactivators. Clin Pharmacokinet 42:619–631

Maisano R, Mare M, Caristi N et al (2005) A modified weekly docetaxel schedule as first-line chemotherapy in elderly metastatic breast cancer: a safety study. J Chemother 17:242–246

Massacesi C, Marcucci F, Boccetti T et al (2005) Low dose-intensity docetaxel in the treatment of pre-treated elderly patients with metastatic breast cancer. J Exp Clin Cancer Res 24:43–48

McLean AJ, Le Couteur DG (2004) Aging biology and geriatric pharmacology. Pharmacol Rev 56:163–184

Muss HB, Woolf S, Berry D et al (2005) Adjuvant chemotherapy in older and younger women with lymph node-positive breast cancer. JAMA 293:1073–1081

Muss HB, Tu D, Ingle JN (2008) Efficacy, toxicity and quality of life in older women with early-stage breast cancer with letrozole or placebo after 5 years of tamoxifen: NCIC CTG intergroup trial MA17. J Clin Oncol 26:1956–1964

Nguyen L, Tranchand B, Puozzo C, Variol P (2002) Population pharmacokinetics model and limited sampling strategy for intravenous vinorelbine derived from phase I clinical trials. Br J Clin Pharmacol 53:459–468

Nuzzo F, Morabito A, De Maio E et al (2008) Weekly docetaxel versus CMF as adjuvant chemotherapy for elderly breast cancer patients: safety data from the multicenter randomised ELDA trial. Crit Rev Oncol Hematol 66:171–180

O'Brien ME, Wigler N, Inbar M et al (2004) Reduced cardiotoxicity and comparable efficacy in a phase III trial of pegylated liposomal doxorubicin HCl (CAELYX/Doxil) versus conventional doxorubicin for first-line treatment of metastatic breast cancer. Ann Oncol 15:440–449

O'Shaughnessy JA, Blum J, Moiseyenko V et al (2001) Randomized, open-label, phase II trial of oral capecitabine (Xeloda®) vs a reference arm of intravenous CMF (cyclophosphamide, methotrexate and 5-fluorouracil) as first-line therapy for advanced/metastatic breast cancer. Ann Oncol 12:1247–1254

Percy CJ, Power D, Gobe GC (2008) Renal ageing: changes in the cellular mechanism of energy metabolism and oxidant handling. Nephrology (Carlton) 13:147–152

Perez EA, Vogel CL, Irwin DH, Kirshner JJ, Patel R (2002) Weekly paclitaxel in women age 65 and above with metastatic breast cancer. Breast Cancer Res Treat 75:85–88

Peyrade F, Frenay M, Etienne MC et al (1996) Age-related difference in tamoxifen disposition. Clin Pharmacol Ther 59:401–410

Pfister CU, Martoni A, Zamagni C (2001) Effect of age and single versus multiple dose pharmacokinetics of letrozole (Femara) in breast cancer patients. Biopharm Drug Dispos 22:191–197

Phillips RJ, Powley TL (2007) Innervation of the gastrointestinal tract: patterns of aging. Auton Neurosci 136:1–19

Pinder MC, Duan Z, Goodwin JS, Hortobagyi GN, Giordano SH (2007) Congestive heart failure in older women treated with adjuvant anthracycline chemotherapy for breast cancer. J Clin Oncol 25:3808–3815

Pritchard KI, Abramson BL (2006) Cardiovascular health and aromatase inhibitors. Drugs 66:1727–1740

Repetto L, Simoni C, Venturino A et al (1995) Mitxantrone in elderly women with advanced breast cancer: a phase II study. Anticancer Res 15:2297–2300

Repetto L, Vannozzi MO, Balleari E et al (1999) Mitoxantrone in elderly patients with advanced breast cancer: pharmacokinetics, marrow and peripheral hematopoetic progenitor cells. Anticancer Res 19:879–884

Repetto L, Comandini D, Mammoliti S, Pietropaolo M, Del Mastro L (2004) Weekly paclitaxel in elderly patients with advanced breast cancer. A dose-finding study. Drugs R D 5:11–15

Robertson JF, Harrison M (2004) Fulvestrant: pharmacokinetics and pharmacology. Br J Cancer 90:S7–S10

Robertson JF, Erikstein B, Osborne KC et al (2004) Pharmacokinetic profile of intramuscular fulvestrant in advanced cancer. Clin Pharmacokinet 43:529–538

Rossi A, Gridelli C, Gebbia V et al (2003) Single agent vinorelbine as first-line chemotherapy in elderly patients with advanced breast cancer. Anticancer Res 23:1657–1664

Rossi A, Colantuoni G, Maione P et al (2005) Chemotherapy of breast cancer in the elderly. Curr Med Chem 12:297–310

Rudek MA, Sparreboom A, Garrett-Mayer ES et al (2004) Factors affecting pharmacokinetic variability following doxorubicin and docetaxel-based therapy. Eur J Cancer 40:1170–1178

Ryberg M, Nielsen D, Cortese G, Nielsen G, Skovsgaard T, Andersen PK (2008) New insight into epirubicin cardiac toxicity: competing risks analysis of 1097 breast cancer patients. J Natl Cancer Inst 100:1058–1067

Salive ME, Cornoni-Huntley J, Phillips CL et al (1992) Serum albumin in older persons: relationship with age and health status. J Clin Epidemiol 45:213–221

Sandstrom M, Lindman H, Nygren P, Johansson M, Bergh J, Karlsson MO (2006) Population analysis of the pharmacokinetics and the hematological toxicity of the fluorouracil-epirubcin-cyclophosphamide regimen in breast cancer patients. Cancer Chemother Pharmacol 58:143–156

Sheth HR, Lord G, Tkaczuk K (2003) Aging may be associated with concentrations of tamoxifen and its metabolites in breast cancer patients. J Womens Health 12:799–808

Siris ES, Brenneman SK, Barrett-Connor E et al (2006) The effect of age and bone mineral density on the absolute, excess, and relative risk of fracture in postmenopausal women aged 50–99: results from the National Osteoporosis Risk Assessment (NORA). Osteoporos Int 17:565–574

Smorenburg CH, ten Tije AJ, Verweij J et al (2003) Altered clearance of unbound paclitaxel in elderly patients with metastatic breast cancer. Eur J Cancer 39:196–202

Sorio R, Robieux I, Galligioni E et al (1997) Pharmacokinetics and tolerance of vinorelbine in elderly patients with metastatic breast cancer. Eur J Cancer 33:301–303

Sotaniemi EA, Anttila MI (1997) Influence of age on toremifene pharmacokinetics. Cancer Chemother Pharmacol 40:185–188

Sugrue MM, Kozloff M, Hainsworth J et al. (2007) Safety and effectiveness of bevacizumab plus chemotherapy in elderly patients with mCRC: results from the BRiTE registry. Am Soc Clin Oncol, Gastrointestinal Cancers Symposium, abstract 345

Takigawa N, Segawa Y, Kishino D et al (2004) Clinical and pharmacokinetic study of docetaxel in elderly non-small-cell lung cancer patients. Cancer Chemother Pharmacol 54:230–236

Ten Tije AJ, Smorenburg CH, Seynaeve C et al (2004) Weekly paclitaxel as first-line chemotherapy for elderly patients with metastatic breast cancer. A multicenter phase II trial. Eur J Cancer 40:352–357

Ten Tije AJ, Verweij J, Carducci MA et al (2005) Prospective evaluation of the pharmacokinetics and toxicity profile of docetaxel in the elderly. J Clin Oncol 23:1070–1077

The Arimidex, Tamoxifen, Alone or in Combination Trialists' Group, Buzdar A, Howell A, Cuzick J et al (2006) Comprehensive side-effect profile of anastrozole and tamoxifen as adjuvant treatment for early-stage breast cancer: long-term safety analysis of the ATAC trial. Lancet Oncol 7:633–643

Toffoli G, Sorio R, Aita P et al (2000) Dose-finding and pharmacologic study of chronic oral idarubicin therapy in metastatic breast cancer patients. Clin Cancer Res 6:2279–2287

Townsley CA, Pond GR, Oza AM et al (2006) Evaluation of adverse events experienced by older patients participating in studies of molecularly targeted agents alone or in combination. Clin Cancer Res 12:2141–2149

Vogel C, O'Rourke M, Winer E et al (1999) Vinorelbine as first-line chemotherapy for advanced breast cancer in women 60 years of age or older. Ann Oncol 10:397–402

Wade JR, Kelman AW, Kerr DJ, Robert J, Whiting B (1992) Variability in the pharmacokinetics of eprirubicin: a population analysis. Cancer Chemother Pharmacol 29:391–395

Wong M, Balleine R, Blair EYL et al (2006) Predictors of vinorelbine pharmacokinetics and pharmacodynamics in patients with cancer. J Clin Oncol 24:2448–2455

Zauderer M, Patil S, Hurria A. (2009) Feasibility and toxicity of dose-dense adjuvant chemotherapy in older women with breast cancer. Breast Cancer Res Treat 117:205–210

Zeeh J, Platt D (2002) The aging liver: structural and functional changes and their consequences for drug treatment in old age. Gerontology 48:121–127

Chapter 7
Impact of Hormone Replacement Therapy on Breast Cancer

Toral Gathani and Valerie Beral

7.1 Introduction

The use of hormone replacement therapy (HRT) and its effect on women's health are contentious issues and have been for as long as HRT has been prescribed. The use of HRT for the treatment of the symptoms of menopause is widespread and well recognized. However, the exposure to exogenous hormones in postmenopausal women and the subsequent risk of cancer in general, and breast cancer in particular, have been of interest.

The reproductive life of women is marked by menarche at puberty and menopause in middle age. The definition of menopause is the cessation of menstruation as a result of ovarian failure and signifies the end of a woman's reproductive life. Ovarian failure in turn leads to decreasing circulating levels of estrogen, and the result of which is the manifestation of the acute symptoms of the menopause. These symptoms most commonly include bleeding irregularities, vasomotor, and urogenital symptoms (Critchley et al. 2005a).

In this chapter, we provide an overview of the use of HRT and the current evidence in relation to the risk of breast cancer.

7.2 Development of HRT and Patterns of Use

In the early part of the twentieth century, with greater understanding of reproductive physiology and hormones, it came to be recognized that replacement of estrogen would alleviate the acute symptoms of the menopause. The use of HRT started to gain widespread popularity in the 1960s and the first mass-produced preparations contained only estrogen. In the 1970s, observational evidence started to emerge of increased incidences of endometrial hyperplasia and carcinoma in postmenopausal

T. Gathani (✉)
Cancer Epidemiology Unit, University of Oxford, Oxford, OX1 2JD, UK
e-mail: toral.gathani@btinternet.com

M.W. Reed and R.A. Audisio (eds.), *Management of Breast Cancer in Older Women*,
DOI 10.1007/978-1-84800-265-4_7, © Springer-Verlag London Limited 2011

users of HRT (Smith et al. 1975; Ziel and Finkle 1975). The response to these findings and others was to develop HRT preparations that contained progesterone in order to confer protection to the uterine lining in postmenopausal women. Observational data have confirmed that the addition of progesterone for at least 10 days per month, together with estrogen, did not increase the risk of endometrial hyperplasia or carcinoma in women with an intact postmenopausal uterus (Pike et al. 1997).

Following the introduction of the combined preparations, the popularity of HRT rose once again, having fallen in the late 1970s. The 1980s saw the publication of observational data suggesting that HRT conferred protection to postmenopausal women against adverse cardiovascular outcomes (Bush and Barrett-Connor 1985). On the background of this evidence, the popularity of HRT grew not only as a treatment for the symptoms of the menopause, but also as a secondary preventative measure against future disease such as cardiovascular disease and osteoporosis in postmenopausal women (Grady et al. 1992).

During the early to mid-1990s, serious doubts had begun to surface in the epidemiological community about the validity of the observation data, which had suggested that HRT provided apparent protection to postmenopausal women against adverse cardiovascular outcomes and suggestions were made that the apparent protective effect seen was due to selection bias and a "healthy user effect," in that HRT was more likely to be prescribed to healthier women compared with less healthy women (Matthews et al. 1996).

The effect of HRT on the health of postmenopausal women was unclear and yet prescription rates continued to rise. By the mid-1990s, one third of women aged 50–64 in the UK were estimated to be using HRT. Furthermore, estimates suggested that somewhere between 20–30% of women aged 45–64 in developed countries were using HRT, and since at that time the population of women in those age groups was about hundred million women, it was estimated that in the 1990s twenty million women were using HRT worldwide (Beral et al. 1999).

An individual woman's gynecological history has a strong bearing on the type of HRT she will use. Broadly, alone-alone therapy is used by women without a uterus following hysterectomy and the combined progesterone-progesterone preparations are used by those with an intact uterus. In the face of the increasing use of HRT and uncertainty regarding its effects on women's health, the 1990s saw the establishment of large scale studies, both randomized controlled trials and observational studies, to try and clarify what effect HRT was having on aspects of women's health, and furthermore, to quantify risk estimates for both only-only HRT and for progesterone-progesterone HRT. These large studies have recently reported results and there has been a substantial rise in the availability of information about the effects of HRT on the risk of major illnesses developing in postmenopausal women including breast cancer. The results of these studies have been widely publicized, and for the most part, accepted. In light of these findings, the prescribing guidance for the use of HRT in postmenopausal women was reviewed and subsequently amended by the Food and Drug Administration in the U.S. (Food and Drug Administration 2002), the Committee for the Safety of Medicines in the U.K. (Medicines and Healthcare Products Regulatory Agency 2002), and the European Union. Subsequently, there has been a significant decrease in the use of HRT worldwide. Since 2002, prescription rates for HRT have fallen substantially, but it is estimated that still about one million UK women continue to use HRT (Hersh et al. 2004).

7.3 Hrt and Risk of Breast Cancer

Evidence from many studies now confirms that postmenopausal women who use HRT have an overall increased risk of developing breast cancer compared to those women who do not use HRT.

7.3.1 Important Studies

There are two studies which are of particular importance and deserve mention.

The first is a randomized controlled trial based in the USA and called the Women's Health Initiative Trial. Briefly, this multicenter US-based study recruited over 1,60,000 healthy postmenopausal women into the trial between 1993 and 1998. The women were randomized into the treatment arms according to their gynecological history. Healthy postmenopausal women with an intact uterus were randomized to receive either progesterone-progesterone combined HRT or placebo. Healthy postmenopausal women who had undergone hysterectomy were randomized to receive either only-only HRT or placebo. The primary outcome measure of both arms of the trial was related to cardiovascular outcomes, including coronary heart disease. Breast cancer was recognized as a primary adverse outcome. The combined arm of the trial was terminated early as an unacceptably high incidence of breast cancer was seen in the treatment arm (hazard ratio 1.26, 95% CI [.00–1.59]) (The Writing Group for the Women's Health Initiative Investigators 2002).

The second study is a prospective cohort study based in the UK and called the Million Women Study. The Million Women Study was set up in the 1990s within the framework of the NHS Breast Screening Programme. Briefly, women aged between 50–64 years of age and registered with a general practitioner were recruited into the study between 1996 and 2001. All participants in the study are flagged on the NHS central registers so that any cases of cancer or deaths are notified to the study organizers. The first results from the study showed an increased risk of breast cancer in current users of HRT (OR 1.66, 95% CI [1.58–1.75]). The results of this study were available to provide information not only about the overall risk of developing breast cancer in users of HRT, but also useful information about the effect of different preparation types and duration of use.

7.3.1.1 Effect of the Type of HRT Preparation on Breast Cancer Risk

Results from both randomized controlled trials and observational data have consistently shown that the risk of breast cancer is greater for current users of combined progesterone-progesterone HRT compared to only-only preparations.

The Million Women Study collected detailed data about HRT preparation use and the results of this study showed that the risk in users of combined HRT (OR 2.00, 95% CI [1.88–2.12]) was substantially greater than for estrogen only users (OR 1.30, 95% CI [1.21–1.40]) (The Million Women Study Collaborators 2003).

In regard to the Women's Health Initiative Trial, a higher risk of breast cancer development was seen in the combined user group. Interestingly, an apparent protective effect of only-only HRT against breast cancer was seen (hazard ratio 0.77, 95% CI (0.59–1.01)), but the result was not significant (The Women's Health Initiative Steering Committee 2004) and was treated with caution as it stood alone and unsupported (Hulley and Grady 2004).

7.3.1.2 Effect of Duration of Use on Breast Cancer Risk

The risk of developing breast cancer increases in current users with increasing duration of use, regardless of the type of preparation. The excess risk associated with increasing duration of use falls once use ceases, suggesting that the HRT has a reversible effect on breast physiology. Within the Million Women Study, the risk of developing breast cancer dropped significantly within 1 year of stopping HRT use. (The Million Women Study Collaborators 2003)

The reversible effect of HRT is further supported by emerging evidence of falling breast cancer incidence in older women in developed societies. In the USA, analysis of cancer registry data has shown that a decrease in incidence of breast cancer in older women started around mid-2002, which coincided with the publication of the first results of the Women's Health Initiative Trial. By the end of that same year, the use of HRT had fallen by 38% in the United States (Ravdin et al. 2007). Similar findings have recently been reported in Australia (Canfell et al. 2008).

7.3.1.3 Effect of HRT on Tumor Pathology

It is unclear as to what the effect of HRT is on the pathology of the cancers that occur on the background of HRT use. Some observational studies, but not all, have suggested that breast cancers that occur on the background of HRT were more likely to have characteristics associated with a favorable prognostic outcome. Data from the Million Women Study showed an increased risk of developing tumors with either tubular or lobular histologies versus ductal morphology (Reeves et al. 2006). However, the tumors diagnosed in the treatment group of the combined progesterone-progesterone arm of the Women's Health Initiative Trial were on average significantly larger and more likely to have spread beyond the breast than the cancers diagnosed in nonusers of HRT (Chlebowski et al. 2003).

7.3.1.4 HRT and Screening for Breast Cancer

Breast cancer represents a very important public health problem and it is widely recognized that treatment of early stage disease significantly improves the chance of disease control and survival. There are mechanisms in place which facilitate the diagnosis of disease in asymptomatic women and provide rapid-access clinics for the diagnosis of disease in symptomatic women.

Interest in screening for breast cancer began in the 1970s and 1980s when results from randomized controlled trials provided evidence that the use of X-ray mammography for the population screening of breast cancer could reduce mortality through early detection by 35%, and as a result of these trials, routine screening mammography is available in most developed countries (Critchley et al. 2005b). As of 1995, at least 22 countries had established national, subnational or pilot population breast cancer screening programs. The common protocol for these programs is that all women within a specified age group are invited at prescribed intervals to undergo mammography. The specification of the age group to be invited and the interval between screens are decided at a national level. All the current programs screen by the age of 50 and repeat intervals are between 1 and 3 years (Stewart and Kleihues 2003). The efficacy of breast screening was questioned in 2000 (Gotzsche and Olsen 2000). Since then the benefit of screening had been re-evaluated and results show that screening can be expected to reduce mortality by 35% in women aged 50–70 years (Tabar et al. 2001; Duffy et al. 2002; Nystrom et al. 2002).

The aim of any screening program is to identify individuals within an asymptomatic population who have or are likely to develop specified disease at a time when intervention may result in the improvement of the disease prognosis. The efficacy of any screening test is dependent on the sensitivity of the test (ability to detect disease in those who have disease) and the specificity of the test (ability to not detect disease in those who do not have disease). The efficacy of mammography as a screening tool for breast cancer is directly related to breast density. Breast density and accuracy of interpretation of mammograms are inversely related: the higher the breast density, the less sensitive and specific the mammogram (Mandelson et al. 2000). Breast density is known to vary with age. With increasing age, the breast density decreases as the glandular elements of the breast regress as the levels of circulating sex hormones fall and these tissue elements are replaced by fat. This leads to an increased radiolucency of the breast, and therefore, greater efficacy of mammography. The sensitivity of mammography in fatty breasts (low breast density) is 98% compared with 48% for breasts of high density (Kolb et al. 2002).

Any factor which increases breast density will, therefore, reduce the sensitivity and specificity of mammography. Two exposures that are known to have this effect are alcohol and hormone replacement therapy. The use of HRT in postmenopausal women increases breast density, thereby resulting in decreased sensitivity and specificity of mammography. The increased breast density is secondary to increased hormone levels causing the breast to remain in its more dense pre-menopausal form

(Banks 2001). Among postmenopausal women who use HRT, breast density is increased (Rutter et al. 2001; Harvey and Bovbjerg 2004). The net effect of HRT on the sensitivity and specificity of mammography is that small cancers may be missed, precisely the ones that screening is designed to detect (Banks et al. 2004a; Laya et al. 1996).

The reduction in sensitivity and specificity of mammography in the setting of a screening program has many effects. Users of HRT are more likely to have 'false-positive' radiological findings compared to nonusers, resulting in the individuals concerned having to undergo further assessment and then subsequently being found not to have cancer (Banks et al. 2004b).

One of the measures of success of a screening program is the interval cancer detection rate, which acts as a surrogate measure of the quality of the cancer screening program. Interval cancers are those cancers that are diagnosed in between screens for cancer and can only be defined for women who have undergone screening. Certainly, the reduction in sensitivity and specificity seen in users of HRT leads to an increase in the interval cancer detection rate (Laya et al. 1996; Wang et al. 2001).

7.4   Current Prescribing Advice

The effect of HRT on the risk of breast cancer is only one part of the recent HRT story. The evidence now shows that users of HRT are at increased risk of developing other cancers and cardiovascular disease. The advice from the central authorities has continually been updated over the last few years, and in light of the recent evidence, HRT should be prescribed to women at the lowest effective dose and for the shortest time. HRT should not be prescribed to prevent secondary disease. It is of much importance that those healthcare professionals involved in the prescribing of HRT are aware of the current evidence base, so that they can inform their patients allowing them to make themselves an informed decision about the management of their own health (MHRA 2007).

7.5   Summary

The use of HRT in postmenopausal women increases the risk of developing breast cancer and the magnitude of the risk is greater for users of combined progesterone-progesterone HRT than estrogen alone preparations. The risk of breast cancer increases with increasing duration of use, but that excess risk reduces very rapidly with cessation of HRT use. Furthermore, the use of HRT increases breast density, thereby reducing the efficacy of mammography for cancer screening resulting in a higher risk of interval cancers.

References

Banks E (2001) Hormone replacement therapy and the sensitivity and specificity of breast cancer screening: a review. J Med Screen 8:29–35

Banks E, Reeves G, Beral V, Bull D, Crossley B et al (2004a) Impact of use of hormone replacement therapy on false positive recall in the NHS breast screening programme: results for the million women study. BMJ 328:1291–1292

Banks E, Reeves G, Beral V, Bull D, Crossley B et al (2004b) Influence of personal characteristics of individual women on sensitivity and specificity of mammography in the Million Women Study: cohort study. BMJ 239:477

Beral V, Banks E, Reeves G, Appleby P (1999) Use of hormone replacement therapy and the subsequent risk of cancer. J Epidemiol Biostat 4(3):191–215

Bush TL, Barrett-Connor E (1985) Noncontraceptive estrogen use and cardiovascular disease. Epidemiol Rev 7:89–104

Canfell K, Banks E, Moa AM, Beral V (2008) Decrease in breast cancer incidence following a rapid fall in hormone replacement therapy in Australia. MJA 188(11):641–644

Chlebowski RT, Hendrix SL, Langer RD (2003) Influence of estrogen plus progestin on breast cancer and mammogrophy in healthy postmenopausal women. The Women's Health Initiative Randomized Trial. JAMA 289(24):3243–3253

Critchley H, Gebbie A, Beral V (2005a) Timing of the menopause and its specific effects on health and wellbeing: epidemiology of the menopause. In: Magnusson C (ed) Menopause and hormone replacement. RCOG press, London

Critchley H, Gebbie A, Beral V (2005b) Hormone replacement therapy and mammographic screening for breast cancer. In: Wilson R (ed) Menopause and hormone replacement. RCOG press, London

Duffy SW, Tabár L, Chen HH, Holmqvist M, Yen MF et al (2002) The impact of organized mammography service screening on breast carcinoma mortality in seven Swedish counties. Cancer 95(3):458–469

Food and Drug Administration (2002). "Questions and Answers for Estrogen and Estrogen with Progestin Therapies for Postmenopausal Women" http://www.fda.gov/cder/drug/infopage/estrogens_progestins/Q&A.htm

Gotzsche PC, Olsen O (2000) Is screening for breast cancer with mammography justifiable? Lancet 355:129–34

Grady D, Rubin SM, Petitti DB, Fox CS, Black D et al (1992) Hormone therapy to prevent disease and prolong life in postmenopausal women. Ann Intern Med 117(12):1016–1037

Harvey JA, Bovbjerg VE (2004) Quantitative assessment of mammographic breast density: relationship with breast cancer risk. Radiology 230(1):29–41

Hersh A, Stefanick M, Stafford R (2004) National use of postmenopausal hormone therapy—annual trends and response to recent evidence. JAMA 291(1):47–53

Hulley S, Grady D (2004) The WHI estrogen-alone trial—do things look any better? JAMA 291(14):1769–1771

Kolb TM, Lichy J, Newhouse JH (2002) Comparison of the performance of screening mammography, physical examination, and breast US and evaluation of factors that influence them: an analysis of 27825 patient evaluations. Radiology 225(1):165–175

Laya MB, Larson EB, Taplin SH, White E (1996) Effect of estrogen replacement therapy on the specificity and sensitivity of screening mammography. JNCI 88(10):643–649

Mandelson MT, Oestreicher N, Porter PL, White D, Finder CA et al (2000) Breast density as a predictor of mammographic detection: comparision of interval and screen-detected cancers. JNCI 92(13):1081–1087

Matthews KA, Kuller LH, Wing RR, Meilahn EN, Plantinga P (1996) Prior to use of estrogen replacement therapy, are users healthier than nonusers? JAMA 143(10):971–978

Medicines and Healthcare Products Regulatory Agency (2002). "Use of Hormone Replacement Therapy in the Prevention of Osteoporosis: Important New Information" <http://www.mhra.gov.uk/home/groups/pl-p/documents/websiteresources/con2032228.pdf>

MHRA (2007) Drug safety update: Hormone-replacement therapy. Drug Safety Update 1(2):2–3

Nystrom L, Andersson I, Bjurstam N, Frisell J, Nordenskjold B et al (2002) Long-term effects of mammography screening: updated overwiew of the Swedish randomized trials. Lancet 359:909–919

Pike M, Peters R, Cozen W, Probst-Hensch N, Felix J et al (1997) Estrogen-progestin replacement therapy and endometrial cancer. JNCI 89(15):1110–1116

Ravdin PM, Cronin KA, Howlader N, Berg CB, Chlebowski RT et al (2007) The Decrease in Breast-Cancer Incidence in 2003 in the United States. JNCI 351(16):1670–1674

Reeves GK, Beral V, Green J, Gathani T, Bull D et al (2006) Hormonal therapy for menopause and breast-cancer risk by histological type: a cohort study and meta-analysis. Lancet Oncol 7(11):910–918

Rutter CM, Mandelson MT, Laya MB, Seger DJ, Taplin S (2001) Changes in breast density associated with initiation, discontinuation and continuing use of hormone replacement therapy. JAMA 285(2):171–176

Smith DC, Prentice R, Thompson DJ, Herrmann WL (1975) Association of exogenous estrogen and endometrial cancer. NEJM 293(23):1164–1167

Stewart BW, Kleihues P (2003) World Cancer Report. IARCPress, Lyon

Tabar L, Vitak B, Chen H-H, Yen M-F, Duffy SW et al (2001) Beyond randomized controlled trials—organised mammographic screening substantially reduces breast carcinoma mortality. Cancer 91(9):1724–1731

The Million Women Study Collaborators (2003) Breast cancer and hormone replacement therapy in the Million Women Study. The Lancet 362:419–427

The Women's Health Initiative Steering Committee (2004) Effects of conjugated equine estrogen in postmenopausal women with hysterectomy. Journal of the American Medical Association 291(14):1701–1712

The Writing Group for the Women's Health Initiative Investigators (2002) Risks and benefits of estrogen plus progestin in healthy postmenopausal women. JAMA 288(3):321–333

Wang H, Bjurstam N, Bjorndal H, Braaten AS, Eriksen L (2001) Interval cancers in the Norwegian breast cancer screening program: frequency, characteristics and use of HRT. Int J Cancer 94:594–598

Ziel HK, Finkle WD (1975) Increased risk of endometrial carcinoma among users of conjugated estrogens. NEJM 293(23):1167–1170

Chapter 8
Experiences of a Multidisciplinary Elderly Breast Cancer Clinic: Using the Right Specialists, in the Same Place, with Time

Anne Stotter, Mohammad Tahir, Robert S. Pretorius, and Thompson Robinson

8.1 Introduction

There is little research evidence that could form the base of breast cancer treatment decisions in the elderly (Wyld and Reed 2003). Few breast cancer trials have included older patients, particularly if they are frail. Evidence for treatment benefit, obtained from trials on a younger patient population, cannot directly apply to frail patients, as such application would under-estimate risk. This means, for example, that a frail patient may not benefit from surgery (Hind et al. 2006). However, thorough treatment is needed for patients who will live long enough to benefit, and in the past there has been a trend, particularly in the UK, toward undue reliance on primary endocrine therapy (PET) in patients over the age of 70.

Recent audits have shown that 40% of breast cancers diagnosed in patients over 70 were treated with endocrine treatment alone (Wyld et al. 2004). Our local audit showed similar figures and the outcome: patients were presenting with persistent or recurrent local disease, sometimes locally advanced and then difficult to treat, months or years after diagnosis. The problem continued despite increasing awareness within the unit. Hence, we set up a special clinic for those patients considered unfit for, or declining, standard treatment for early breast cancer. We aimed to improve the management of early breast cancer in the elderly and, as we did so, we learnt about the underlying causes of undertreatment in this population.

Patients are referred to this special clinic by any of the consultants responsible for symptomatic or screen detected breast cancer patients in the unit. We ask for a core biopsy confirming invasive cancer, with tumor hormone receptor status, breast imaging, simple staging investigations (blood count, serum biochemistry, and chest radiograph), and an ECG.

A. Stotter (✉)
Department of Breast/General Surgery, Glenfield Hospital, University Hospitals
Leicester NHS Trust, Leicester, UK
e-mail: anne.stotter@uhl-tr.nhs.uk

M.W. Reed and R.A. Audisio (eds.), *Management of Breast Cancer in Older Women*, 109
DOI 10.1007/978-1-84800-265-4_8, © Springer-Verlag London Limited 2011

8.2   The Geriatrician's Role

The proportion of the United Kingdom's population over the age of 65 years continues to increase, with an estimated total life expectancy of 19.4 years for a female currently aged 65 years (Jagger et al. 2007). With increasing age comes an increased risk of comorbidity and associated disability and functional dependence, such that disability-free life expectancy for a female aged 65 years is currently only 11.0 years (Jagger et al. 2007). This has important implications for surgical oncology, with 50% of cancer diagnoses being made in patients aged 70 years or older (Gosney 2005), where an assessment of biological rather than chronological age will play an important part in the determination of the most appropriate treatment for the patient's cancer.

A comprehensive geriatric assessment (CGA) comprises the evaluation of a patient in her (or his) environment, encompassing medical, functional, and psychosocial elements, and, presumably via subsequent intervention, leads to overall reductions in mortality and institutionalization, as well as benefits in physical and cognitive function (Stuck et al. 1993). There are a number of different models for the application of CGA, which can be used in different health care settings and adapted for disease-specific management programs. However, to date, there is limited evidence of survival benefit in outpatient populations, and little evidence that they inform surgical management, particularly the assessment of suitability for treatment (Gosney 2005). Nonetheless, the recent Preoperative Assessment of Cancer in the Elderly (PACE) study of 460 elderly elective surgical patients, of whom 47% had breast cancer, identified that increasing dependency (assessed by an activities of daily living (IADL) scale) and disability (assessed by personal and IADL scales, and performance status) were predictive of postsurgical complications and increased length of hospital stay, respectively (PACE Participants 2008).

Therefore, it is intuitive that treatment decisions in respect of breast cancer management of the older, often frail, patient should include an assessment of the key domains of CGA. The concept of "frailty" is increasingly recognized, and refers to the accumulation of acute and chronic, often subclinical, conditions, including weakness, fatigue, weight loss, poor balance, reduced physical activity, reduced motor processing and performance, social withdrawal, cognitive change, and increased vulnerability to stressors, such as surgery (Walston et al. 2006). However, the assessment of frailty is not easy in a busy breast diagnostic clinic, hence we established a separate clinic. Most importantly, the assessments are undertaken by a multidisciplinary team using common documentation to avoid duplication in information gathering, and these assessments cover the following domains:

8.3   Functional Assessment

A number of scales are available that assess the older person's ability to function in a personal, as well as in a global setting, though evidence is often limited to the elderly without cancer (e.g., Katz index, Walter et al. 2001) or nonelderly cancer patients (e.g., Karnofsky performance status, Karnofsky and Burchenal 1949). For assessment of ADL, we have selected the Barthel index (Mahoney and Barthel 1965), which was originally developed for the assessment of patients with neurological disorder, but has been recommended by the Royal College of Physicians and British Geriatrics Society (1992). The Barthel Index comprises ten sections and uses direct health care professional or caretaker observations to assess dependence in personal ADL, including washing, dressing, mobility, transfers, feeding, toileting, and continence, and is useful for identifying specific care needs. In addition, the instrumental activities of daily living index (IADL) (Lawton and Brody 1969) is used to assess function in more global domains, for example, shopping, cleaning, driving, drug management, finances, etc.

8.4 Comorbidity Assessment

It is also important to assess the presence of other diseases, which often have a negative effect on physical and cognitive function greater than the individual effects of the single diseases, and are an important determinant of treatment selection and cancer survival. Again, a number of scales exist, which have been validated in elderly, noncancer patients (e.g., Greenfield individual disease severity index (Greenfield et al. 1987), or developed in the elderly, but subsequently validated in a cancer population. In particular, the Charlson Index is an easily applied rating system, which uses standardized criteria to identify the presence or absence of prognostic comorbidity, though not its severity (Charlson et al. 1994). The Satariano Index has been assessed in older breast cancer patients, and reports that patients with three or more comorbidities have an increased risk of death over the 3-year follow-up period, independent of age, breast cancer staging, and treatment type, though again the time course and severity of comorbidity were not accounted for (Satariano and Ragland 1994). Finally, the Medical Research Council Cognitive Function and Ageing Study, a population-based longitudinal study of health in the older population, has identified prevalent comorbidities associated with incident disability and mortality over a 10-year follow-up period (Spiers et al. 2005), and calculated the effect on disability-free and total life expectancy (Jagger et al. 2007).

Initially, we collected data on medical diagnoses for the Satariano Index, but did not document the degree of associated ill-health. More recently we have used a structured questionnaire in our clinic to determine the presence and severity of comorbidities associated with a reduced disability-free and total life expectancy, but enabling the calculation of a score on the basis of the validated Charlson Index.

8.5 Multidimensional Assessment

Any assessment of an older person must acknowledge the importance of cognitive impairment, not only through its impact on reduced disability-free and total life expectancy (Jagger et al. 2007), but also its effect on the patient's ability to participate fully in an informed discussion and consent process regarding best management, and cooperate with treatments. The Folstein mini-mental state (MMS) examination is a well-validated tool, which is commonly used in everyday clinical practice in geriatric medicine (Folstein et al. 1975). In addition, the psychological ability to adapt to illness and treatment is an important aspect of the management of any patient, and the geriatric depression score (GDS) is a well-validated screening tool to identify those patients requiring further assessment for depression (Van Marwijk et al. 1995).

8.6   Anesthetic Assessment/The Role of the Anesthetist

Advancing age and the presence of comorbidities raise a plethora of issues pertinent to the conduct of safe anesthesia. The increasing prevalence and severity of comorbidities and the age-related reduction in the functional reserve of organs lead to an increased incidence of intraoperative and postoperative problems in the elderly surgical patient (Sielenkamper and Booke 2001; Murray and Dodds 2004).

Ordinarily, the patient might not be assessed by an anesthetist until shortly before surgery, often behind a curtain on the ward, while other health care professionals clamor for their share of a patient's time and attention to complete vital parts of the admission and preparation rituals. The anesthetist may feel pressurized to proceed with his task of administering anesthesia despite concerns about the risks that un-investigated comorbidity may hold. Or he (or she) might feel obliged to cancel the case in the patient's best interests pending further investigations. This results in patient distress and wasted theater time, and deterioration in the surgeon-anesthetist relationship.

The advantages of including the anesthetic assessment in the multidisciplinary elderly breast clinic assessment include those of time and privacy. The precise nature, onset and duration, severity, and impact of comorbidity can be assessed by a thorough history, usually verifiable or elaborated by an accompanying family member. The anesthetic assessment includes previous surgical history, medical and drug history, and examination, including that of the airway and the teeth. Investigation results are reviewed and further investigations or other specialist opinion may be requested as appropriate, avoiding a hurried request on the day of surgery. Alterations to management for optimization of medical conditions may be made at the clinic, and passed on to the patient's GP for follow up. Special arrangements that may be needed, such as temporary changes in medication or physiotherapy, can be anticipated and organized. The inclusion of the anesthetist at the clinic allows for an exchange of information and perspective between the anesthetist, physician, and the surgeon, and minimizes the risk that any operation will be canceled on the day. Patient's fears in relation to anesthesia can be discussed and allayed.

Since breast cancer surgery has a low mortality and morbidity, we rarely find a patient who is considered physically unfit. However, we have found that an assessed American Society of Anesthesiologists (ASA) grade of 4 or the apparent need for an ITU bed immediately postoperatively are associated with a short life expectancy, with the associated implication that an operation may not benefit the patient.

The smooth passage of events around surgery makes for improved patient confidence and reduced anxiety, which lead to a better response to anesthetic. The anesthetist can work confidently with a complete picture of the patient's physiological status, and take necessary steps to improve the quality of anesthetic and perioperative care. The list goes ahead as planned. The time spent and the shared expertise in the clinic benefit not only the patient, but also the clinical team (Wise and Thomas 2002).

8.7   Surgical Assessment

A breast specialist surgeon (with experience of endocrine therapy) sees the patient to assess the cancer clinically, and review the breast imaging, core biopsy histology, and staging investigations. It is usually then possible to write a standard treatment plan for the patient's cancer, using the protocols that apply to young, fit patients. This may include treatment choices such as conservative surgery with radiotherapy versus mastectomy (± radiotherapy). There may be special practical problems that need oncology input: a patient with limited arm movement, for example, would need assessing to learn whether radiotherapy would be possible, and in an ideal world, an oncologist/radiotherapist would be available in the clinic.

The tumor hormone receptor status is a crucial piece of information. Most cancers are receptor positive, the proportion increasing to 90% with increasing age (Diab et al. 2000) and 80% of these can be expected to respond to endocrine treatment. (Hormone receptor negative cancers are very unlikely to benefit from endocrine treatment, and so the treatment decisions are simpler.) There is, however, at present no way of predicting which receptor-positive cancers will prove insensitive to hormone manipulation, or the duration of the response in those that do respond. The median response duration that can be expected is about two years, with wide variation, extending to many years in a few cases. Systemic endocrine treatment, of course, treats the micrometastatic disease that is often present at the time of diagnosis (especially in the older patient who tends to present with later stage disease) and will determine the disease-specific survival. In the majority of cases, therefore, the question is whether local treatment should be offered in addition to endocrine treatment.

Tamoxifen has been used to treat breast cancer, and studied, for decades. Important side effects in the elderly are the long-term ones of thrombosis and endometrial cancer. Acquired tumor resistance to tamoxifen is well recognized (Normanno et al. 2005), but second-line endocrine therapy with an aromatase inhibitor (AI) is known to be often effective. There is evidence, particularly from studies of locally-advanced disease, that first-line endocrine treatment with an AI may be more effective than tamoxifen (Howell et al. 2005; Ingle and Suman 2003). However, the osteoporosis associated with AI use is a particular problem for the very elderly, with a high baseline incidence, in whom a hip fracture has a 50% risk of mortality or subsequent institutional care (Cummings and Melton 2002) (which is feared by many elderly women more than death itself). There is little direct evidence, yet, that bone thinning can be prevented or reversed by any particular therapy in patients on AIs. Also, disabling musculo-skeletal pain is not uncommon. After first-line AI therapy has failed, tamoxifen can be used, but there is little data, yet, on its efficacy in this situation. All these factors mean that we cannot, at the present time, be dogmatic about which endocrine agent is best used first. In practice, in patients for PET, we check for contra-indications to either (e.g. deep venous thrombosis for tamoxifen, severe renal failure for AIs) and then decide which to start with, weighing up the risks and benefits. Research evidence should soon make this decision less arbitrary.

8.8 Multidisciplinary Team Discussion

When the assessments of the patient are complete, the team members meet and discuss their findings to decide what recommendations should be made.

Modifications from the "standard" treatment plan may be needed because of reduced fitness and/or life expectancy. Putting it simply: a patient who dies from a cancer operation has not benefited from that operation; similarly a patient who dies soon after a cancer operation (of something else) has not benefited from the surgery. This is particularly true with breast cancer, since the local disease rarely causes life-threatening problems, contrasting with, for example, lung or colon cancer. Mortality from breast cancer surgery is low, so deaths directly due to surgery are rare, and therefore, life expectancy is more important than fitness for surgery. With increasing age and comorbidity, patients with breast cancer are likely to die as a result of problems other than the breast cancer (Diab et al. 2000).

Breast cancer is usually slow growing. We estimate that a life expectancy of two years or less means that recommending primary endocrine treatment should be safe; five years or more and effective local treatment is likely to be important; between two and five years and the pros and cons should be discussed in detail.

Different malignancies need different decisions. Where the potential cure comes from an operation with a significant associated morbidity and mortality, as for colorectal or lung cancer, the problem is one of preoperative assessment to determine the chance of the patient surviving the treatment with an acceptable quality of life, especially the avoidance of institutional care for the rest of their life. A value judgment is, of course, required as to what risk is acceptable; the patient may wish to accept a different level of risk from their family or carers (see communication issues, below). Other malignancies, where toxic chemotherapy provides the potential cure, present similar decisions except that there is the option to start a course of treatment and then stop; this is not an option with surgery, except occasionally when the disease proves more advanced than expected.

Malignancies where a potential treatment is easily tolerated, such as endocrine treatment for breast or prostate cancer, can make the decisions more difficult – should the easy option be selected, or is it better to argue for more aggressive treatment if it might be tolerated, and would improve the chance of disease control?

If aggressive treatment is to be offered, it is usually better offered soon after diagnosis, when the patient is at their youngest and, usually, most fit, rather than months or years down the line. The exception to this is the patient who is diagnosed with cancer when they are recovering from a serious event such as a myocardial infarct or pulmonary embolus, where it is safer to use endocrine treatment first, until recovery is complete.

8.9   Discussion with the Patient

Conversation with an older patient can be a very slow process. To communicate successfully, the clinician must allow the patient to set the pace, difficult though that is when the conversation repeatedly goes off at a tangent, or round in circles. Busy cancer clinics are very difficult places in which to find the necessary time and patience.

Older patients decline treatments more frequently than do the young. Our experience indicates that here are many reasons for saying no (in marked contrast to young patients), and these reasons are very varied and often unpredictable. Since many older people will not easily discuss personal issues with a stranger, it may not be straightforward to discover the reasoning behind a decision. Time and patience may allow a proper discussion, since the clinician or nurse may eventually become familiar. Spending such time should not be seen as an unaffordable luxury in the NHS – we do not hesitate to provide long and detailed consultations to discuss the risks, complications, and potential benefits from cosmetic reconstructive surgery for breast cancer patients.

Communication is more difficult (and the issues are unfortunately more complex) in the older cancer patient. Poor hearing is an obvious barrier. Poor sight means that visual clues, an important component of doctor-patient communication, cannot be used and, of course, written information is less valuable. Interactive computer software is unpopular and we find relatively few "silver surfers."

Cognitive impairment is an important problem. Without formal evaluation, for example, by Mini Mental State assessment, even quite severe dementia can be missed in someone who is good at confabulation. Research staff and others may be reluctant to formally assess cognitive function, feeling that the necessary questions are insulting to the patient and if the questionnaire is not applied thoroughly and with confidence, the score will not be valid. However, geriatricians use these assessment tools regularly and patient acceptance is known to be high.

It is now well recognized that a cancer patient should be encouraged to bring a relative or other companion to a consultation. This person acts as a moral support, will help remember what was said, and may help ensure that all the questions are asked. The family, or companion, of an older patient may take on the further role of advocate. This can be helpful, but can also create an extra problem since they may take over and dominate the conversation, failing to recognize the patient's wishes and priorities. The older patient is likely to be less well educated, less assertive, and less vocal. Sometimes he or she is unable to find a voice at all (Cummings and Melton 2002; Fentiman 2007).

Possibly the most important communication difficulty stems from the fact that the medical team does not know what is important for the patient and cannot know how he or she thinks about the medical problem. A young woman wants to know her breast cancer diagnosis and what treatments are recommended, including any choices she might have. She may ask about why the various treatments are recommended and about side effects. She may have concerns about her dependents, her job, her relationships, and her appearance. She will usually be able to accept the offered treatments, co-operate with the medical team, and get through it all reasonably cheerfully.

Older patients have had life experiences we know nothing about, and often could not guess at, since we are, always, younger. We do not, for example, know what it was like to be born before the last war and to have lived through it. How many clinicians ask about an older patient's past, even just their employment? We tend to forget that education teaches everyone, these days, the rudiments of biology and science, so that most younger patients have a fair understanding of cancer biology. Education teaches logical thinking, and without much education there may be little logic and more emotion dictating responses. Indecision is common, together with a desire to be told what should be done and sometimes a deep reluctance to be involved in the decision-making process.

When the clinician is uncertain of the best treatment, that uncertainty is picked up by the patient and she is likely to decline anything unpleasant. The multidisciplinary team discussion enables a confident approach to the patient. Nevertheless, more than one visit and more than one long discussion may be needed before a decision is made and the treatment plan is complete.

8.10   Audit of the Function of the Clinic

With over three years of clinic activity, over 250 patients assessed, and prospective collection of detailed data, meaningful audit is possible, though outcome information is limited at present. This patient population is particularly liable to default from follow-up because of physical illness, dementia, and moves into another catchment area for residential care or to be closer to family. Also, of the first 250 patients seen, only 152 proved to have newly-diagnosed "early" invasive breast cancer; 108 (72%) of these were advised to have surgery, of whom 103 accepted it.

Looking at the documented comorbidities, 41% had ischemic heart disease, 12% congestive cardiac failure, 36% stroke, 8% peripheral vascular disease, 11% diabetes, 24% chronic obstructive pulmonary disease, and 10% another cancer. There was no significant correlation between any of the individual comorbidities and 2 year survival. Figure 8.1 shows the distribution of scores for the components of the geriatric assessment.

Do we have evidence that our advice has been sound? Patients with "early" breast cancer are very unlikely to die of this disease within 2 years, so survival at

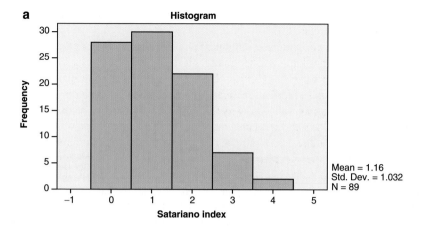

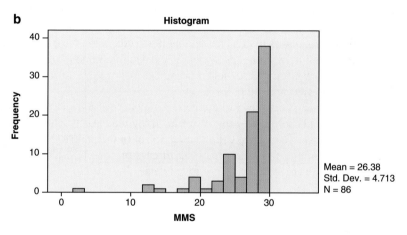

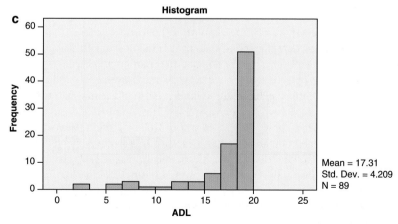

Fig. 8.1 Components of comprehensive geriatric assessment (CGA) and their original scores. (**a**) Satariano index of comorbidities; (**b**) mini mental state examination score; (**c**) activities of daily living (ADL) (Barthel index)

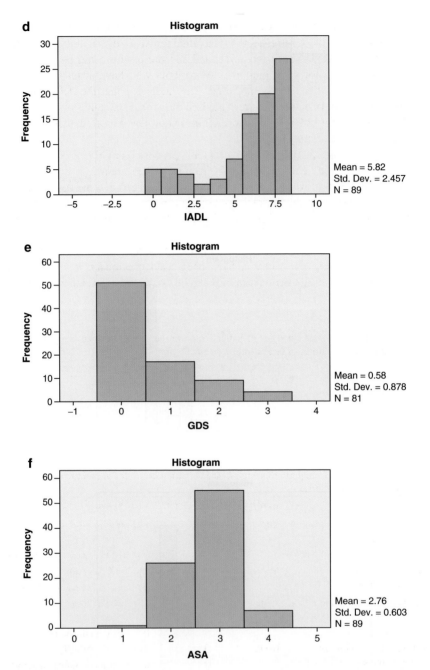

Fig. 8.1 (continued) (d) IADL; (e) geriatric depression score (GDS); and (f) American Society of Anesthesiologists (ASA) scale

2 years is largely determined by comorbidity and functional status. Survival at 2 years can, therefore, be used retrospectively to distinguish between those for whom surgery should not have been recommended and those who could be expected to benefit. Table 8.1 shows the outcomes of patients who have at least 2 years of follow-up, or who died within that time. This indicates that the decisions were roughly right, with patients who were advised surgery significantly more likely to live beyond 2 years ($p < 0.001$). However, it also shows, as expected, that life expectancy cannot be accurately predicted.

Having confirmed that our assessment process roughly predicts which patients will live long enough to benefit from local treatments, we then set about to document how that was achieved. That is, we sought to determine whether the numerical scores from the geriatric assessment might be combined to produce a summary score that predicted survival. This could then be used by others to help in decision-making.

Firstly, we dichotomized each of the components of the geriatric assessment into two categories, using cut-offs that have been used previously, in other studies (Table 8.2). Each contributes a score of 0, "good" or 1, "poor." Logistic regression

Table 8.1 Two-year outcomes of patients seen in the specialist clinic: 89 patients followed up to 2 years or dead within 2 years

n	Advised surgery (declined)	Advised PET
Alive 71	56 (1)	14
Dead 18	10 (1)	8
Total 89		

Chi-squared $p < 0.001$

Table 8.2 The scores from the components of the geriatric assessment dichotomized into "good" (0) and "poor" (1) categories

Component of CGA	Acronym	Score range	Categorization
Satariano's index of comorbidities	SIC	0–7	1–2=0 (2 or less comorbidities)
			3–7=1 (3 or more comorbidities)
Mini-mental state examination	MMS	0–30	24–30=0 (normal)
			0–23=1 (cognitive impairment)
Activities of daily living (Barthel index)	ADL	0–20	12–20=0 (mild or no dependence)
			0–11=1 (significant dependence)
Instrumental activities of daily living	IADL	0–8	8=0 (no disability)
			0–7=1 (one or more disability)
Geriatric depression score	GDS	0–4	0=0 (normal)
			1–4=1 (depression)
American Society of Anesthesiologists score	ASA	1–4	1–3=0 (mild to moderate risk)
			4=1 (severe risk)

analysis was then used to look for any correlation between the dichotomized scores and 2-year survival. Three components showed significant correlation: MMS, ADL, and ASA. If the dichotomized scores for these three are then combined, we have a summary score with a range between 0 and 3, which proves useful. Logistic regression analysis shows that patients with a score of 0 have a more than 84% chance of surviving 2 years or more; those with a score of 1 or more have a less than 34% chance of 2-year survival. Essentially this means that cognitive impairment, significant dependence, or an ASA grade above 3 are each associated with reduced life-expectancy in this elderly patient population, which is what a geriatrician could have predicted without the analysis. However, as we accrue longer follow-up on larger numbers of patients, we should be able to improve on this initial analysis. With more data, it should become clear whether the other components of the geriatric assessment contribute significantly, and whether weighting of the components might improve on the predictive value of the summary score. It is interesting that comorbidities have not proved significant in this, as in other studies: a diagnostic label is, perhaps, less useful in this context than the degree of ill-health it produces. For this reason we are now collecting information on disease and its level of control, using the Charlson Index. Depression seems uncommon in our patients, so this seems unlikely to prove useful. Prospective validation of the final summary score, preferably including a similar patient population from a different Unit, will be needed in due course.

Has our approach to frail patients made a difference to the overall management of our breast cancer patient population? Comparing the rates of uptake of breast cancer treatments in the years preceding the setting up of the clinic with the subsequent period, we find an increase in acceptance (Table 8.3). Early surgery rates have increased in all the older age groups, overall radiotherapy use has increased, and chemotherapy and Herceptin are starting to be used in patients in their seventies. The small reduction in the use of endocrine therapy is due to the fact that its use is now more closely linked to proof of tumor hormone receptor status; in the past it might be used for receptor negative or unknown status cancers in the hope of a response. We have the impression that the increase in uptake of local treatments has resulted in a reduction in the incidence of locally advanced disease, though we have no hard data on this, locally-advanced disease having been poorly documented in the past.

Two things have contributed to the increase in uptake of surgery. The first, with the patients seen in the clinic, is that the detailed assessment allows confident communication of risks and benefits (with time available for this) and patients then feel more positive about the offered treatment and are able to accept it. The second is that the success of treatment of our clinic patients has led to a shift in approach among other breast surgeons in Leicester, with a move toward offering surgery with or without radiotherapy to most patients regardless of chronological age, keeping PET for those who are really very frail.

Table 8.3 Proportion of newly diagnosed older Leicester early breast cancer patients having treatments by age decade at diagnosis, 2003–2004 (gp 1) compared to 2005–2007 (gp 2)

Age at diagnosis	n		% Surgery		% xrt		% Endo		% Chemo		% Her	
	Gp 1	Gp 2	Gp 1	Gp 2	Gp 1	Gp 2	Gp 1	Gp 2	Gp 1	Gp 2	Gp 1	Gp 2
70–79	196	308	68	86	64	70	90	83	2	6	0	3
80–89	104	158	28	53	42	47	91	91	0	0	0	0
90+	15	26	7	12	7	19	93	79	0	0	0	0
Total	315	492	52	71	54	60	90	86	1	3	0	1

Surgery = operation within 90 days of diagnosis, excluding salvage operations (the special clinic was started in January 2005

xrt = local ± egional radiotherapy

Endo = endocrine therapy (tamoxifen or an aromatase inhibitor (AI))

Chemo = neo adjuvant (7) or adjuvant chemotherapy

Her = adjuvant herceptin

8.11 Summary and Conclusions

We have audited the function of this clinic since its inception and it has helped us to understand why undertreatment of breast cancer in the elderly was so common.

Firstly, frailty was overestimated. The patient in a wheelchair with bandaged legs was thought to be unfit, where thorough assessment showed that arthritis and varicose veins were major problems for her, but her cardiac and respiratory function were good.

Secondly, life expectancy was underestimated. It is not generally known that a 70-year-old woman has an anticipated further 16 years of life, an 80-year-old has 9 years, and a woman who is fit enough to have lived up to 90 has on average another 4 years of life. Old age itself should not be considered a good reason for effective treatment to be withheld, except where extreme old age or frailty predicts a short future life span. The aging process, however, does reduce functional reserve, so that while a patient may be fit enough to cope with an anesthetic and an operation, she may cope less well with any complications: a postoperative bleed may lead to hypotension, then myocardial infarct or stroke.

Thirdly, communication of the need for treatment(s), making proposed treatments acceptable, is considerably more complex and difficult, and takes much longer, than in the young, fit patient. There are multiple barriers to the acceptance of treatment in the elderly. This is an important area for future research.

References

Wyld L, Reed MW (2003) The need for targeted research into breast cancer in the elderly. Br J Surg 90:388–399

Hind D, Wyld L, Beverley CB, Reed MW (2006) Surgery versus primary endocrine therapy for operable primary breast cancer in elderly women (70 years plus). Cochrane Database Syst Rev 1:CD004272

Wyld L, Garg DK, Kumar ID, Brown H, Reed MW (2004) Stage and treatment variation with age in postmenopausal women with breast cancer: compliance with guidelines. Br J Cancer 90:1486–1491

Jagger C, Matthews R, Matthews F, Robinson T, Robine J-M, Brayne C, and the MRC-CFAS Investigators (2007) The burden of diseases on disability-free life expectancy in later life. J Gerontol Med Sci 62A:408–414

Gosney M (2005) Clinical assessment of elderly people with cancer. Lancet Oncol 6:790–797

Stuck A, Siu A, Wieland G, Adams J, Rubenstein L (1993) Comprehensive geriatric assessment: a meta-analysis of controlled trials. Lancet 342:1032–1036

PACE Participants (2008) Shall we operate? Preoperative assessment in elderly cancer patients (PACE) can help – a SIOG surgical task force prospective study. Crit Rev Oncol Hematol 65:156–163

Walston J, Hadley E, Ferrucci L et al (2006) Research agenda for frailty in older adults: toward a better understanding of physiology and etiology: summary from the American geriatrics society/ National Institute on aging research conference on frailty in older adults. J Am Geriatr Soc 54:991–1001

Walter L, Brand R, Counsell S (2001) Development and validation of a prognostic index for a 1-year mortality in older adults after hospitalisation. J Am Med Acad 285:2987–2994

Karnofsky D, Burchenal J (1949) The clinical evaluation of chemotherapeutic agents in cancer. In: Macleod C (ed) Evaluation of chemotherapeutic agents. Columbia University Press, New York, pp 199–205

Mahoney F, Barthel D (1965) Functional evaluation: the Barthel index. MD State Med J 14:61–66

Royal College of Physicians and the British Geriatrics Society (1992) Standardized assessment scales for elderly people. Royal College of Physicians and the British Geriatrics Society, London

Lawton M, Brody E (1969) Assessment of older people: self-maintaining and instrumental activities of daily living. Gerontologist 9:179–186

Greenfield S, Blanco D, Elashoff R (1987) Development and test of a new index of comorbidity index. Clin Res A35:346

Charlson M, Szatrowski T, Peterson J, Gold J (1994) Validation of a combined comorbidity index. J Clin Epidemiol 47:1245–1251

Satariano W, Ragland D (1994) The effect of comorbidity on 3-year survival of women with primary breast cancer. Ann Inter Med 120:104–110

Spiers N, Matthews R, Jagger C, Matthews F, Boult C, Robinson T (2005) Diseases and impairments as risk factors for onset of disability in the older population in England and Wales: findings from the medical research council cognitive function and ageing study. J Gerontol Biol Med Sci 60:248–254

Folstein M, Folstein S, McHugh P (1975) Mini mental health for grading the cognitive status of patients for the clinicians. J Psychiatr Res 12:189–198

Van Marwijk H, Wallace P, de Bock G, Hermans J, Kaptein A, Mulder J (1995) Evaluation of the feasibility, reliability and diagnostic value of shortened versions of the geriatric depression scale. Br J Gen Pract 45:195–199

Sielenkamper AW, Booke M (2001) Anesthesia and the elderly. Curr Opin Anaesthesiol 14:679–684

Murray D, Dodds C (2004) Perioperative care of the elderly. Contin Educ Anesth Crit Care Pain 4:193–196

Wise H, Thomas M (2002) Elderly anesthesia as part of a multidisciplinary team. Anesthesia 57:926–927

Diab SG, Elledge RM, Clark GM (2000) Tumor characteristics and clinical outcome of elderly women with breast cancer. J Natl Cancer Inst 92:550–556

Normanno N, Di Maio M, De Maio E et al (2005) Mechanisms of endocrine resistance and novel therapeutic strategies in breast cancer. Endocr Relat Cancer 12:721–747

Howell A, Cuzick J, Baum M et al (2005) Results of the ATAC (arimidex, tamoxifen, alone or in combination) trial after completion of 5 years' adjuvant treatment for breast cancer. Lancet 365:60–62

Ingle JN, Suman VJ (2003) Aromatase inhibitors versus tamoxifen for management of postmenopausal breast cancer in the advanced disease and neoadjuvant settings. J Steroid Biochem Mol Biol 86:313–319

Cummings SR, Melton LJ (2002) Epidemiology and outcomes of osteoporotic fractures. Lancet 359:1761–1767

Fentiman IS (2007) Communication with older breast cancer patients. Breast J 13:406–409

Part III
Therapeutics

Chapter 9
Mammographic Breast Screening in Elderly Women

Lynda Wyld

9.1 Mammographic Breast Screening

The National Health Service Breast Screening Programme (NHS BSP) was established in 1987 following publication of the Forrest Report (Forrest et al. 1986). This advocated mammographic breast screening for all UK women between ages 50 and 64, based on evidence from a number of large screening trials from the USA, UK, Sweden, and Canada (Table 9.1). There were three reasons cited for the upper age cut off at 65: other cause mortality, lower attendance rates with increasing age, and breast cancer running a less aggressive course in older women.

Data from these studies, now with very mature follow up, demonstrate that screening is associated with a reduction in breast cancer specific mortality of between 30 and 40% (Tabar et al. 2003).

The NHS BSP has now been running for over 20 years and its data suggest an improvement in the survival for screened UK women in line with the predictions of the trials: 5-year survival for UK screen detected breast cancer is 96.5%, compared to 70% for symptomatic cancer (BASO 2006), though some of this striking difference will be due to lead time bias.

It is likely that these figures will improve over the next 5 years with the introduction of routine 2-view mammography, double film reading, and the increased quality of mammograms (digital mammography). In addition, the upper age limit for screening in the UK has just increased from 64 to 69, which will permit more women to benefit. There are also proposals to increase the upper age limit still further, to 73, in the next few years. What of women over this age, who make up one third of all breast cancer diagnoses (Sader et al. 1999)? In the UK, at present, women over 70 may continue to have mammograms, but have to self refer as they are no longer routinely invited. In practice, this means that uptake rates are very low.

L. Wyld (✉)
Academic Unit of Surgical Oncology, University of Sheffield, Sheffield, UK
e-mail: l.wyld@sheffield.ac.uk

M.W. Reed and R.A. Audisio (eds.), *Management of Breast Cancer in Older Women*, 127
DOI 10.1007/978-1-84800-265-4_9, © Springer-Verlag London Limited 2011

Table 9.1 Review of large mammographic breast screening randomized trials

Trial name	Age range	Number patients	Mammographic frequency (year)	Follow-up (years)	Relative risk death	Confidence interval (95%)	Reference
Health insurance plan	40–64	60,995	1	18	0.78	0.61–1.0	Shapiro (1988)
Edinburgh trial	45–64	44,268	2	14	0.79	0.60–1.02	Alexander et al. (1999)
Canadian National	50–59	39,405	1	13	1.02	0.78–1.33	Miller et al. (2000)
Finnish National	50–64	158,755	2	4	0.76	0.53–1.09	Hakama et al. (1997)
Swedish Malmo 1	45–70	42,283	2	19.2	0.81	0.66–1.00	Nystrom et al. (2002)
Swedish 2 Counties	40–74	133,065	2–3	20	0.68	0.59–0.8	Tabar et al. 2000

Breast cancer mortality has fallen in most age groups in the past 20 years partly due to the effect of screening and partly due to improvements in adjuvant therapies such as chemotherapy, endocrine therapies, and new drugs such as Trastuzumab. This survival improvement has not been seen in older women who are rarely treated with adjuvant chemotherapy or Trastuzumab. In addition, older women present with later stage disease than their younger counterparts. The size of the primary tumor is larger (Golledge et al. 2000; Diab 2000; Daidone et al. 2003), and there is a higher incidence of locally advanced (Eaker et al. 2006) and metastatic disease (Wyld et al. 2004; Yancik et al. 1989). This tendency to present with later stage disease is partly due to reduced levels of breast awareness (Siapush and Singh 2002), lower rates of regular self examination (Mah and Bryant 1992), and reduced levels of mammographic screening.

With this in mind, this chapter will explore the issue of screening women over the age of 70.

9.2   Attitudes of Older Women to Breast Screening

Old age has been repeatedly shown to be a contributing factor to poor mammography uptake rates (Bynum et al. 2005; Bryant and Mah 1992).

In the UK, uptake rates for those over 70 are poor, with only half of all older women in the UK being aware that they are eligible for screening. In addition, most (81%) are unaware of how they can access this service (Kumar et al. 2004). However, when asked, 95% of older women were keen to have mammograms. Knowledge about breast cancer is poor in older women (Gunnfeld et al. 2002; Dolan et al. 1997), with low levels of knowledge about breast cancer symptoms and their own level of risk of developing the disease. Many believe they are less susceptible than younger women (Mah and Bryant. 1992), an impression fostered by the fact that they are no longer invited for screening once they are over 70. There may also be a perception that other health issues assume more importance, and there is a widely held belief that mammography is not helpful if there are no cancer symptoms, which denotes a lack of understanding of the principles of screening (Mah and Bryant 1992).

Some women may be deterred from attending by difficulty with traveling to the screening center.

9.3   Is Mammography Effective in Older Women?

Data from the NHS BSP (2006) demonstrate that mammography attendance is low in women over the age of 70 (Table 9.2). However, the pickup rate for cancer is much higher in this group than in younger age cohorts (Table 9.2), demonstrating that screening is effective in diagnosing cancers in this age

Table 9.2 NHS BSP data by age group (BASO 2006)

Age group	50–54	55–59	60–64	65–70	70+
Number screened per year	418,300	448,800	359,500	326,100	42,600
Number recalled for assessment	26,540	16,347	13,705	13,882	2,326
Percentage recalled	6.3%	3.6%	3.8%	4.3%	5.5%
Number with cancer	2,625	3,039	3,160	3,768	723
Percentage cancer diagnosis	0.62%	0.67%	0.87%	1.15%	1.7%

Table 9.3 Comparison of screened and symptomatic cancers by age group (BCCOM 2006)

Prognostic factor	Method of presentation	Age range (years)		
		<50 (%)	50–64 (%)	65+ (%)
Nodal disease present (% of cases where known)	Screen detected	20	29.2	21.2
	Symptomatic	46.6	41.3	40.6
Nottingham prognostic index, % in excellent prognostic group	Screen detected	33	26.7	26.9
	Symptomatic	6.7	9.6	8.3
Mastectomy rate %	Screen detected	33	27.2	26.5
	Symptomatic	45.9	45.3	56.1

group. The rate of cancer diagnosis is 0.62% in the 50–54 year age cohort compared to 1.7% in the 70+ cohort. Whether this translates into an improved survival in this age group is not known.

There is little doubt that mammographic breast screening improves survival for younger (50–70 years) women with breast cancer: mature trial data from the large screening studies now include absolute survival data, which are not subject to biases such as lead time, lag time, and length bias. Most authors estimate a survival benefit in the region of 20–39% (Tabar et al. 2003).

There is a lack of direct randomized controlled trial (RTC) data for older women who were excluded from most of the large trials (see Table 9.1). We have, therefore, little direct evidence of benefit and have to look at different forms of evidence such as extrapolation of the RCT data from younger cohorts, uncontrolled case series, the use of surrogate markers (i.e., stage reduction at diagnosis as a surrogate of improved prognosis, reduced incidence of metastatic disease as a surrogate of mortality), modeling, and cohort study data.

Screening does result in the diagnosis of earlier stage cancers in older women. A recent (2002) UK audit of symptomatic cancers demonstrated that screening results in a lower average Nottingham Prognostic Index for older women with screened vs. symptomatic cancers (BCCOM Project Report 2006). The rate of node positivity is almost halved, as is the mastectomy rate (Table 9.3). There is, therefore, little doubt that screen detected breast cancers should be associated with an improved prognosis in older women. However, there are confounding factors, which may mean that these improvements in surrogate outcome measures do not translate into improved survival. These include the risks of screening which include psychological distress, pain, unnecessary procedures, and the very substantial costs to health care providers. There is also a risk that the radiation dose of the mammogram may contribute to the development of some cancers, though the risk of such low dose radiation exposure is extremely low (often quoted in the order of two additional radiation induced breast cancers per million mammograms), and the risk is lower in postmenopausal women (IARC Breast Screening Handbook 2002). There is also a higher rate of breast cancer diagnosis in screened women (Tabar et al. 2003), which implies that for screened women some of their cancers would never have affected them during their lifetime and were, therefore, clinically insignificant (Smith-Bindman et al. 2000).

9.4 Evidence for Screening Efficacy in Older Women

9.4.1 Randomized Controlled Trials

Most of the large RCTs performed in the 1970s and 1980s recruited women up to age 64 or 70, with only 2 of the trials recruiting up to age 74 (Swedish 2 Counties Trial and the Swedish Malmo Trial) and none beyond this age (Nystrom et al. 2002). In a joint analysis of the Swedish studies, there was insufficient power to determine whether there was a survival advantage for the cohort of screened women between age 70 and 74 (Nystrom et al. 2002).

9.4.2 Cohort Studies

There have been retrospective cohort studies of older women who have had screening vs. those who have not. For example, one US study examined the risk of death from breast cancer and the incidence of stage 1 or 2 disease in regular users or nonusers of mammography in 3 age cohorts: 67–74, 75–85, and over 85. They found that in the 2 youngest age cohorts, the risk of breast cancer death was significantly less in regular users (RR 3.69, CI 2.58–5.27 for the 75–84 group, RR 3.18, CI 2.27–4.46, 67–74 age group) (McCarthy et al. 2000). A significant difference persisted even after allowing for a 1.25 year lead time bias (this was based on the lead time for the 70–74 year age group found in the Swedish 2 Counties Trial, though some suggest that a longer lead time bias is appropriate in older women due to less aggressive disease biology. Boer et al. 1998). The trial also used a modified Charlson Index of comorbidity (Charlson et al. 1987) to correct for comorbidity variance between cohorts and found the results continued to show a survival advantage when this was corrected for. Another cohort study showed a survival advantage for screened vs. nonscreened women in an age cohort from 68–83 years (Van Dijck et al. 1997). They found a relative survival rate of 0.8 in favor of screening, though this was not significant (CI 0.53–1.22), and no subgroup analysis by age group was possible due to small sample size.

A further retrospective cohort study found a direct survival benefit for older screened women vs. non-screened (McPherson et al. 2002). There was a significant relative survival difference in all age subgroups over 70 (70–74, RR survival 1.0 screened vs. 0.66 nonscreened, P<0.001, 75–79, 1.0 vs. 0.54, P<0.001, 80–84, 0.89 vs. 0.76, P< 0.039, >85, 1.0 vs. 0.39, P<0.007). However, on testing their data for selection bias (women in poor health not being referred for screening), they found this had occurred in the 75–79 year age group, but not other age groups, though the accuracy of such assessments on retrospective data is questionable. The data were not corrected for lead or length time bias, which may also have had an influence.

Data from existing screening programs have also been reported and demonstrate that screening in the 70–75 year age group is associated with a reduction in breast cancer specific mortality of 29.5% compared to a cohort of women prior to the introduction of screening into this age group (1986–1997 vs. 1997–2003) (data from the Netherlands Screening Programme, Otten et al. 2008). These data may be somewhat flawed as there may have been other treatment differences to account for some of the change (e.g., less use of tamoxifen and chemotherapy).

9.4.3 Surrogate Markers

Studies that have used surrogate markers of survival have found that older women (66–79 years) who have regular breast screening have a relative risk of having metastatic disease at diagnosis of 0.57 compared to their nonscreened counterparts (CI 0.45–0.72), and a relative risk of 3.3 of having localized breast cancer (CI 3.1–3.5) (Smith-Bindman et al. 2000).

The data relating to prognostic factors at diagnosis are presented above.

9.4.4 Modeling Studies

As data from RCTs in this age group are very limited and few good quality cohort studies are available, many researchers have used modeling techniques to estimate the potential benefit from screening to older age groups. All of these studies have indicated that the relative benefit of screening older women, compared to screening in the 50–69 year age group, decreases with increasing age (Barratt et al. 2002). For example, Mandelblatt and colleagues (1992) found that the relative benefit was 83% for the 70–74 cohort, 61% for the 75–79 group, 45% for 80–84, and only 32% for the over 85s. Other workers have drawn similar conclusions (Rich and Black 2000; Eddy 1989). In terms of advising on the upper age cut off, some suggest that there is still likely to be cost effective benefit up to at least the age of 80 years, but the increase in negative effects means the relative cost efficacy is lower in this older age group (Boer et al. 1995).

9.5 Why is Screening Potentially Different in Older Women?

There are a number of reasons why it is not appropriate to simply extrapolate RCT trial data on screening efficacy to the elderly population.

9.5.1 Mammographic Sensitivity

Screening in older women will detect more cancers per 10,000 mammograms than in younger women due to a higher incidence of cancer and a greater mammographic sensitivity with age (Faulk et al. 1995; Rosenberg et al. 1998). A US study reported a cancer detection rate of 9.2/1,000 mammograms in women over 65 vs. 5.7/1,000 in women between 50 and 64 (Carney et al. 2003). The sensitivity of mammograms varies from 68% in 40–44 year olds to 83% in 80–89 year olds (Carney et al. 2003), with similar figures reported by other authors (Rosenberg et al. 1998).

9.5.2 Competing Risks of Death

For a woman to benefit from earlier detection of breast cancer, she must survive for long enough to see this benefit. Life expectancy is related to age, with the average 70 year old having a life expectancy of 15 years and the average 80 year old 7 years. However, the elderly are very heterogeneous and comorbid disease has a major impact on life expectancy. The incidence of comorbidity increases with age. Once a woman is over the age of 80, even if she has breast cancer, she has a higher chance of dying of non-breast cancer causes. For example, 73% of deaths in breast cancer patients in the 50–54 year age group are due to their breast cancer, compared to only 29% of deaths in the over 85 age group (Diab et al. 2000). A large study of older women with breast cancer showed that those with 3 or more comorbid diseases had a 20 times higher rate of non-breast cancer death which was independent of the stage of their disease, and therefore, earlier diagnosis for these women conferred no survival advantage (Satariano and Ragland 1994). Similar findings were published by Siegelmann-Danielli et al. (2004), who demonstrated a progressively diminishing impact of stage on prognosis as age and comorbidity levels increase. In the screening setting, regardless of age, screening no longer confers a survival advantage in women with severe comorbid disease and the influence of moderate comorbid disease lessens the impact of screening on survival in an age dependant manner (McPherson et al. 2002).

Cognitive impairment is also very common in older women, with a prevalence of 50% at age 85. This includes a wide spectrum of severities, varying from mild impairment which will have little influence on life expectancy but may compromise a women's ability to weigh up the pros and cons of screening and make an informed choice, to the severely impaired where life expectancy will be markedly shortened (Raik et al. 2004).

In the frail elderly, much harm may be done by screening women inappropriately. One study offered mammographic screening to 216 women who were nursing home candidates with an average age of 81 years, 91% of whom had dependency in at least one activity of daily living and 49% had some degree of cognitive impairment (Walter et al. 2001). Of these 216 women, 18% were recalled and two thirds of these recalls were for false positives, which required further tests (further imaging, biopsy or surgery). Four women were diagnosed with cancer and treated, but 2 of these died within 15 months of unrelated diseases, one of whom had severe wound infection problems postoperatively and had chronic wound pain. Only 2 of the patients with treated cancers might have derived some benefit (0.9% of the total cohort). Of the women who were recalled, almost half had documented anxiety or depression as a result of the process.

As a result of these competing causes of death, the effect of any cancer-directed interventions is diluted and its benefit more difficult to prove. In addition, it has been suggested that there is little value in screening women with a predicted life expectancy of less than 5 years as for most screening interventions, cancer specific survival curves do not start to diverge until at least 5 years after the start of screening (Walter and Covinski, 2001). The maximal effect of most screening interventions is not seen until 10 years after screening commences (Nystrom et al. 2002).

From a health economics perspective, which is important in the assessment of any mass screening intervention, the usual means of assessing cost efficacy is to determine the number of life years gained per unit cost. Clearly in this older population where life expectancy is much lower, the gain in life years per unit cost will automatically be lower.

Because older women differ in their likely benefit from screening according to their life expectancy, some authors have explored alternate strategies for selection based either on breast cancer risk or on life expectancy. Although absolute age and life expectancy are linked, a more refined prediction can be achieved by the use of scoring systems which take into account comorbid disease, functional status, dementia, or a combination of all of these factors (Gosney 2005). Kerlikowske et al. (1999) used a modeling technique to examine what the cost to benefit ratio of screening all women up to the age of 79 would be compared to the use of a selection technique for identification of high breast cancer risk. (High bone mineral density was taken as a marker for increased risk.) They found that while screening of all women up to age 79 had some benefit, this was enhanced if only the higher risk cohort was offered screening. They also suggested that screening up to the age of 79 would only result in a gain in life expectancy of 7 h per woman screened, compared to 48 h if screening was stopped at the age of 69.

9.5.3 Over Diagnosis of Cancer

As mentioned above, breast screening results in the over diagnosis of cancer, that is, it identifies a higher rate of cancer than the non-screened population, implying that these additional cancers would never have caused problems during the women's lifetime. This effect is likely to be more significant in older women due to their reduced life expectancy, and therefore, the treatment related costs, side effects, and detrimental effects on quality of life of these clinically insignificant cancers must be taken into account in performing the cost benefit analysis. The rate of over diagnosis is variably quoted between 10 and 40% (Zackrisson et al. 2006; Zahl et al. 2004; Jonsson et al. 2005). In addition, there is a 3.5 times greater incidence of diagnosis of in situ disease in women aged 66–79 who have screening vs. those who do not (Smith-Bindman et al. 2000). For women with a short life expectancy, and especially those with small areas of low grade ductal carcinoma in situ (DCIS), it is unlikely that this disease would ever become significant or symptomatic in the patient's lifetime.

The risk of DCIS progressing to invasive disease is dependent on the size and grade. While large areas of high grade disease have a risk of progression, if untreated, of 75% over 4 years (Dean and Geshchicter 1938), small low grade disease has a progression rate of only 40% at 30 years (Page et al. 1995). Not surprisingly, the incidence of DCIS falls sharply once screening stops (Kaplan and Saltzstein 2005).

9.5.4 Different Disease Biology with Age

Breast cancer in older women tends to express different markers of disease aggression than that in younger women with higher levels of ER expression (McCarty et al. 1983; Diab 2000), lower rates of HER 2 receptor expression (Diab 2000), lower tumor grade (Erbas et al. 2004; Gajdos et al. 2001; Schaefer et al. 1984), and lower markers of proliferation (S phase fraction) (Wenger et al. 1993). As a result, the lead time bias that should be factored into screening studies to allow for the presymptomatic period gained through screening may need to be longer in older women. This has not always been considered in studies of screening in the elderly.

9.5.5 Cost

Most of the data indicate that there is still chance for cost-effective benefit at all ages (Mandelblatt et al. 1992, 2003; Barratt et al. 2002; Broeders et al. 2002), though the benefits are smaller in the older age groups and the cost per life saved is much greater (Stout et al. 2006). For example, Mandelblatt (1992) studied women in 5 age cohorts over age 65, and factored in 3 different levels of comorbidity (average health, mild hypertension, or congestive cardiac failure). They found that the cost per year of life saved was $23,212 for a women in the 65–69 year age group, $27,983 in the 70–74 year age group, and $73,000 for a women of over 85 years (all in the average health category). Factoring in poor health status made these costs even greater.

There are several reasons for this increased cost. The number of life years gained will be less due to the reduced life expectancy of this age group and competing causes of death, the increased rate of clinically insignificant cancers, and the increased cost of treatment for older women who may require longer inpatient stays and suffer increased side effects from surgery and anesthesia (Wyld and Reed 2007).

Data on quality adjusted life year costs relating to screening older women are very difficult to obtain due to a lack of studies, though Mandelblatt et al. (1992) found in their modeling study that adverse quality-of-life effects in the oldest (85+) and least healthy (congestive cardiac failure) cohort in their model probably outweighed the small gain in survival.

Another issue to be considered in screening older women is that the actual process of screening may be more costly, with frailer women taking more time to screen and requiring more assistance. Up to age 69, this does not appear to be a major factor (Brown et al. 2002), but as the age range is extended, more difficulties may be encountered

9.6   Risks of Screening in Older Women

Breast screening is associated with risks which include psychological distress, unnecessary biopsies (both percutaneous and surgical), and the slight risk posed by the radiation exposure itself. The radiation dose of the mammogram may contribute to the development of some cancers, though the risk of such low dose radiation exposure is extremely low. A single mammogram exposure of 2 mGy may cause 4.5 cases of breast cancer per million women screened in 40–49 year olds and 1.5 per million in 50–59 year olds (Sabel et al. 2001). For the older group of women, the radiation risk is smaller still and may be negligible for women over 70 due to their reduced life expectancy, the increased sensitivity of mammograms which may require lower radiation doses to achieve good quality films, and reduced breast sensitivity to radiation due to lower rates of breast epithelial proliferation in the postmenopausal state (Jansen and Zoetelief 1997). For those diagnosed with cancer, screening may affect quality of life both negatively and positively. The quality of life may have been low initially due to earlier awareness (prolonged knowledge of disease, knowledge of disease that would never have become symptomatic), but it improved later due to a reduced rate of metastatic disease and increased rates of breast conservation.

9.7 Who Should be Screened and What Selection Criteria Could be Used

There is evidence that the benefits of screening probably extend beyond the age of 70. But does this effect extend to all women and at what age does efficacy cease? Some work has been done to show that cost effectiveness only extends up to age 75, while others suggest that the age cut off should be at age 79 (Mandelblatt et al. 2005), with screening beyond this age only for women in the top 25% of life expectancy for age. This is based on a presumption that screening only benefits people with a life expectancy of over 5–10 years. The life expectancy of a 79 year old will be 10 years for 75% of women, compared to only 25% of women of 85 and over (Mandelblatt et al. 2005). It is, therefore, apparent that the health status of the individual will have a significant effect. McPherson and colleagues (2002) studied women of 65–101 years and found that at all ages, for women with no comorbidity or mild to moderate comorbidity, screening was of some benefit, even for women over 80. They found that only when a woman had severe comorbid disease, screening lost its efficacy.

However, restricting mammography to fit women over 70 would pose substantial logistical problems related to the fitness level at which to set the cut off. Who should determine this and most importantly, what do older women think of this type of selection process? In the US, where physician recommendation is a strong predictor of screening uptake, selection of appropriate older women tends to favor fitter older women and age itself is an independent negative predictor of referral, with older women less likely to be advised to attend (Bynum et al. 2005). There are also a significant number of inappropriate referrals, suggesting a lack of understanding of those likely to benefit from screening. Nursing home residency and dementia have a negative impact on the likelihood of referral, but chronic medical problems do not (Marwill et al. 1996). In another US study, more than 50% of women having mammograms at age 80 or over were in the worst quartile of health status, suggesting that they would be unlikely to benefit from screening (Walter et al. 2004). A further study in the US found that women with greater levels of comorbid disease were more likely to be advised to have screening, a fact ascribed to increased levels of physician contact in those with other health problems (Heflin et al. 2002). In short, decision making by the US physicians, the main determinant of screening uptake in a voluntary system, is poor with both over and underscreening occurring.

In the UK, women over 70 self select for screening. If physicians find this decision difficult, how can we expect patients themselves to make the correct decision?

There are validated methods of assessing patient fitness and use of these to predict life expectancy. These models are becoming more sophisticated, and computerized models are being developed. It has been suggested that rather than basing the offer of screening on comorbidity per se, or age cut-offs, it should be based on a women having a predicted life expectancy of over 5–10 years. There are now large datasets which link comorbidity and age with life expectancy, and prediction accuracy is improving (MRC-CFAS dataset for example) (Spiers et al. 2005). Linking this data with NHS screening data on outcomes would enable us to model the results of various selection techniques to determine which cut off would be most practical and result in reasonable cost to benefit ratios. It would seem sensible to issue guidelines to clinicians to enable them to better decide whom to refer for screening and to channel screening requests in women over age 79 through family physicians.

The current system of screening on request for the over 70 cohort in the UK may already provide some filter to ensure that fitter women attend for screening, but uptake is low. Women in better health may be more concerned with health maintenance and their physicians may be more likely to advise them to attend for screening when they attend for routine health checks.

It appears that practice relating to who should be screened is converging internationally. In the US, the American Geriatrics Society advocates no upper age limit, but that screening should be offered to all women with an estimated life expectancy of greater than 4 years (AGS 2004). In practice, this places the onus for decision making on the physician and such estimates can be difficult. The American Cancer Society is even less specific and suggests no upper age limit, but to screen as long as the patient is in good health and fit for treatment (Smith et al. 2007). In Europe, practice varies between countries, but most screen to age 69 or 75 (Table 9.4).

Table 9.4 Summary of national screening practices in western countries

Country	Age range offered screening	Periodicity (year)	National program	Comments
UK	50–69	3	Yes	Screening on request after age 70
USA	40+	1–2	No	No upper age limit: recommended to screen until life expectancy less than 4 years
Sweden	50–74	2	Yes	
Finland	50–69	2	Yes	For over 70s, no formal screening but may be accessed by private clinics and family physicians
Hungary	45–65	2	Yes	
Australia	50–69	2	Yes	Over 70s can elect to attend if wished
Iceland	40–69	2	Yes	
Italy	Variable by region, 25–70	2	No, regional	
Netherlands	50–75	2	Yes	No screening for over 75s. Under legal challenge at present
Canada	50–69	2	Yes	
France	50–74	2	Yes	
Norway	50–69	2	Yes	
Portugal	50–69	2	No, regional	

The International Society for Geriatric Oncology recommends screening be available up to age 75, with individualized decision making beyond this based on patient preference, physiological age, and life expectancy (Wildiers et al. 2007).

The planned extension of the NHS BSP upper age limit to 73 will put the UK more in line with this, but steps need to be taken to educate older women and their health care providers about the availability of screening on demand beyond this age so that they, in conjunction with their health care providers, can make an informed choice about whether to continue to attend.

9.8 Summary

Screening women over age 70 is controversial. It will almost certainly be beneficial to healthy older women, but may do more harm than good to those with a life expectancy of less than 5 years. National screening programs must also consider the cost to benefit ratio of screening older women, and while benefit can still be had screening up to the age of 80, costs for population screening become prohibitive beyond this age. Screening, therefore, needs to be targeted at those older women who are more likely to benefit, by education of both patients and their health care professionals about who is likely to benefit. This will optimize benefits and costs and minimize harms.

References

AGS (2004) American geriatrics Society position statement: Breast cancer screening in older women. http://www.americangeritrics.org/staging/products/positionpapers/brstcncrPF.shtml

Alexander FE, Anderson TJ, Brown HK et al (1999) Lancet 353:1903–1908

Barratt AL, Irwig LM, Glasziou PP, Salkeld GP, Houssami N (2002) Benefits, harms and costs of screening mammography in women 70 years and over: a systematic review. Med J Aust 176:266–272

BASO (2006) NHS Breast Screening Programme and Association of Breast Surgery at the British Association of Surgical Oncology. An audit of screen detected breast cancers for the year of screening April 2005 to March 2006. At: http://www.cancerscreening.nhs.uk/breastscreen/publications/ba05-06.html. Accessed 21 Apr 2009

BCCOM (2006) Breast Cancer Clinical Outcome Measures (BCCOM) project. Analysis of the management of symptomatic breast cancers diagnosed in 2002. At: http://www.wmpho.org.uk/wmciu/documents/BCCOM_annual_report.pdf. Accessed 21 Apr 2009

Boer R, de Koning HJ, van Oortmarssen GJ, van der Maas PJ (1995) In search of the best upper age limit for breast cancer screening. Eur J Cancer 31A(12):2040–2043

Boer R, de Koning HJ, Threlfall A, Warmerdam P, Street A, Friedman E, Woodman C (1998) Cost effectiveness of shortening screening interval or extending the age range of NHS breast screening programme: computer simulation study. Br Med J 317:376–379

Broeders MJ, Verbeek ALM, Straatman H, Peer PGM, Pasker de Jong PCM, Beex LVAM, Hendriks JHCL, Holland R (2002) Repeated mammographic screening reduces breast cancer mortality along the continuum of age. J Med Screen 9:163–167

Brown J, Garvican L, Moss S (2002) An investigation into the effect of extending routine mammographic screening to older women in the United Kingdom on the time it takes to screen. J Med Screen 9:15–19

Bryant H, Mah Z (1992) Breast cancer screening attitudes and behaviours of rural and urban women. Prev Med 21:405–418

Bynum JPW, Braunstein JB, Sharkey P, Haddad K, Wu AW (2005) The influence of health status, age, and race on screening mammography in elderly women. Arch Intern Med 165:2083–2088

Carney PA, Miglioretti DL, Yankaskas BC, Kerlikowske K, Rosenberg R, Rutter CM, Geller BM, Abraham LA, Taplin SH, Dignan M, Cutter G, Ballard-Barbash R (2003) Individual and combined effects of age, breast density and hormone replacement therapy use on the accuracy of screening mammography. Ann Intern Med 138:168–175

Charlson ME, Pompei P, Ales KL, McKenzie CR (1987) A new method of classifying prognostic comorbidity in longitudinal studies: development and validation. J Chronic Dis 40(5):373–383

Daidone MG, Coradini D, Martelli G, Veneroni S (2003) Primary breast cancer in elderly women: biological profile and relation to clinical outcome. Crit Rev Oncol Haematol 45:313–325

Dean L, Geshchicter CF (1938) Comedocarcinoma of the breast. Arch Surg 36:225–235

Diab SG, Elledge RM, Clarke GM (2000) Tumor characteristics and clinical outcome of elderly women with breast cancer. J Natl Cancer Inst 92:550–556

Dolan NC, Lee AM, McDermott MM (1997) Age related differences in breast carcinoma knowledge, beliefs and perceived risk among women visiting and academic general medicine practice. Cancer 80(3):413–420

Eaker S, Dickman PW, Bergkvist L, Holmberg L (2006) Differences in management of older women influence breast cancer survival: Results from a population-based database in Sweden. PloS Med 3(3):e25

Eddy DM (1989) Screening for breast cancer. Ann Inter Med 111(5):389–399

Erbas B, Amos A, Fletcher A, Kavanagh AM, Gertig DM (2004) Incidence of invasive breast cancer and ductal carcinoma in situ in a screening program by age: should older women continue screening. Cancer Epidemiol Biomarkers Prev 13(10):1569–1573

Faulk RM et al (1995) Clinical efficacy of mammographic screening in the elderly. Radiology 194(1):193–197

Forrest P et al (1986) Breast cancer screening. Report to health ministers of England, Wales, Scotland and Northern Ireland. HMSO, London

Gajdos C, Tartter PI, Bleiweiss IJ, Lopchinski RA, Bernstein JL (2001) The consequences of undertreating breast cancer in the elderly. J Am Coll Surg 192:698–707

Golledge J, Wiggins JE, Callam MJ (2000) Age-related variation in the treatment and outcomes of patients with breast carcinoma. Cancer 88:369–374

Gosney MA (2005) Clinical assessment of elderly people with cancer. Lancet Oncol 6(10):790–797

Gunnfeld EA, Ramirez AJ, Hunter MS, Richards MA (2002) Women's knowledge and beliefs regarding breast cancer. Br J Cancer 86:1373–1378

Hakama M, Pukkala E, Heikkila M, Kallio M (1997) Effectiveness of the public health policy for breast cancer screening in Finland: population based cohort study. Br Med J 314:864–867

Heflin MT, Oddone EZ, Pieper CF, Burchett BM, Cohen HJ (2002) The effect of co-morbid illness on receipt of cancer screening by older people. J Am Geriatr Soc 50:1651–1658

IARC (International Agency for Research on Cancer) handbook: breast cancer screening (2002) Vaino H and Bianchini F (eds) IARC Press, Lyon, pp 87–117

Jansen JThM, Zoetelief J (1997) Assessment of lifetime gained as a result of mammographic breast cancer screening using a computer model. Br J Radiol 70:619–628

Jonsson H, Johansson R, Lenner P (2005) Increased incidence of invasive breast cancer after the introduction of service screening with mammography in Sweden. Int J Cancer 117(5):842–847

Kaplan RM, Saltzstein SL (2005) Reduced mammographic screening may explain declines in breast carcinoma in older women. J Am Geriatr Soc 53:862–866

Kerlikowske K, Salzmann P, Phillips KA, Cauley JA, Cummings SR (1999) Continuing screening mammography in women aged 70 years: Impact on life expectancy and cost effectiveness. JAMA 282(22):2156–2163

Kumar ID, Reed MWR, Wyld L (2004) Breast screening in the older woman. Efficacy and awareness of availability. Eur J Surg Oncol 30(9):1012

Mah Z, Bryant H (1992) Age as a factor in breast screening knowledge, attitudes and screening behaviours. Can Med Assoc J 146(12):2167–2174

Mandelblatt JS, Wheat ME, Monane M, Moshief RD, Hollenberg JP, Tang J (1992) Breast cancer screening for elderly women with and without co-morbid conditions: A decision analysis model. Ann Intern Med 116:722–730

Mandelblatt J, Saha S, Teutsch S, Hoerger T, Siu AL, Atkins D, Klein J, Helfand M and the Cost Work Group of the US Preventative Task Force (2003) The cost effectiveness of screening mammography beyond age 65 years. A systematic review for the US preventative services task force. Ann Intern Med 139:835–842

Mandelblatt JS, Schechter CB, Yabroff R, Laurence W, Dignan J, Extermann M, Fox S, Orosz G, Silliman R, Cullen J, Balducci L as the Breast Cancer in Older Women Consortium (2005) Towards optimal screening strategies for older women. J Gen Inter Med 20:487–496

Marwill SL, Freund K, Barry PP (1996) Patient factors associated with breast cancer screening amongst older women. J Am Geriatr Soc 44(10):1210–1214

McCarthy EP, Burns RB, Freund KM, Ash AS, Shwartz M, Marwill SL, Moskowitz MA (2000) Mammography use, breast cancer stage at diagnosis and survival among older women. J Am Geriatr Soc 48:1226–1233

McCarty KS, Silva JS, Cox EB, Leight GS, Wells SA, McCarty Sr KS (1983) Relationship of age and menopausal status to oestrogen receptor content in primary carcinoma of the breast. Ann Surg 197:123–127

McPherson CP, Swenson KK, Lee MW (2002) The effect of mammographic detection and comorbidity on the survival of older women with breast cancer. J Am Geriatr Soc 50:1061–1068

Miller AB, To T, Baines CJ, Wall C (2000) Canadian National breast screening study-2: 13-year results of a randomized trial in women aged 50–59 years. J Natl Cancer Inst 92:1490–1499

NHS Breast Screening Programme (2006) Audit of breast cancer in women aged 50 to 74. April 2006. NHS Breast Screening Programme Pub No 62

Nystrom L, Andersson I, Bjurstam N, Frisell J, Nordenskjold B, Rutqvist LE (2002) Long-term effects of mammography screening: updated overview of the Swedish randomised trials. Lancet 359:909–919

Otten JD, Broeders MJ, Fracheboud J, Otto SJ, de Koning HJ, Verbeek AL (2008) Impressive time related influence of the dutch screenig programme on breast cancer incidence and mortality 1975-2006. Int J cancer 123(8):1929–1934

Page DL, Dupont WD, Rogers LW et al (1995) Cancer 76:1197–1200

Raik BL, Miller FG, Fins JJ (2004) Screening and cognitive impairment: Ethics of foregoing mammography in older women. J Am Geriatr Soc 52:440–444

Rich JS, Black WC (2000) When should we stop screening. Eff Clin Pract 3:78–84

Rosenberg RD, Hunt WC, Williamson MR, Gilliland FD, Wiest PW, Kelsey CA, Key CR, Linver MN (1998) Effects of age, breast density, ethnicity and oestrogen replacement therapy on screening mammographic sensitivity and cancer stage at diagnosis: review of 183, 134 screening mammograms in Albuquerque, New Mexico. Radiology 209:511–518

Sabel M, Aichinger U, Schultz-Wendtland R (2001) Radiation exposure in X-ray mammography. Fortschr Rontgenstr 173:79–91

Sader C, Ingram D, Hastrich D (1999) Management of breast cancer in the elderly by complete local excision and tamoxifen alone. Austr N Z J Surg 69:790–793

Satariano WA, Ragland DR (1994) The effect of co-morbidity on 3-year survival of women with primary breast cancer. Ann Inter Med 120:104–110

Schaefer G, Rosen PP, Lesser ML, Kinne DW, Beatie EJ (1984) Breast carcinoma in elderly women: pathology, prognosis and survival. Pathol Annu 19:195–218

Shapiro S, Venet W, Strax P, Venet L (1988) Current results of the breast cancer screening randomised trial. The Health Insurance Plan (HIP) of greater New York study. In: Day NE, Miller AB, Bern A (eds) Screening for breast cancer. Hans Huber, Toronto, pp 3–15

Siapush M, Singh G (2002) Sociodemographic variations in breast cancer screening behaviour among Australian women: Results from the 1995 national health survey. Prev Med 35:174–180

Siegelmann-Danielli N, Khandelwal V, Wood GC (2004) Breast cancer in elderly women: combined effect of tumor feature, age, comorbidities and treatment approach. Poster at the San Antonio breast cancer conference, p 20

Smith RA, Cokkinides V, Eyre HJ (2007) Cancer screening in the United States 2007: a review of current guidelines, practices and prospects. CA Cancer J Clin 57:90–104

Smith-Bindman R, Kerlikowske K, Gebretsadik T, Newman J (2000) Is screening mammography effective in elderly women. Am J Med 108:112–119

Spiers NA, Matthews RJ, Jagger C, Brayne C, Matthews FE, Boult C, Robinson TG and MRC-CFAS (2005) Diseases and impairments as risk factors for disability onset in the older population in England and Wales: findings from the MRC cognitive function and ageing study (MRC CFAS). J Gerontol (Med Sci) 60A:248–254

Stout NK, Rosenberg MA, Trentham-Dietz A, Smith MA, Robinson SM, Fryback DG (2006) Retrospective cost effectiveness analysis of screening mammography. J Natl Cancer Inst 98:774–782

Tabar L, Vitak B, Chen HH (2000) The Swedish two counties trial twenty years later. Updated mortality results and new insights from long-term follow-up. Radiol Clin North Am 38:625–651

Tabar L, Yen M-F, Vitak B, Chen H-HT, Smith RA, Duffy SW (2003) Mammography service screening and mortality in breast cancer patients: 20 year follow-up before and after introduction of screening. Lancet 361:1405–1410

Van Dijck J, Verbeek ALM, Beex LVAM, Hendriks JHCL, Holland R, Mravnac M, Straatman H, Were JM (1997) Breast cancer mortality in a non randomised trial on mammographic screening in women over age 65. Int J Cancer 70:164–168

Walter L, Covinski KE (2001) Cancer screening in the elderly: a framework for individualized decision making. JAMA 285(21):2750–2756

Walter LC, Eng C, Covinski KE (2001) Screening mammography in frail older women. J Gen Intern Med 16:779–784

Walter LC, Lindquist K, Covinski KE (2004) Relationship between health status and use of screening mammography and papanicolaou smears amongst women older than 70 years of age. Ann Intern Med 140:681–688

Wenger CR, Beardslee S, Owens MA, Pounds G, Oldaker T, Vendely P, Pandian MR, Harrington D, Clark GM, McGuire WL (1993) DNA ploidy, S-phase and steroid receptors in more than 127, 000 breast cancer patients. Breast Cancer Res Treat 28:9–20

Wildiers H, Kunkler I, Biganzoli L, Fracheboud J, Vlastos G, Bernard-Marty C, Hurria A, Extermann M, Girre V, Brain E, Audisio RA, Bartelink H, Barton M, Giordano SH, Muss H, Aapro M (2007) Management of breast cancer in elderly individuals: recommendations of the international society of geriatric oncology. Lancet Oncol 8:1101–1115

Wyld L, Garg DK, Brown H, Reed MWR (2004) Stage and treatment variation with age in post-menopausal women with breast cancer: compliance with guidelines. Br J Cancer 90(8):1486–1491

Wyld L, Reed MW (2007) Surgery for the older women with breast cancer. Eur J Cancer 43:2253–2263

Yancik R, Ries LG, Yates JW (1989) Breast cancer in ageing women. A population based study of contrasts in stage, surgery and survival. Cancer 63:976–981

Zackrisson S, Andersson I, Janzon L, Manjer J, Garne JP (2006) Rate of over diagnosis of breast cancer 15 years after end of Malmo mammographic screening trial: follow up study. Br Med J 332:689–690

Zahl P-H, Strand BH, Maehlen J (2004) Incidence of breast cancer in Norway and Sweden during introduction of Nationwide screening: prospective cohort study. BMJ 328:921–924

Chapter 10
Primary Endocrine Therapy for the Treatment of Early Breast Cancer in Older Women

Lynda Wyld and Daniel Hind

10.1 Introduction

The standard treatment for operable breast cancer is some form of surgery followed by a combination of adjuvant therapies, such as radiotherapy, endocrine therapy, chemotherapy, and Trastuzumab. Primary endocrine therapy (PET), by comparison, is the use of an antiestrogen as the sole method of treatment for early stage, operable, estrogen receptor (ER) positive breast cancer in women who may be less able to tolerate standard therapy.

PET is widely used in the treatment of older, frailer women in the UK. It has much to recommend it from the perspective of both the patients and their health care professional. From the patients' point of view, it may allow the complete avoidance of surgery with all its physical and psychological morbidity. From the perspective of the health care professional, it may be as effective at systemic disease control, with no significant mortality disadvantage in women over the age of 75. It may also be less costly, though a formal health economic assessment has never been undertaken to compare PET with standard surgical care. Local disease control rates, however,are inferior as some women will develop endocrine resistant disease and require surgery at a later stage.

10.2 History

Approximately 60–80% of breast cancers express the ER on their nuclear membrane (McCarty et al. 1983; Wenger et al. 1993). Stimulation of this receptor causes cellular proliferation. Antagonism inhibits cell proliferation and may cause cell death. The rate of ER positivity is related to the age of the patient (McCarty

L. Wyld (✉)
Academic Unit of Surgical Oncology, University of Sheffield, Western Bank,
Sheffield, S10 2TN, UK
e-mail: l.wyld@sheffield.ac.uk

M.W. Reed and R.A. Audisio (eds.), *Management of Breast Cancer in the Elderly*,
DOI 10.1007/978-1-84800-265-4_10, © Springer-Verlag London Limited 2011

et al. 1983; Diab et al. 2000). For example, in patients younger than 35, 26% of tumors express the ER, 74% for those over 75, and 90% at age 85 and above. (McCarty et al. 1983; Diab et al. 2000). Tamoxifen is a selective ER modulator, which acts as an ER antagonist in breast cancer cells. Aromatase inhibitors (AIs) act by reducing the peripheral conversion of androgens to estrogens (the only endogenous source of estrogen in postmenopausal women), and reduce circulating estrogen levels to almost undetectable levels. They, therefore, both act as antiestrogens and may be used for PET, though to date there has been no research into the use of AIs in PET.

The first report of the use of tamoxifen as the sole treatment for operable breast cancer in older women was by Preece and colleagues (1982) in Dundee, Scotland. Based on reports of good tamoxifen response rates in women with advanced cancer (Mouridsen et al. 1978), they used the drug in a series of 67 women over the age of 75 years. Tumors were not analyzed for ER expression. They found that 73% had either a partial or complete response. They categorized static disease (SD) as failure of treatment (9/76), as was truly progressive disease (9/67). Their results were sufficiently interesting to stimulate the conduct of a number of randomized clinical trials and cohort studies in the UK and Europe (Table 10.1).

The results of these trials demonstrated that while rates of local disease control were inferior in PET-treated women, there was no disadvantage in terms of overall survival.

The studies were all flawed by modern standards (but appropriate for standard management at the time they were undertaken). All but one of the studies did not test for the ER status of the cancer, and therefore, in this age cohort, up to 20% of women would have had ER-negative tumors. These women would, therefore, have been disadvantaged by their initial trial of PET as effective treatment would have been delayed by many months while awaiting response to PET. Hence, the rates of local disease control and potentially also overall survival would have been inferior in the PET arm of these studies.

All the randomized trials prespecified that the patients be fit for surgery under general anesthesia, and therefore, the least fit women, who are by current standards most likely to be offered PET, would have been excluded. The average age of the women in these trials was mid-70s, an age at which median life expectancy would be predicted to be over 10 years (Jagger and Matthews 2002; Sauvaget et al. 2001). Again this would tend to disadvantage women in the PET arm, as we now know that endocrine resistance develops after a median of 2–3 years, and thus, we would expect many of these fit older women to outlive the control of tamoxifen.

Longer-term follow-up of these studies to 8 and 10 years similarly found inferior rates of local control, but no survival disadvantage. However, analysis of one of the larger trials at 12 years did demonstrate a small but significant survival disadvantage in the PET arm (Fennessy et al. 2004). This could perhaps have been predicted with the information we now have about the design of these studies: the selected women who were fittest, survived for 10–15 years and outlived the efficacy of the antiestrogen. This does not suggest that PET should never be used, but merely that the criteria for selection used in these trials were inappropriate, as will be discussed below.

Table 10.1 Cohort studies and randomized clinical trials of tamoxifen primary endocrine therapy (PET)

Trial reference	Study type	# of patients	ER receptor status assessed	Stage range	Length of follow-up, months median	Rate of complete response	Rate of partial response	Rate of static disease	Rate of progressive disease	Rate of failure of local control	Age range and mean
Cohort studies											
Horobin et al. 1991	Cohort	113	No	1–3	60	38/113	17/113	34/113	24/113	62%	70–93
Bergman et al. 1995	Cohort	85	Largely unknown (59/84) plus 10 ER negative	1–3a	28 (3–97)	12/85	20/85	39/85	13/85	34/84	75–96
Gaskell et al. 1992	Cohort	66	Yes. 11 ER neg/weak +ve 33 ER mod/strong +ve	1–3	24	0/13 12/33	2/13 15/33	1/13 4/33	10/13 3/33	Not stated	>70
Akhtar et al. 1991	Cohort	100	incomplete	1–3	59	40/100	28/100	22/100	10/100	Not stated	>70
Preece et al. 1982	Cohort	67	Not assessed	1–3	36	18/67	14/67	17/67	18/67	21/67	78.3, range 67–95
Randomized Trial comparing PET with surgery alone											
Fentiman et al. 2003	RCT	82	No	Up to T3, N1	120	NS	NS	NS	NS	62%	76.3 mean
Willsher et al. 1997	RCT	94	Yes, all moderate or strongly positive. H score >100	1–2	36	28/94 (as assessed at 6 months)	41/94	23/94	3/94	32%	78
Willshire et al. 1997	RCT	66	Not assessed	1–2	120	28/66	11/66	10/66	26/66	62%	>70

(continued)

Table 10.1 (continued)

Trial reference	Study type	# of patients	ER receptor status assessed	Stage range	Length of follow-up, months median	Rate of complete response	Rate of partial response	Rate of static disease	Rate of progressive disease	Rate of failure of local control	Age range and mean
Gazet et al. 1994	RCT	116	Not assessed	T1–4	36	NS	NS	NS	NS	25%	75.4
Fennessy et al. 2004	RCT	230	Not assessed	1–3	151	NS	NS	NS	NS	53.4%	Median 76, range 70–87
Mustacchi et al. 2003	RCT	473	Not assessed	T1–3, N0–1	80	21/228	74/228	125/228	2/228	45.2%	77

10.3   Overview of the Current Use of Primary Endocrine Therapy

In the UK at present, the use of PET is widespread with 55% of women over 80 (British Association of Surgical Oncology 2003) and 40% of women over 70 (Wyld et al. 2004; Golledge et al. 2000) being treated solely with hormone therapy. The rate of nonsurgical treatment increases with increasing age (Lavelle et al. 2007aBJC). Elsewhere in Europe, PET is used less frequently and it is rarely used in the US. An audit of practice in Southern Ireland (Eire) found 26% (79/302) of women over 70 with operable breast cancer received PET (Hooper et al. 2002). A French review of 1,143 older breast cancer cases showed that only 11% did not undergo surgery (Garbay et al. 1998), a Dutch review showed only 16% of older women did not have surgery (Van Dalsen and de Vries 1995), and an Italian study found that only 3% of older women did not undergo surgery (Crivellari et al. 1991). A number of audit studies in the US have shown very low rates of nonsurgical treatments: Diab and colleagues (2000), in a massive review of the surveillance, epidemiology, and end results database (SEER), found that of 7,873 women aged 75–84, 7,838 had surgery (99.5%), and in the over 85 age group, 2,043 out of 2,057 (99.3%) had surgery.

In the UK, detailed analysis of why PET is selected for certain women has been undertaken (Wyld et al. 2004; Lavelle et al. 2007b). In 45% of cases, the women were judged to be high risk for general anesthesia due to comorbidity: in 8.5% of cases, they were offered PET on the basis of extreme old age (over 85 years); in 10.6%, they were significantly cognitively impaired; and in 36% of cases they were offered a choice of PET or surgery and chose PET (Wyld et al. 2004). Functional status and chronological age are more likely to predict the use of PET than comorbidity (Lavelle et al. 2007b). Similar figures were quoted by Hooper and colleagues (2002), with 62% offered PET based on the presence of significant comorbidity (including dementia), 14% based on age, and 11% based on patient preference.

10.4   Local Disease Control Rates with Tamoxifen PET

Local disease control with PET is inferior to that provided by surgery, with significant numbers requiring second-line therapy, with either surgery, radiotherapy, or alternate antiestrogens. Metaanalysis of randomized trials comparing surgery alone with PET (tamoxifen) demonstrates an odds ratio for the failure of local control by PET of 0.28 (CI 0.23–0.35). Trials comparing surgery plus adjuvant endocrine therapy with PET show an odds ratio of 0.54 (95% CI 0.4–0.74) (Hind et al. 2006). Despite this, there is no mortality difference and many women have excellent disease control, avoiding surgery completely, and eventually dying of comorbid disease.

Rates of local disease control vary between studies (Table 10.1). Local control can be categorized according to the best clinical response achieved (either complete response [CR], partial response [PR], static disease [SD], or progression [PD] from the outset). In general, the studies report an overall clinical benefit rate (i.e., CR plus PR plus SD) of between 74% and 84% in ER-untested tumors, rising to 91–97% in confirmed ER-positive tumors (Table 10.1). The duration of response is also variable, with SD cases progressing within a few months and some complete responders enjoying 10 years or more of disease control. Obviously, in most of the PET trials, these data have to be viewed with the knowledge that the ER status of the tumor was unknown. In addition, all of these studies used tamoxifen. Better response rates may be achieved with AIs, but here we have to extrapolate from neo-adjuvant studies to infer superiority.

10.5 The Role for Aromatase Inhibitors in PET

Neoadjuvant studies differ from PET studies as the patients are usually younger, and therefore, may have different disease biology (i.e., a higher rate of HER-2 positivity which tends to predict a poorer response to antiestrogens); they may have more locally advanced disease and the aim of neoadjuvant therapy is short-term response, not long-term disease control.

Comparison of letrozole with tamoxifen in the neo-adjuvant setting in 337 post-menopausal women demonstrated a significantly higher clinical response rate in the letrozole group (55% vs. 36%, P<0.001) at follow-up of 4 months (Eiermann et al. 2001). Of interest was the fact that letrozole was superior to tamoxifen regardless of the level of ER positivity, even inducing response in only weakly ER-positive tumors, where tamoxifen was ineffective.

Another neo-adjuvant letrozole study found that letrozole was effective in reducing the size of large primary cancers considered unsuitable for breast conserving surgery. The study also found that while in most women the best response had been achieved by 4 months of therapy, further benefit was seen at up to 8 months on letrozole, which was the maximum period of neoadjuvant therapy (Krainick-Strobel et al. 2008). They found a 62% reduction in tumor volume at 4 months and 70% at 8 months. This is the only study to look at longer-term response rates in the neoadjuvant setting.

Similarly, anastrozole is superior to tamoxifen in the neoadjuvant setting and has been studied in two trials: IMPACT and PROACT. In the IMPACT study (IMmediate Pre-operative Arimidex, Tamoxifen or Combined with Tamoxifen), 330 women with a median age of over 70 found a significantly higher rate of breast conservability with anastrozole compared to tamoxifen when used for only 3 months prior to surgery (46% vs. 22%), though the actual clinical response rates were not statistically significantly different (Smith et al. 2005).

In the PROACT (PRe-Operative Arimidex Compared to Tamoxifen) study comparing anastrozole and tamoxifen in women with large operable or potentially operable breast cancer, 12 weeks of preoperative neoadjuvant endocrine treatment demonstrated superior efficacy for anastrozole in terms of increased rates of breast conservation versus tamoxifen (43 vs. 31%), and numerically superior clinical and ultrasound response rates (36 vs. 26% ultrasound response rates, though this failed to reach statistical significance, P<0.07) (Cataliotti et al. 2006).

Exemestane has also been used in the neoadjuvant setting and has a similar efficacy rate to anastrozole (Semiglazov et al. 2007; Mlineritsch et al. 2008).

There are no long-term neo-adjuvant data or PET data on the use of AIs at present. While it is likely that AIs will give better outcomes from PET than tamoxifen in terms of breast cancer control rates based on extrapolation of the above neoadjuvant data and a generally improved side effect profile, uncertainty about the use of these agents in frailer older women remains. This relates to the known adverse effect of AIs on bone mineral density, which tends to reduce by 1–2% per year (Eastell et al. 2008). As the baseline rate of osteoporosis is high in women over 70, this may result in an increased risk of fractures, which may nullify any overall benefit. Recently issued guidelines have recommended bone density monitoring for older women on AIs and prophylactic use of calcium, vitamin D, and bisphosphonates in high-risk women (Reid et al. 2008). This strategy may offset any increased fracture risk in younger women on AIs (Bundred et al. 2008), but direct trial data in this older age group is urgently needed.

10.6   Clinical Response Prediction

Clinical factors which predict a good quality and long duration of response include a small initial tumor size and a good initial clinical response. Women with SD at their 3–6 month assessment are less likely to have good long-term disease control than women with a complete or partial response. There is a correlation between early-stage disease and good response, with one study reporting a 100% clinical benefit rate for stage 1 disease, 83% for stage 2 disease, and 66% for stage 3 disease (Horobin et al. 1991). Other studies have shown similar findings, with only a 53% response rate in T4 tumors compared to an 80–86 % response in T2 and T3 disease (Akhtar et al. 1991). In addition, the type of initial response predicts response duration, with initial CR being associated with a 50-month response duration, PR 18 months, and SD 21 months (Horobin et al. 1991).

The time taken to reach a best response is quite variable, ranging from 3 to 37 months, with a median of 9 months (Horobin et al. 1991). In fact, for women who have an initial complete response, up to 90–100% will still be controlled at 5 years in some studies (Horobin et al. 1991; Bergman et al. 1995). Others studies have shown less favorable results, with only 42% of complete responders in remission at 47 months, but the range of response duration was from 5–96 months in this study, which included a high proportion (47%) of T4 tumors (Akhtar et al. 1991).

Most studies of the long-term rate of local control report that local disease progression, requiring a change of management, occurs in between 32 and 62% of women. The longest reported follow-up trial (Fennessy et al. 2004), with follow-up of over 12 years, found a failure of local control rate of 53.4%, with the median time for failure to occur being at 1.69 years (range 1.43–1.82 years). This was substantially worse than women in the surgical arm of the trial, where local failure occurred in only 15.6% of women. Most of these local failures were treated with surgery (64%), with 29% having a change of hormonal therapy or radiotherapy (19%). As with most of the studies of PET, these data have to be viewed in the knowledge that they do not mirror current PET practice, as approximately 20% of all patients would have had ER-negative cancers, and would have, thus, inevitably progressed on PET and effectively had a delay in stating any effective therapy for a significant period. Moreover, in view of the knowledge accrued from these studies, most clinicians would reserve PET for older and frailer women (unlike most of the trials which recruited women over 70 who were fit for general anesthesia).

One of the risks of PET is loss of local control due to deteriorating patient fitness for surgery with advancing age and worsening health status. One study of PET found that of the 43% of patients who required a change of management, 59% were unfit for surgery at progression and required alternate endocrine therapies or radiotherapy (Bergman et al. 1995).

10.7   Molecular Response Prediction

There have been significant advances in our understanding of the biology of breast cancer, and in particular, of the complex interplay of estrogen responsive pathways and other cellular regulatory pathways. The molecular features of a tumor that predict a good response to endocrine therapy are now better understood and there have been new insights into the development of endocrine resistance.

In practical terms, clinical management is currently based largely on the level of ER expression. Prediction may be refined further by knowledge of progesterone receptor (PgR) expression and Her-2 expression as these are now routinely measured in most units in the UK. Both of these latter receptors may aid in prediction of both the likelihood of antiestrogen response and which antiestrogen (tamoxifen or an AI) may be more likely to be effective. In future, as technology advances, response prediction may be further refined by a panel of other molecular markers and even gene expression array. These markers will now be briefly summarized.

10.7.1   The Estrogen Receptor

The best predictor of response remains the ER status of the tumor. Tumors which are ER negative will almost all progress from the outset, weakly positive tumors will usually show partial response, stasis, or initial progression, whereas moderately or strongly positive tumors will have a 90% clinical benefit rate (CR, PR, or stasis) (Gaskell et al. 1992). The presence of the ER usually indicates a 70–90% rate of antiestrogen response.

Conversely, therefore, up to 30% of ER+ve tumors display primary or de-novo resistance and of those tumors that do respond to antiestrogens initially, most will eventually develop resistance after a variable period of time: the so-called secondary or acquired resistance. Use of additional markers may help in the identification of these resistant tumors.

The ER is now known to exist as two forms, ERα [alpha] (or classical ER) and ERβ [beta]. Both are transcription factors regulating the expression of estrogen target genes in the nucleus. ERα [alpha] is the receptor commonly measured in clinical practice. It is thought that phosphorylation of ERα [alpha] at serine 118 may predict a better disease outcome (Murphy et al. 2004), though this is not routinely tested for in clinical practice.

The clinical value of the second form of ER, ERβ [beta], is unclear and there are conflicting data concerning its potential role as a predictive factor. ERβ [beta] may be an independent predictor of response to tamoxifen (Hopp et al. 2004) and may also be up-regulated in tamoxifen resistant tumors, (Speirs et al. 1999).

10.7.2   The Progesterone Receptor

The progesterone receptor (PgR) has been recognized for many years as an indicator of response to endocrine therapy since PgR induction requires the ER to be functional, (Anderson 2002; Clark et al. 1983; Gelbfish et al. 1988). However, there is now emerging data that ER+ve, PgR+ve cancers are more likely to respond to both tamoxifen and AIs, whereas for ER+ve, PgR-ve cancers, AIs are more effective (Ellis et al. 2001). This may enable better selection of antiestrogen for PET.

10.7.3   The Epidermal Growth Factor Receptor Family

10.7.3.1   EGFR-1

Cancers overexpressing epidermal growth factor receptor (EGFR)-1 are usually ER-ve. Cancers that are ER+ve and overexpress both EGFR and HER-2 are highly sensitive to the effects of letrozole, with 88% response rates compared with 54%

for ER+ve EGFR−ve, HER-2−ve and 21% response rates to tamoxifen (Ellis et al. 2003; Ellis and Ma 2007). Unfortunately, EGFR-1 is not routinely measured by UK Breast Units at present.

10.7.3.2 EGFR-2 (HER-2)

As with its family member EGFR-1, HER-2 overexpressing cancers are more likely to be ER−ve, with only 14–18% being ER+ve (Konecny et al. 2003). Most, but not all, studies indicate that HER-2 overexpression predicts for some degree of endocrine resistance (Houston et al. 1999; Ring and Dowsett 2003), but with letrozole being more effective than tamoxifen in inducing regression in ER+ve, HER-2+ve cancers (Ellis et al. 2001). Her-2 status is now routinely tested in UK Breast Units which may enable improved selection of antiestrogen for PET.

10.7.3.3 Cell cycle regulatory proteins

ERK-1 and 2 play a central role in cell proliferation. Breast cancers with a low level of ERK1 and 2 respond well to endocrine agents, while those with high levels exhibit de novo resistance. These associations are present within ER+ve cancers (Gee et al. 2001).

The stress activated MAP kinase p38 pathway acts in an opposite manner to ERK1 and 2, inducing apoptosis and negatively regulating growth through its action on cyclin D1. Significant expression of activated p38 confers an advantage on endocrine response (Gee et al. 2000). Most data relate to tamoxifen rather than AIs.

Expression of cyclin D1 is directly correlated with that of the ER and is thought to be an estrogen-regulated gene (Hui et al. 1996). Overexpression of cyclin D1 confers a poor response to endocrine therapy specifically in ER+ve breast cancer (Kenny et al. 2001).

None of these cell cycle regulatory proteins are routinely tested in clinical practice so are of limited usefulness at present.

10.7.3.4 Ki67/MIB1

Changes in the level of Ki67, a marker of cell proliferation, may give a good early indication of endocrine responsiveness. In neoadjuvant AI studies, an early reduction in proliferation occurs to a greater extent with AIs than with tamoxifen (Dixon et al. 2004) and may predict improved treatment outcomes (Dowsett et al. 2007). In a previous tamoxifen PET study in elderly patients, greater reduction in MIB1 in a tumor biopsy after 6 weeks of therapy correlated with a longer duration of response (Kenny et al. 2001). Undertaking a biopsy shortly after PET has commenced is one potential strategy for improved response prediction, but in a cohort of frail older women might be seen as overly invasive by some.

10.7.3.5   Bcl-2

Increased expression of the antiapoptotic protein, bcl-2 is associated with hormone-responsiveness, (Gee et al. 1994; Hellemans et al. 1995; Kobayashi et al. 1997). Bcl-2 protein is down-regulated during treatment with tamoxifen. A greater extent of down-regulation of bcl-2 is associated with improved quality and longer duration of response (Kenny et al. 1999).

10.7.3.6   P13K/AKT

AKT is a serine/threonine kinase which is up-regulated in a number of human cancers including some breast cancers. It may protect breast cancer cells from tamoxifen-induced apoptosis (Faridi et al. 2003). There is increasing evidence that activation of this enzyme is important in the development of tamoxifen resistance (deGraffenried et al. 2004; Jordan et al. 2004).

10.7.3.7   P53 mutation

Breast cancers that are ER+ve and p53+ve have a higher rate of nonresponse or relapse on endocrine therapy, suggesting that p53 mutation could be a useful marker for resistance (Martin et al. 2006).

10.7.4   Gene Expression Profiling

Gene expression profiling permits the simultaneous study of messenger RNA expression from thousands of genes from human tumors and whether they are up or down-regulated. Gene expression profiling is being used for breast cancer characterization and prediction of outcome, (Paik et al. 2004van 't Veer LJ et al. 2002; van de Vijver et al. 2002). There is evidence that different gene expression profiles may predict response to antiestrogens.

For example, after 2 weeks of neoadjuvant treatment of ER+ve breast cancers with letrozole, marked changes in gene expression were observed compared to baseline samples (Miller et al. 2008).

Such studies are starting to identify estrogen dependent genes and how these interact with genes involved in cellular proliferation, but at present there is still no easily identifiable signature for endocrine resistance as there appears to be a high level of heterogeneity in gene expression in endocrine resistance suggesting a number of different mechanisms. There are emerging 'gene signatures' that may be accurate in predicting disease recurrence after adjuvant endocrine therapy, with similar levels of accuracy as the Nottingham Prognostic Index or Adjuvant! Online, but these do not specifically relate purely to endocrine resistance and reflect disease aggression and metastatic potential (Chanrion et al. 2008; Dobbe et al. 2008)

There is some early work on differences in gene expression between patients with AI resistant and sensitive tumors in terms of gene expression profiling. One group studied anastrozole-treated tumors which either progressed or responded and identified 298 genes whose expression patterns differed significantly between groups, (Kristensen et al. 2005). It was possible to differentiate ER+ve and ER-ve tumors using this technology. However, the small sample size prevented the study determining which gene profiles were specific for responders and nonresponders and the authors suggested that a larger study would be needed. In addition, the real interest would be to determine which subgroup of ER positive tumors is likely to be nonresponsive or to progress early.

10.8   Mortality Rates with Pet

Metaanalysis of the PET versus surgery trials has demonstrated that there is no significant difference between women treated with PET and women treated with surgery and adjuvant endocrine therapy (Hind et al. 2007). There have been six randomized trials of PET versus either surgery alone or surgery plus adjuvant tamoxifen (Table 10.1). The mortality in the two treatment arms does not differ significantly (Fig. 10.1) (Hind et al. 2007). There is a trend in favor of surgery and adjuvant tamoxifen. Of all the trials, only one reported a significant survival advantage to surgery (Fennessy et al. 2004). This study reported overall survival rates at 5 years of 67% in the surgery arm vs. 59.5% in the PET arm. Similarly at 10 years follow-up, rates were 37.7 vs. 28.8%, respectively. These differences were statistically significant. However, the trial recruited women with ER-unknown tumors, and in the age group of the study, approximately 20% of the women would have had ER-negative cancers. In the surgery arm, these ER-negative cases would have had immediate tumor removal, whereas in the PET arm no effective antitumor therapy would have been given for many months, which would have skewed the mortality in favor of the surgery arm significantly. If metaanalysis of the 2 PET versus surgery plus adjuvant endocrine therapy is undertaken including only women over age 75, there is no survival difference between the 2 groups (Mustacchi et al. 1998).

10.9   Quality-of-Life and Patient Preference

There has been a considerable amount of research on quality-of-life (QoL) in breast cancer patients, but very little has specifically focused on the comparative outcomes of surgery or PET in older patients. In fact, there has only been one such study (Bates et al. 1991; Fallowfield et al. 1994). This study was performed as part

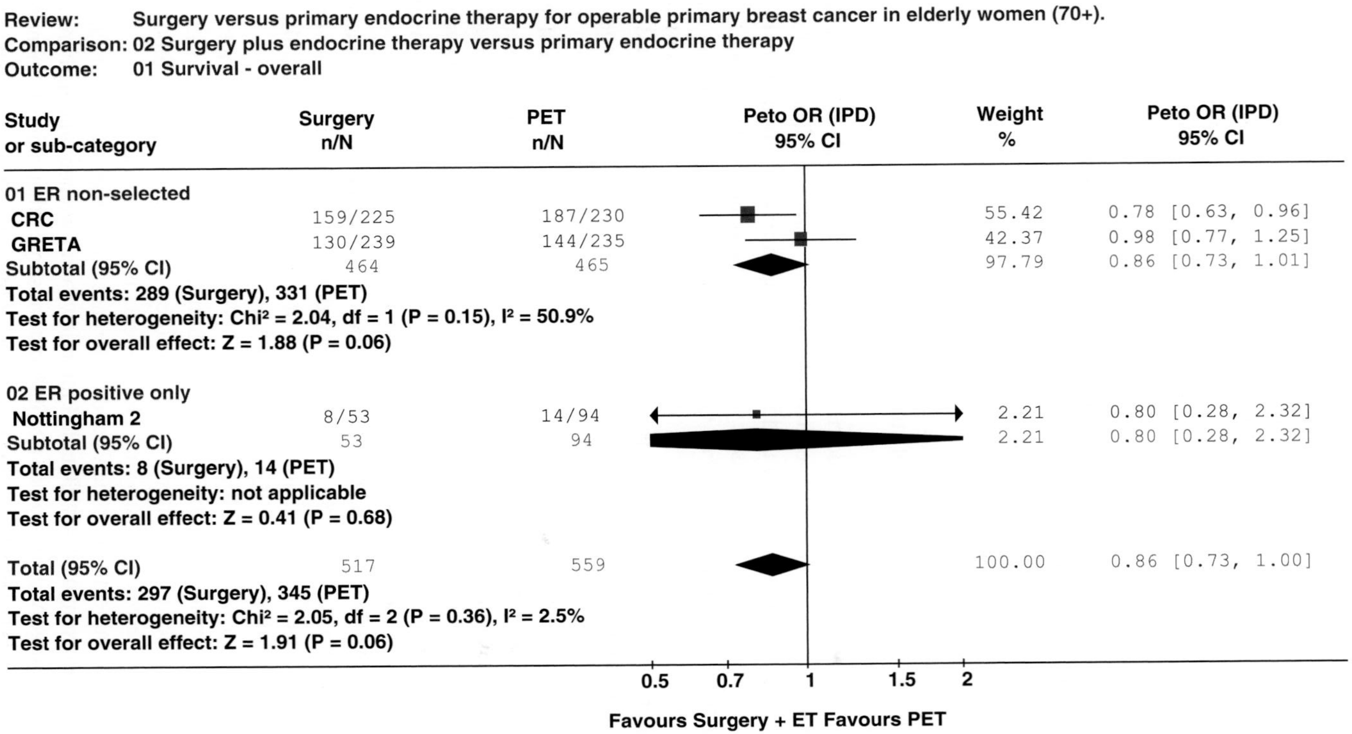

Review: Surgery versus primary endocrine therapy for operable primary breast cancer in elderly women (70+).
Comparison: 02 Surgery plus endocrine therapy versus primary endocrine therapy
Outcome: 01 Survival - overall

Fig. 10.1 Metaanalysis of randomized trials of primary endocrine therapy vs. surgery plus adjuvant tamoxifen. Reproduced with permission (Hind et al. 2006)

of the CRC Trial (Fennessy et al. 2004), using the General Health Questionnaire-28 (GHQ-28) and assessing patients at two time points: at 3 months and at 2 years after surgery or PET commencement. While finding that women in the surgical arm had worse QoL scores at the 3-month assessment, this difference had disappeared by 2 years. This study, however, did not perform long-term follow-up, and therefore, nothing is known about the effect of late treatment failures or the need to change therapy in the two treatment arms. In addition, the main study found a late (12 year FU) small but significant difference in overall survival with surgery being superior, but no QoL data were collected at this time. Therefore, late effects due to adverse disease outcomes may have had an impact on long-term QoL. It is also worth bearing in mind that the GHQ-28 is a generic measure of QoL and may not have been as sensitive for cancer effects and treatment side effects as a breast cancer specific instrument (for example, the EORTC QLQ-30 plus BR23 or the FACT B). Such a specific study has never been performed in this context. One would expect that breast cancer surgery would have a detrimental effect on QoL as has been shown in a number of studies where breast cancer specific instruments have been used.

Breast cancer surgery has a detrimental effect on QoL, with adverse effects at 1 month postoperatively (fatigue, loss of function, and pain). These effects may persist for a long time, with up to 45% still complaining of fatigue and 15% still struggling with household chores at 12 months (Shimozuma et al. 1999).

The type of surgery influences QoL. The most significant factor is whether an axillary lymph node dissection (ALND) is performed. This results in significant short- and long-term side effects with a detrimental effect on QoL. Up to 38% of women still experience problems at 5 year follow-up (Engel et al. 2003), including neuropathic pain, lymphedema, and arm movement restrictions. These effects are less severe in patients undergoing limited axillary surgery, such as axillary sampling or sentinel node biopsy (Mansell et al. 2006; Fleissig et al. 2006).

Similarly, women undergoing mastectomy have a worse QoL than those treated with breast conservation surgery (BCS), due in part to improved body image and cosmesis (Curran et al. 1998; Caffo et al. 2003).

Overall, chronic wound pain may affect 75% of women following breast cancer surgery, regardless of type (50% mild, 25% moderate), which may impact on QoL. In 35% of breast cancer patients, the pain is of neuropathic origin, and therefore, relatively difficult to control (Grond et al. 1996).

In contrast for women on PET, there may be additional concerns about treatment failure or recurrence due to the sometimes continued presence of the palpable lump: fear of cancer recurrence affects quality-of-life (Kuehn et al. 2000), though how this compares between surgery and PET patients is not known.

In terms of patient's own views and preferences for either surgery or PET, only one study has examined this. Detailed interviews with women who had previously had PET or surgery in this older age group have shown that older women tolerate both therapies very well (Hussain et al. 2008). Women on PET are unconcerned by the persistence of a palpable lump in the breast. In fact, the reverse is true and most are reassured that they can feel the lump themselves and know that the endocrine therapy is still working. Older women find PET a simple and attractive option, despite awareness that the treatment may not control their disease indefinitely. They are concerned that there be as little disruption to their normal daily life as possible. Surgery mandates a hospital visit which many older women have anxieties about. Surgery for some older women will take the form of a mastectomy, and for most, the loss of a breast is a source of great distress. Many older women are concerned about the risks of surgery and anesthesia. Of those women who do have surgery, however, most find the experience tolerable. Overall, the overwhelming perception of these ladies was that they were happy to accept the treatment advised for them by their doctor, which reflected the passive decision-making style of many older women, which has been confirmed by others working in this area of study (Petrisek et al. 1997; Degner et al. 1997; Maly et al. 2004).

10.10   Patient Selection Criteria

At present, there is no direct evidence base to help in the selection of women for PET or those that will do best with surgery. Indirect evidence suggests that we should be offering PET for women with a likely median survival, based on age and comorbidity of 3 years, the median duration of response of PET.

There are two issues to consider:

- Is the patient fit for surgery under gerneral, regional, or local anesthesia?
- Does the patient need surgery or will PET suffice?

This article will not discuss the many methods available for deciding about the risks of anesthesia and surgery (such as the ASA and POSSUM scores). In terms of whether surgery is needed at all in someone who is potentially able to withstand it, is that of life expectancy and whether PET is likely to control their breast cancer for the remainder of it.

The science of prediction of life expectancy has been progressing in recent years and we now have well-validated geriatric scoring systems, which enable prediction of likely life expectancy. There is an interaction of factors, however, and such assessment can be complex with age interacting with comorbidity, functional status, cognitive function, and the breast cancer itself.

A number of authors have tried to look at using these factors in women with breast cancer to predict outcomes. Perhaps the most well known is the Charlson Index (Charlson et al. 1987), a weighted index of the number and severity of a panel of comorbid diseases which may then be used to predict mortality. The method was validated in a cohort of women with breast cancer and is fairly simple and reliable, though limited in the range of diseases it takes into account.

Another similar system was proposed by Satariano and Ragland (1994), which again used a limited number of key comorbidities to devise a simple scoring system to predict life expectancy.

Such systems have become more complex and now more detailed geriatric assessment systems are available, which cover not only a broader range of comorbidities, but also functional status and cognitive function. While these systems are more accurate, they are perhaps unwieldy, and therefore, less likely to be used in daily clinical practice. The reality of current UK practice is that most surgeons use no formal system at all (Audisio et al. 2004).

With simplicity in mind, an elegant piece of work was done by Siegelmann-Danielli who looked at cohorts of women aged 70 or 80 with varying numbers of comorbid diseases, in addition to breast cancer (type is not specified). As can be seen from Fig. 10.2, a woman of 70 with no comorbidity will have an average life expectancy of 16 years, whereas one with four comorbid diseases will have a life expectancy of 2–3 years. Clearly, the second lady would be a candidate for PET.

The scientific community is also increasingly using web-based technology. Many are familiar with the Adjuvant! On-Line web site <http://www.adjuvantonline.com/online.jsp> (Ravdin et al. 2001) for calculating the benefits of different adjuvant therapies for women with varying stages and grades of cancer. This program presumes that surgery has already been performed, and therefore, has no facility to predict whether surgery would be of benefit, but it does have age and comorbidity adjustment functions which can display life expectancy and death rate from breast and nonbreast cancer causes. Thus, it may help in estimating life expectancy, and therefore, whether PET may be appropriate. Another web-based program enables the interaction of breast cancer stage, grade, and age, but does not factor in comorbidity <http://cancer.lifemath.net/>. Clearly, there is an opening for a more detailed tool where age, comorbidity, and breast cancer factors can be taken into account to decide about optimal treatment in older women.

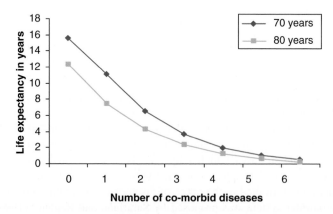

Fig. 10.2 The effect of age and number of comorbidities on life expectancy of women with breast cancer (Modified from Siegelmann-Danielli et al. 2004)

10.11   Summary

Primary hormone therapy for women with primary, operable breast cancer should be reserved for women with moderately or strongly ER positive tumors and who have a predicted life expectancy of less than 5 years (i.e., women of over 85 or those over 75 with significant comorbid disease). Close monitoring during the first year of therapy should aim to identify those who have a complete or PR who may be predicted to have a long duration of local disease control. For those with disease stasis or progressive disease, early consideration should be given to surgery, either under local or general anesthesia as these tumors are unlikely to have a long duration of disease control. For frailer women or those who refuse surgery on progression, second line endocrine therapy may be offered (switching between tamoxifen and an AI).

For ER+ve, PgR+ve, and Her-2 negative tumors, tamoxifen may be an appropriate first choice as this avoids the need for bone density monitoring and osteoporosis prophylaxis. In women with weakly ER positive or PgR negative or Her-2 positive tumors, there are theoretical advantages of using upfront AIs, but bone density will need to be monitored and treated. The strongest evidence of efficacy relative to tamoxifen is from letrozole, but all AIs have been demonstrated to be effective in the short-term neoadjuvant setting.

References

Akhtar SS, Allen SG, Rodger A, Chetty UDI, Smythe JF, Leonnard RCF (1991) A ten year experience of tamoxifen as primary treatment of breast cancer in 100 elderly and frail patients. Eur J Surg Oncol 17:30–35

Anderson E (2002) The role of estrogen and progesterone receptors in human mammary development and tumorigenesis. Breast Cancer Res 4:197–201

Audisio RA, Osman N, Audisio MM, Montalto F (2004) How do we manage breast cancer in the elderly patients? A survey among members of the British Association of Surgical Oncologists (BASO). Crit Rev Oncol/Haematol 52:135–141

Bates T, Riley DL, Houghton J, Fallowfield L, Baum M (1991) Breast cancer in elderly women: A cancer research campaign trial comparing treatment with tamoxifen and optimal surgery with tamoxifen alone> The elderly breast cancer working party. Bri J Surg 78(5):591–594

Bergman L, van Dongen JA, van Ooijen B, van Leeuwen FE (1995) Should tamoxifen be a primary treatment choice for elderly breast cancer patients with loco-regional disease. Breast Cancer Res Treat 34:77–83

British Association of Surgical Oncology (2003) Monypenny I. UK Symptomatic breast audit 1.4.2001–31.3.2002

Bundred NJ, Campbell ID, Davidson N, DeBoer RH, Eidtmann H, Monnier A, Neven P, von Minckwitz G, Miller JC, Schenk NL, Coleman RE (2008) Cancer 112(5):1001–1010

Caffo O, Amichetti M, Ferro A, Lucenti A, Valduga F, Galligioni E (2003) Pain and quality of life after breast cancer. Breast Cancer Res Treat 80(1):39–48

Cataliotti L, Buzdar AU, Noguchi S, Bines J, Takatsuka Y, Petrakova K, Dube P, Oliveira CTD (2006) Comparison of anastrozole versus tamoxifen as pre-operative therapy in postmenopausal women with hormone receptor-positive breast cancer. Cancer 106:2095–2103

Chanrion M, Negre V, Fontaine H, Salvetat N, Bibeau F, Mac Grogan G, Mauriac L, Katsaros D, Molina F, Theillet C, Darbon JM (2008) A gene expression signature that can predict the recurrence of tamoxifen treated primary breast cancer. Clin Cancer Res 14(6):1744–1752

Charlson ME, Pompei P, Ales KL, McKenzie CR (1987) A new method of classifying prognostic comorbidity in longitudinal studies: development and validation. J Chronic Dis 40(5): 373–383

Clark GM, McGuire WL, Hubay CA, Pearson OH, Carter AC (1983) The importance of estrogen and progesterone receptor in primary breast cancer. Prog Clin Biol Res 132E:183–190

Curran D, van Dongen JP, Aaronson NK, Kiebert G, Fentiman IS, Mignolet F, Bartelink H (1998) Quality of life of early stage breast cancer patients treated with radical mastectomy or breast conserving procedures: results of the EORTC Trial 10801. The European Organisation for Research and Treatment of Cancer (EORTC), Breast Cancer Co-operative Group (BCCG). Eur J cancer 34(3):307–313

Degner LF, Kristjanson LJ, Bowman D, Sloan JA, Carriere KC, O'Neil J, Bilodeau B, Watson P, Mueller B (1997) Information needs and decisional preferences in women with breast cancer. JAMA 277(18):1485–1492

deGraffenried LA, Friedrichs WE, Russell DH, Donzis EJ, Middleton AK, Silva JM, Roth RA, Hidalgo M (2004) Inhibition of mTOR activity restores tamoxifen response in breast cancer cells with aberrant Akt Activity. Clin Cancer Res 10:8059–8067

Diab SG, Elledge RM, Clarke GM (2000) Tumor characteristics and clinical outcome of elderly women with breast cancer. J Natl Cancer Inst 92:550–556

Dixon JM, Jackson J, Hills M, Renshaw L, Cameron DA, Anderson TJ, Miller WR, Dowsett M (2004) Anastrozole demonstrates clinical and biological effectiveness in estrogen receptor positive breast cancer, irrespective of the erbB2 status. Eur J Cancer 40:2742–2747

Dobbe E, Gurney K, Kiekow S, Lafferty JS, Kolesar JM (2008) Gene expression assays: new tools to individualise treatment of early stage breast cancer. Am J Health Syst Pharm 65(1):23–28

Dowsett M, Smith IE, Ebbs SR, Dixon JM, Skene A, A'Hern R, Salter J, Detre S, Hills M, Walsh G (2007) Prognostic value of Ki67 expression after short term pre-surgical endocrine therapy for primary breast cancer. J Natl Cancer Inst 99:167–170

Eastell R, Adams JE, Coleman RE, Howell A, Hannon RA, Cuzick J, Mackey JR, Beckmann MW, Clack G (2008) Effect of anastrozole on bone mineral density: 5-year results from the anastrozole, tamoxifen, alone or in combination trial 18233230. J Clin Oncol 26(7):1051–1057

Eiermann W, Paepke S, Appfelstaedt J, Llombart-Cussac A, Eremin J, Vinholes J, Mauriac L, Ellis M, Lassus M, Chaudri-Ross HA, Dugan M, Borgs M (2001) Preoperative treatment of postmenopausal breast cancer patients with letrozole: A randomized double-blind multicenter study. Ann Oncol 12:1527–1532

Ellis MJ, Ma C (2007) Letrozole in the neoadjuvant setting: the P024 trial. Breast Cancer Res Treat 105:33–43

Ellis MJ, Coop A, Singh B, Mauriac L, Llombert-Cussac A, Janicke F, Miller WR, Evans DB, Dugan M, Brady C, Quebe-Fehling E, Borgs M (2001) Letrozole is more effective neoadjuvant endocrine therapy than tamoxifen for ErbB-1- and/or ErbB-2-positive, estrogen receptor-positive primary breast cancer: evidence from a phase III randomized trial. J Clin Oncol 19:3808–3816

Ellis MJ, Rosen E, Dressman H, Marks J (2003) Neoadjuvant comparisons of aromatase inhibitors and tamoxifen: pre-treatment determinants of response and on-treatment effects. J steroid biochem mol biol 86:301–307

Engel J, Kerr J, Schlesinger-Raab A, Sauer H, Holzel D (2003) Quality of life following breast conserving therapy or mastectomy: Results of a 5 year prospective study. Breast J 10(3):223–231

Fallowfield LJ, Hall A, Maguire P, Baum M, A'Herne RP (1994) Psycological effect of being offered choice of surgery for breast cancer. Bri Med J 309:448

Faridi J, Wang L, Endemann G, Roth RA (2003) Expression of constitutively active Akt-3 in MCF-7 breast cancer cells reverses the estrogen and tamoxifen responsivity of these cells in vivo. Clin Cancer Res 9:2933–2939

Fennessy M, Bates T, MacRae K, Riley D, Houghton J, Baum M (2004) Late follow up of a randomized trial of surgery plus tamoxifen versus tamoxifen alone in women aged over 70 years with operable breast cancer. Bri J Surg 91(6):699–704

Fentiman IS, Christiaens M-R, Paridaens R et al (2003) Treatment of operable breast cancer in the elderly: a randomized clinical trial EORTC 10851 comparing tamoxifen alone with modified radical mastectomy. Eur J Cancer 39:309–316

Fleissig A, Fallowfield LJ, Langridge CI et al (2006) Post operative arm morbidity and quality of life. Results of the ALMANAC randomized trial comparing sentinel node biopsy with standard axillary treatment in the management of patients with early breast cancer. Breast Cancer Res Treat 95(3)):279–293

Ganz PA, Lee JJ, Sim M-S, Polinsky ML, Schag AC (1992) Exploring the influence of multiple variables on the relationship of age to quality of life in women with breast cancer. J Clin Epidemiol 45:473–485

Garbay JR, Bertheault-Cvitkovic F, Cohen Solal Le Nir C, Stevens D, Cherel P, Berlie J, Rouesse J (1998) Treatment of breast cancer after 70 years of age. Report of 1143 cases. Chirurgie 123(4):379–385

Gaskell DJ, Hawkins RA, de Carteret S, Chetty U, Sangster K, Forrest APM (1992) Indication for primary tamoxifen therapy in elderly women with breast cancer. Bri J Surg 79:1317–1320

Gazet JC, Ford HT, Coombes RC, Bland JM, Sutcliffe R, Quilliam J, Lowndes S (1994) Prospective randomized trial of tamoxifen vs surgery in elderly patients with breast cancer. Eur J Surg Oncol 20:207–214

Gee JM, Robertson JF, Ellis IO, Willsher P, McClelland RA, Hoyle HB, Kyme SR, Finlay P, Blamey RW, Nicholson RI (1994) Immunocytochemical localization of BCL-2 protein in human breast cancers and its relationship to a series of prognostic markers and response to endocrine therapy. Int J Cancer 59:619–628

Gee JM, Robertson JF, Ellis IO, Nicholson RI (2000) Impact of activation of MAP kinase family members on endocrine response and survival in clinical breast cancer. Eur J Cancer 36(4):105

Gee JM, Robertson JF, Ellis IO, Nicholson RI (2001) Phosphorylation of ERK1/2 mitogen-activated protein kinase is associated with poor response to anti-hormonal therapy and decreased patient survival in clinical breast cancer. Int J Cancer 95:247–254

Gelbfish GA, Davidson AL, Kopel S, Schreibman B, Gelbfish JS, Degenshein GA, Herz BL, Cunningham JN (1988) Relationship of estrogen and progesterone receptors to prognosis in breast cancer. Ann Surg 207:75–79

Golledge J, Wiggins JE, Callam MJ (2000) Age-related variation in the treatment and outcomes of patients with breast carcinoma. Cancer 88(2):369–374

Grond S, Zech D, Diefenbach C, Radbruch L, Lehmann KA (1996) Assessment of cancer pain: a prospective evaluation in 2266 cancer patients referred to a pain service. Pain 64(1):107–114

Hellemans P, van Dam PA, Weyler J, van Oosterom AT, Buytaert P, Van Marck E (1995) Prognostic value of bcl-2 expression in invasive breast cancer. Br J Cancer 72:354–360

Hind D, Wyld L, Reed MW, Beverley CB (2006) Surgery versus primary endocrine therapy for operable primary breast cancer in elderly women (70+). The Cochrane Library, Issue 1. John Wiley, Chichester, UK

Hooper SB, Hill ADK, Kennedy S, Dijkstra B, Kelly LM, McDermott EWM, O'Higgins N (2002) Tamoxifen as the primary treatment in elderly patients with breast cancer. Irish J Med Sci 171(1):28–30

Hopp TA, Weiss HL, Parra IS, Cui Y, Osborne CK, Fuqua SA (2004) Low levels of estrogen receptor beta protein predict resistance to tamoxifen therapy in breast cancer. Clin Cancer Res 10:7490–7499

Horobin JM, Preece PE, Dewar JA, Wood RAB, Cushieri A (1991) Long term follow-up of elderly patients with loco-regional breast cancer treated with tamoxifen only. Bri J Surg 78:213–217

Houston SJ, Plunkett TA, Barnes DM, Smith P, Rubens RD, Miles DW (1999) Overexpression of c-erbB2 is an independent marker of resistance to endocrine therapy in advanced breast cancer. Br J Cancer 79:1220–1226

Hui R, Cornish AL, McClelland RA, Robertson JF, Blamey RW, Musgrove EA, Nicholson RI, Sutherland RL (1996) Cyclin D1 and estrogen receptor messenger RNA levels are positively correlated in primary breast cancer. Clin Cancer Res 2:923–928

Husain LS, Collins K, Reed M, Wyld L (2008) Choices in cancer treatment: a qualitative study of the older woman's (over 70) perspective. Psycho-oncology 17(4):410–416

Jagger C, Matthews F (2002) Gender differences in life expectancy free of impairment at older ages. J women ageing 14(1–2):85–97

Jordan NJ, Gee JM, Barrow D, Wakeling AE, Nicholson RI (2004) Increased constitutive activity of PKB/Akt in tamoxifen resistant breast cancer MCF-7 cells. Breast Cancer Res Treat 87:167–180

Kenny FS, Hui R, Musgrove EA, Gee JM, Blamey RW, Nicholson RI, Sutherland RL, Robertson JF (1999) Overexpression of cyclin D1 messenger RNA predicts for poor prognosis in estrogen receptor-positive breast cancer. Clin Cancer Res 5:2069–2076

Kenny FS, Willsher PC, Gee JM, Nicholson R, Pinder SE, Ellis IO, Robertson JF (2001) Change in expression of ER, bcl-2 and MIB1 on primary tamoxifen and relation to response in ER positive breast cancer. Breast Cancer Res Treat 65:135–144

Kobayashi S, Iwase H, Ito Y, Yamashita H, Iwata H, Yamashita T, Ito K, Toyama T, Nakamura T, Masaoka A (1997) Clinical significance of bcl-2 gene expression in human breast cancer tissues. Breast Cancer Res Treat 42:173–181

Konecny G, Pauletti G, Pegram M, Untch M, Dandekar S, Aguilar Z, Wilson C, Rong HM, Bauerfeind I, Felber M, Wang HJ, Beryt M, Seshadri R, Hepp H, Slamon D (2003) Wuantitative association between HER-2/neu and steroid hormone receptor-positive primary breast cancer. J Natl Cancer Inst 95(2):142–153

Krainick-Strobel UE, Lichtenegger W, Wallwiener D, Tulusan AH, Janicke F, Bastert G, Kiesel L, Wackwitz B, Paepke S (2008) Neoadjuvant letrozole in postmenopausal estrogen and/or progesterone receptor positive breast cancer: A phase iib/iii trial to investigate optimal diration of pre-operative endocrine therapy. BMC Cancer 8:62

Kristensen VN, Sorlie T, Geisler J, Langerod A, Yoshimura N, Karesen R, Harada N, Lonning PE, Borresen-Dale AL (2005) Gene expression profiling of breast cancer in relation to estrogen receptor status and estrogen-metabolizing enzymes: clinical implications. Clin Cancer Res 11:878s–883s

Kuehn T, Klauss W, Darsow M et al (2000) Long term morbidity following axillary dissection in breast cancer patients- clinical assessment, signifiicance for life quality and the impact of demographic and therapeutic factors. Breast Cancer Res Treat 64:275–286

Lavelle K, Todd C, Moran A, Howell A, Bundred N, Campbell M (2007a) Non-standard management of breast cancer increases with age in the UK: a population based cohort of women ≥65 years. Bri J Cancer 96:1197–1203

Lavelle K, Moran A, Howell A, Bundred N, Campbell M, Todd C (2007b) Older women with operable breast cancer are less likely to have surgery. Bri J Surg 94:1209–1215

Maly RC, Umezawa Y, Leake B, Silliman RA (2004) Determinants of perticipation in treatment decision making by older breast cancer patients. Breast Cancer Res Treat 85(3):201–209

Mansell RE, Fallowfield L, Kissin M et al (2006) Randomized multicentre trial of sentinel node biopsy versus standard axillary treatment in operable breast cancer: the ALMANAC trial. J Natl Cancer Inst 98:599–609

Martin CV, Stotter A, Kenny F, Walker RA (2006) Tumor markers predictive of response to primary endocrine therapy for breast cancer-a prospective study. Eur J Surg Oncol 32:1050–1051

McCarty KS, Silva JS, Cox EB, Leight GS, Wells SA, McCarty KS Sr (1983) Relationship of age and menopausal status to estrogen receptor content in primary carcinoma of the breast. Ann Surg 197:123–127

Miller WR, Larionov A, Anderson TJ, Walker JR, Krause A, Evans DB, Dixon JM (2008) Predicting response and resistance to endocrine therapy. Profiling patients on aromatase inhibitors. Cancer 112(3):689–694

Mlineritsch B, Tausch C, Singer C, Luschin-Ebengreuth G, Jakesz R, Austrian Breast, Colorectal Cancer Study Group (ABCSG) et al (2008) Exemestane as primary systemic therapy for hormone receptor positive post-menopausal breast cancer patients: a phase II trial of the Austrian Breast, Colorectal Cancer Study Group (ABCSG-17). Breast Cancer Res Treat 112(1):203–213

Murphy LC, Niu Y, Snell L, Watson P (2004) Phospho-serine-118 estrogen receptor-alpha expression is associated with better disease outcome in women treated with tamoxifen. Clin Cancer Res 10:5902–5906

Mustacchi G et al (1998) Tamoxifen versus surgery plus tamoxifen as primary treatment for elderly patients with breast cancer: combined data from the "GRETA" and "CRC" trials. In: Proceedings of Am Soc Clin Oncol 17:99a.

Mustacchi G, Ceccherini R, Milani S et al (2003) Tamoxifen alone versus adjuvant tamoxifen for operable breast cancer of the elderly: Long-term results of the phase III randomized controlled multicenter GRETA trial. Ann Oncol 14:414–420

Paik S, Shak S, Tang G, Kim C, Baker J, Cronin M, Baehner FL, Walker MG, Watson D, Park T, Hiller W, Fisher ER, Wickerham DL, Bryant J, Wolmark N (2004) A multigene assay to predict recurrence of tamoxifen-treated, node-negative breast cancer. N Engl J Med 351:2817–2826

Petrisek AC, Laliberte LL, Allen SM, Mor V (1997) The treatment decision-making process: Age differences in a sample of women recently diagnosed with non-recurrent, early stage breast cancer. Gerontologist 37:598–608

Preece PE, Wood RAB, Mackie CR, Cushieri A (1982) Tamoxifen as initial sole treatment of localised breast cancer in elderly women: a pilot study. Bri Med J 284:869–870

Ravdin PM, Siminoff LA, Davis GJ, Mercer MB, Hewlett J, Gerson N, Parker H (2001) Computer program to assist in making decisions about adjuvant therapy for women with early breast cancer. J Clin Oncol 19:980–991

Reid DM, Doughty J, Eastell R, Heys SD, Howell A, McCloskey EV, Powles T, Selby P, Coleman RE (2008) Guidance for the management of breast cancer treatment-induced bone loss: a consensus position statement from a UK Expert Group. Cancer Treatment Reviews 34(1):S3–18

Ring A, Dowsett M (2003) Human epidermal growth factor receptor-2 and hormonal therapies: clinical implications. Clin Breast Cancer 4(Suppl 1):S34–41

Satariano WA, Ragland DR (1994) The effect of co-morbidity on 3-year survival of women with primary breast cancer. Ann Intern Med 120:104–110

Sauvaget C, Jagger C, Arthur AJ (2001) Active and cognitive impairment-free life expectancies: results from the Melton Mowbray 75+ health checks. Age Ageing 30(6):509–515

Semiglazov VF, Semiglazof VV, Dasyan GA, Ziltsova EK, Ivanov VG, Bozhok AA, Melnikova OA, Paltuev RM, Kletzel A, Bernstein LM (2007) Phase 2 randomized trial of primary endocrine therapy versus chemotherapy in post menopausal patients with estrogen receptor positive breast cancer. Cancer 110(2):244–254

Shimozuma K, Ganz PA, Petersen L, Hirji K (1999) Quality of life in the first year after breast cancer surgery: rehabilitation needs and patterns of recovery. Breast Cancer Res Treat 56(1):45–57

Siegelmann-Danieli N, Khandelwal V, Wood GC, et al (2004) Breast cancer in elderly women: Combined effect of tumor feature, age, co-morbidities and treatment approach. Poster at the San Antonio Breast Cancer Conference,

Smith IE, Dowsett M, Ebbs SR, Dixon JM, Skene A, Blohmer JU, Ashley S, Francis S, Boeddinghaus I, Walsh G (2005) Neoadjuvant treatment of post menopausal breast cancer with anastrozole, tamoxifen or both in combination: The immediate pre-operative anastrozole, tamoxifen or combined with tamoxifen (IMPACT) multicentre double blind randomized trial. J Clin Oncol 23(22):5108–5116

Speirs V, Malone C, Walton DS, Kerin MJ, Atkin SL (1999) Increased expression of estrogen receptor beta mRNA in tamoxifen-resistant breast cancer patients. Cancer Res 59:5421–5424

Van Dalsen AD, de Vries JE (1995) Treatment of breast cancer in elderly patients. J Surg Oncol 60(2):80–2

van de Vijver MJ, He YD, van't Veer LJ, Dai H, Hart AA, Voskuil DW, Schreiber GJ, Peterse JL, Roberts C, Marton MJ, Parrish M, Atsma D, Witteveen A, Glas A, Delahaye L, van der Velde T, Bartelink H, Rodenhuis S, Rutgers ET, Friend SH, Bernards R (2002) A gene-expression signature as a predictor of survival in breast cancer. N Engl J Med 347:1999–2009

Veer LJ van 't, Dai H, van de Vijver MJ, He YD, Hart AA, Mao M, Peterse HL, van der Kooy K, Marton MJ, Witteveen AT, Schreiber GJ, Kerkhoven RM, Roberts C, Linsley PS, Bernards R, Friend SH (2002) Gene expression profiling predicts clinical outcome of breast cancer. Nature 415:530–536

Wenger CR, Beardslee S, Owens MA et al (1993) DNA ploidy, S-phase and steroid receptors in more than 127, 000 breast cancer patients. Breast Cancer Res Treat 28:9–20

Willsher PC, Robertson JFR, Jackson L, Al-Hilaly M, Blamey RW (1997) Investigation of primary tamoxifen therapy for elderly patients with operable breast cancer. Breast 6:150–154

Wyld L, Reed M (2007) The role of surgery in the management of older women with breast cancer. European Journal of Cancer 43(15):2253–2263

Wyld L, Garg DK, Brown H, Reed MWR (2004) Stage and treatment variation with age in postmenopausal women with breast cancer: compliance with guidelines. Br J Cancer 90(8):1486–1491

Chapter 11
Peroperative Radiotherapy

Roberto Orecchia, Giovanni Battista Ivaldi, and Maria Cristina Leonardi

11.1 Introduction

Breast-conserving surgery (BCS) consists of the surgical removal of the tumor mass plus a margin, followed by postoperative whole-breast irradiation (WBI). This combination of treatments has proven to obtain equivalent results in terms of local control and survival rates to those of mastectomy in women with comparable tumor size and stage, and therefore, is currently accepted as the standard approach for most women with early-stage breast cancer (Veronesi et al. 2002). In postoperative radiation therapy (RT), the whole breast tissue left by the surgeon is irradiated up to a dose of 45–50 Gy delivered over 5–6 weeks. The treatment is then completed within 1–2 weeks by a boost dose of 10–15 Gy to the tumor bed.

Radiotherapy significantly reduces local recurrence (LR), 15-year breast cancer mortality, and overall mortality, as shown by a meta-analysis of the most relevant randomized trials recently published (Clarke et al. 2005). Meanwhile, several institutions further investigated different aspects of adjuvant radiation treatment such as the fractionation, the overall treatment time, and the target volume. The concept of minimum effective treatment in breast radiotherapy is exploited by PBI, which consists of the irradiation of the site of surgical excision and adjacent tissues only. PBI can be performed using different approaches, including brachytherapy (BRT), intraoperative RT (IORT) with electrons or low-energy X-rays, 3D conformal external beam (CRT), and particle beams. With PBI, it is possible to reduce the irradiation only to the involved quadrant of the breast plus a margin. The drastic reduction of both target volume and nontarget tissue allows changing the RT course from 40 to 50 days to a shorter intensive schedule of fractionation.

R. Orecchia (✉)
Department of Radiation Oncology, European Institute of Oncology, University of Milan,
Milan, Italy
e-mail: roberto.orecchia@ieo.it

M.W. Reed and R.A. Audisio (eds.), *Management of Breast Cancer in Older Women,*
DOI 10.1007/978-1-84800-265-4_11, © Springer-Verlag London Limited 2011

11.2   Rationale for PBI in Older Women

It is still not clear whether, after BCS, the irradiation of the entire breast is needed or not and this is the main concern over the adequacy of PBI as a standard treatment in BCT. Long-term studies that independently either added EBRT or not to BCS reported that local relapses occur at the original tumor site at a rate of 85% or more, and this is the rationale for the use of segmental irradiation in place of WBI. The optimal treatment of elderly patients is debated. Clinical studies showed that post-menopausal women have lower failure rates than premenopausal women, even though these differences could result from the higher percentage of low-risk factors in this age group: better-differentiated tumors, poor extensive intraductal compo-nent (EIC), and minimal lymph vascular invasion.

In elderly patients, the results of radiotherapy trials showed small absolute difference, as low as 3%, in breast recurrence rate when WBI was added to con-servative surgery. In the Milan III trial, patients over 65 who received quadran-tectomy plus conventional WBI did not show any difference in the rate of intrabreast tumor reappearances compared to same-age patients who received only quadrantectomy. However, these data were not conclusive because of the limited number of patients in this age group (Veronesi et al. 2001). For the majority of patients and particularly for the elderly, traveling distance from home to hospital or long waiting times to begin radiation is often detrimental to the number that actually receive the recommended local treatment. It has also been demonstrated that the 4–6 weeks of conventional external beam radiother-apy could be associated with a higher incidence of psychological morbidity (e.g., depression, anxiety). With PBI techniques, it is possible to reduce the radiation field to the single involved quadrant of the breast plus a margin. This downsizing of the target volume greatly reduces the amount of normal tissue irradiated, allowing a shorter intensive treatment schedule. The conventional course of 40–50 days can be reduced to less than 10 days. For postmenopausal women with small, low-grade, hormone receptor-positive, node-negative tumors, it is justified to investigate a shorter and less damaging course of RT. A significant shortening of the treatment time is, in any case, a major issue in favor of PBI, because it minimizes some constraints and setbacks that affect adjuvant RT compliance, particularly in the elderly such as traveling distance from the patient's home to hospital and long waiting times to begin the treatment.

An overview of 40 trials has confirmed an increase in death from cardiac and other causes for patients receiving radiotherapy, mostly in the 1970s and early 1980s with outmoded techniques, nullifying the long-term reduction of breast cancer mortality obtained by the local treatment. Contemporary radiotherapy techniques can involve substantially lower cardiac and lung exposures than those used previously. The decreased morbidity of modern radiotherapy could improve this therapeutic ratio, particularly when it is administered to older patients who are frequently affected by chronic concurrent cardiopulmonary illness. PBI could further reduce the "intensity" of RT by diminishing the spread of irradiation to nontarget tissues. In the use of the electron intraoperative technique, PBI avoids any dose to the skin and subcutaneous tissue. For these reasons elderly patients with early breast cancer could be considered as ideal candidates for PBI.

The EORTC trial 22881/10882 demonstrated that a higher radiation dose to the primary tumor area significantly reduced the rate of LR at 5 years. These data suggest the relevance of delivering a high dose of irradiation to the surgical bed as PBI does (Bartelink et al. 2001). However, there are no conclusive current data to support the use of PBI in the routine management of early-stage breast cancer. Clinical outcome can be strongly influenced by patient selection. The results in terms of safety and efficacy should be managed with caution because of major differences in technical approach, fractionation schedules, and skills between difference centers. Uncertainties in clinical outcome are mainly due to the too short follow-up time of some institutional experiences (often with small numbers of patients treated) and the need for definitive results from several large randomized trials that are still underway. Nevertheless, while surgery shifted from mastectomy to lumpectomy and from axillaries dissection to sentinel node biopsy, PBI is headed in the same direction, reducing the "intensity" of RT by reducing the volume of nontarget tissue irradiated. The importance of proper patient selection should be stressed. It is well known that age is an independent risk factor for local relapse. The American Brachytherapy Society and the American Society of Breast Surgeons recently proposed guidelines to select appropriate patients for PBI. They both chose age, respectively older than 45 and older than 50, as the first criteria for selection, underlining that postmenopausal women could be the most suitable candidate for this customized treatment.

11.3   Clinical Peroperative Methodologies

Peroperative radiotherapy can be performed with several different techniques. Six main modalities are currently in use in clinical and research settings:

Intraoperative RT (IORT) and IORT with electrons (IOERT)
Intraoperative RT with low energy x-rays (Intrabeam)
Multicatheter-based interstitial brachytherapy
MammoSite Radiation Therapy System
3D conformal external beam RT (3D CRT)
Protons

11.4   Intraoperative Radiation Therapy

IORT consists of a single-fraction treatment targeted at the tumor bed during the surgical procedure immediately following the removal of the tumor mass. Mobile accelerators that can be brought to the operating room solved the logistic problem of bringing the radiation source and the patient together. In modern IORT, two kinds of beams are used: either megavoltage electrons or kilovoltage photons.

In IOERT, the electron beams with variable energies (from 3 up to 10–12 MeV) are produced by a specialized linear accelerator mounted on a robotic arm. After the excision of the tumor, the surgeon separates the remaining parenchyma from the thoracic wall and inserts an aluminum-lead shielding disc behind the gland to protect deep-seated organs. The breast anatomy is temporarily restored and the radiation oncologist visually identifies the tumor bed and, together with the medical physicists, measures the depth of the tissue to be irradiated in order to select the most appropriate beam energy. Irradiation is delivered through Perspex cylindrical applicators with different diameters (4–10 cm) and angles of the head: perpendicular or oblique from 15 to 45° respect to their axis (Fig. 11.1).

IOERT has been extensively employed at the European Institute of Oncology (EIO) in Milan. Between 1999 and 2000, a pilot phase I-II trial was conducted on 101 patients. Dose was escalated from 10 to 15 Gy (as anticipated boost) up to 21 Gy, as sole treatment. After a median follow up of 42 months, 16% of the patients had developed transient breast fibrosis that was mild in 15% and severe in 1% and resolved within 24 months (Luini et al. 2005). Postoperative infections (2%) and liponecrosis (4%) were observed in the sample. The Santa Chiara Hospital, in Trento, Italy, between October 2000 and November 2002, enrolled 47 early-stage breast cancer patients into a phase I/II study to investigate IORT as sole radiation treatment after conservative surgery (Mussari et al. 2006). Three different dose levels prescribed at Dmax were used: 20 Gy (7 patients), 22 Gy (20 patients), and 24 Gy (20 patients). After a median follow up of 48 months, 15 (30%) patients developed breast fibrosis (14 G2 and one G3). Only one clinical liponecrosis was recorded, but mammographic signs of fat necrosis were observed in 25% of the treated patients. Two patients showed a permanent G3 alteration of the skin with pigmentation change and telangiectasia. No LR was observed. Overall cosmesis

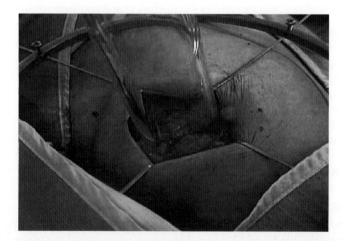

Fig. 11.1 Intraoperative radiotherapy with electrons. The collimator of a dedicated linear accelerator is placed directly in contact with the breast target

was judged good/excellent in 44 (94%) patients, while a bad score was assigned only to one patient.

From 2000 to 2007, the EIO randomized 1,306 patients in a prospective phase III trial (ELIOT trial) to receive conventional EBRT (50 Gy to the whole breast plus a 10 Gy boost to the tumor bed) or a single dose of 21 Gy of IOERT. All patients received quadrantectomy followed by sentinel node biopsy and, in cases of positive nodes, axillary dissection. The primary endpoint for analysis was the rate of LR within a 5-year observation period. Patients are now actively followed (median follow up is now 33.8 months) in order to evaluate chronic toxicity and to determine whether ELIOT can replace conventional radiotherapy in that subgroup of women.

IORT has been used as a boost also by Reitsamer and his group (Reitsamer et al. 2006) that demonstrated that IORT as immediate supplementary dose yields excellent local control in patients with invasive breast cancer who had been treated with BCS and postoperative RT to the whole breast up to 51–56.1 Gy in 1.7 Gy/fractions. Boost to the tumor bed was performed either with postoperative electrons of 12 Gy (188 pts – group 1) or with intraoperative boost (IORT) of 9 Gy (190 pts – group 2). During a median follow up of 81 months in group 1 and 51.1 in group 2, LR was observed in 12 of 188 pts (6.4%) in group 1 and no event was observed in group 2. Distant metastases occurred in 15 patients (7.9%) in group 1 and 2 patients in group 2 (1.1%). The 5-year actuarial rates of recurrence were 4.3 and 0.0% (p 0.0018) and the 5-year actuarial rates of distant metastases were 8.6 and 4.2% (p 0.08). The 5-year disease free survival rates were 90.9% in group 1 and 95.8% in group 2 (p 0.064).

A nonrandomized "ELIOT boost" study for premenopausal women after BSC was started at the EIO in June 2004. After a 12 Gy intraoperative boost, patients received hypofractionated external beam radiotherapy (HEBRT) to the whole breast in 13 fractions over a period of 2.5 weeks to a total of 37.05 Gy (Ivaldi et al. 2008). Eligible patients are premenopausal women below 48 years of age, affected by invasive breast cancer cT1-T2, clinically cN0-1, who are candidates for BCS. Available data on the first 211 consecutive patients showed a high compliance to treatment: 99.5% of the patients completed the whole treatment schedule including HEBRT. Maximum acute side effects were observed at the end of HEBRT with a grade 3 skin toxicity in 3.8% and grade 2 in 29% of patients. At a median follow up of 11 months, 6 patients complained of symptomatic edema, one patient suffered from grade 3 fibrosis, and one grade 4 event was recorded. Overall, 4.4% of patients experienced liponecrosis of the surgical area within the first month from surgery. Thus, IOERT as a boost appears to be a possible alternative to the conventional EBRT. By giving the boost in a single intraoperative session, when a dedicated IORT unit is available, operative time increases only modestly (15–20 min). This technique reduces the total time of external treatment by 1–2 weeks, with consequent economic savings and improvement in the general well-being of the patient. Preliminary data are promising, but median follow-up is still too short to draw conclusions on the efficacy.

At the EIO, breast surgeons and radiation oncologists combined the subcutaneous mastectomy with IORT to the preserved nipple areola complex (NAC). The aim of this approach would be to maintain the blood supply and the sensitivity of the NAC and avoid the feeling of mutilation carried by mastectomy, while reducing the risk of recurrence in the central area of the breast. A total dose of 16 Gy at a 90% isodose is delivered in a single fraction to the clinical target volume that includes the remaining glandular tissue behind the NAC. Breast reconstruction is performed immediately after irradiation with the use of prosthesis or a myocutaneous flap. Results of 579 skin-sparing mastectomies (NSM) plus IORT performed at EIO in 570 patients from March 2002 to November 2006 (Petit et al. 2008) report the good feasibility of the procedure and a high level of satisfaction. The rate of local relapse (LR) was 0.9% per year: this incidence was consistent with the rate of LR after modified mastectomy. Most relapses were observed near to the primary tumor bed, while no event occurred underneath the preserved NAC. From this experience the authors conclude that for large or multicentric tumors and/or diffuse microcalcifications far from the NAC, NSM with IORT of the NAC obtains good local control and satisfactory cosmetic results.

11.5   Intrabeam – TARGIT

The targeted intraoperative radiotherapy (TARGIT) is another approach to perform PBI. It is delivered through the INTRABEAM (INTRABEAM, Photoelectron Corp, Lexington, MA), a low-energy (50 KV) X-ray tube that delivers radiation from the tip of a probe with sphere-shaped applicators of different diameters. Intraoperatively, after tumor excision, the device is inserted into the surgical cavity with a sterile cover. Tungsten-impregnated rubber sheets are placed on the chest wall to protect heart and lungs. Skin dose is monitored with thermoluminescence detectors. The applicator size has to properly match the size of the surgical cavity in order to yield a uniform dose to the tumor bed. Because of its physical characteristics, Intrabeam provides a limited spherical distribution of the dose without any possibility to adapt the depth of dose penetration to individual risk situation. The dose usually prescribed is 20 Gy on the applicator surface. Due to tissue attenuation of radiation, which is proportional to the distance from the source, 20 Gy at 10 mm depth corresponds physically to a dose of 5 Gy. The treatment takes 20–30 min. The use of a low-energy x-ray source has the advantage of not requiring specifically shielded operating room because the dose drops rapidly away from the source. The main concern about this treatment modality is the possibility that 5 Gy at 1 cm from the surface of the applicator could not be adequate to eradicate occult carcinoma.

In 1999,Proulx et al. (2001) started one of the earliest experiences with low-energy x-rays as boost followed by WBRT, using 120 kVp-x-rays (Picker Zephyr, modified at Roswell Park Cancer Institute, Buffalo, NY). In the pilot study, seven women with stage I and II breast cancer were treated delivering 15–20 Gy at the surface of the applicator. At a median follow-up of 6 years, the author reported no toxicity and 2 LRs (one with < 2 mm margin and one node positive).

IORT is more popular in Europe than in the US. Vaidja performed a pilot trial including 25 patients with T1-T3 any N (Vaidya et al. 2001) treated with the INTRABEAM device used as sole therapy or as a boost and observed no LR.

After this initial experience, Vaidja initiated an international randomized trial (Great Britain, Australia, US, Germany) to investigate whether the outcome with IORT using INTRABEAM is equivalent to conventional WBRT with the endpoints of local control, cosmetic outcome, patient satisfaction, and cost analysis. Clinically, low-risk patients are considered eligible for TARGIT: age > 50 years, < 2 cm unifocal carcinoma, ductal invasive, free margins ≥ 10 mm, no lymphatic vessel invasion. The protocol provides the possibility, according to each center's decision, to add 46 Gy of external WBRT in case further risk factors (tumor size > 2 cm, close surgical margin, extensive intraductal component, etc.) are found at the final pathologic examinations (Holmes et al. 2007).

11.6 Multiple Catheters for Interstitial Brachytherapy

BRT is able to deliver high doses to a small volume confined to the tumor bed while sparing the surrounding breast tissue and the overlying skin. The main indication for BRT using the multiple-catheter technique in early breast cancer is to boost the site of the primary tumor after BCS and EBRT of the entire breast. Interstitial BRT as sole RT after BCS has been exploited recently. Several centers have evaluated the feasibility and efficacy of tumor bed irradiation alone in phase I and II trials: results in selected patients suggest that a similar local tumor control for early breast cancer can be achieved with interstitial BRT compared to conventional EBRT. By following strict inclusion criteria and rigorous quality assurance procedures, a local failure rates as low as 0–1.5 per year can be achieved with BRT, comparable to the present standard of whole breast RT. In the William Beaumont Hospital's trial (US), 199 women with early breast cancer treated by interstitial BRT alone reported local tumor control rates of 97% and an OS of 99% with an excellent cosmetic results. Polgar in a recent review of the literature shows an overall rate of breast failure of only 1.9% in a cohort of 887 patients treated with multicatheter BRT (Polgár et al. 2004). The main series that recorded late effects on normal tissues report a low rate of in-field fibrosis (4–9%) and a high overall rate of good/excellent cosmetic outcome (80–99%) (Arthur et al. 2003).

The technique consists of placing multiple afterloading catheters into the tissue surrounding the lumpectomy cavity, either during surgery with the evident advantage of directly seeing the tumor bed, or after, when the histopathologic parameters are already known. Catheters are uniformly positioned at 1–1.5 cm intervals to ensure proper coverage of the target volume along with a 2–3 cm margin around it (Fig. 11.2). Total number and catheter configuration depend on the size and shape of the surgical cavity and are geometrically adjusted based on dosimetric consideration in order to uniformly cover the tumor bed. These implants routinely require 14–20 catheters. In interstitial BRT, critical structures can be spared by a differential loading of the catheters. The complexity of the treatment planning requires considerable training and experience. Radiation dose to the implant can be delivered by means of sources at low dose-rate that deliver 45–60 Gy over 4–6 days on

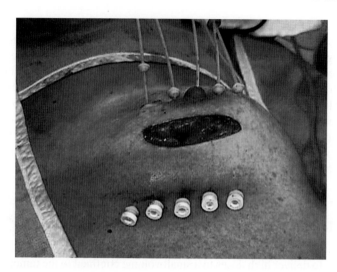

Fig. 11.2 Multiple afterloading catheters placed into the tissue surrounding the lumpectomy cavity for interstitial brachytherapy (BRT) treatment

hospitalized patients or by means of high dose-rate sources, usually in an outpatient setting. The most used fractionations are either 3.4 or 5.2 Gy per fraction usually delivered twice daily (with a minimum 6-h interfraction interval) to a total dose of 32–37 Gy over 4–5 days. High-dose rate interstitial BRT may be preferred over low-dose rate because it allows better control of the dose and delivers less exposure to radiation to the operators.

The RTOG 95-17 phase I/II cooperative group trial compared 66 patients treated with high-dose rate BRT with 33 treated with low-dose rate BRT. At a median follow-up of 73 months, relapse rates of 3% and 6% for the high and low dose rates, respectively, and corresponding 5-year disease free survival rates of 86 and 94% were observed. Kuske reported an incidence of breast erythema (51%) and edema (40%) in the high-dose rate patients, while the incidence in the low-dose rate patients was 42 and 27%, respectively. G3 late toxicity involving skin thickening, fibrosis, breast tenderness, and telangiectasia was seen in 4% of patients receiving high dose rate and 18% for the low dose rate group. The phase III randomized Hungarian National Institute Trial study using implant BRT enrolled 258 selected patients (T1 N0-1, G1-2, not lobular histotype, no presence of extended intraductal component, free margin) to receive WB vs. interstitial BRT, and is now closed. Long-term results, with a minimum follow-up of 5 years, do not show any difference in local control, overall survival, cancer-specific, and disease-free survival in the two groups (Polgár et al. 2006). Other phase III trials using wide implant BRT after BCS are ongoing. The international phase III trial under the direction of the European Brachytherapy Breast Cancer GEC-ESTRO Working group (Strnad et al. 2004) will randomize 1,170 patients to either conventional WBERT vs. PBI using either HDR (32 Gy/8 × 4 Gy twice a day or 30.3 Gy/7 × 4.3 Gy twice a day) or PDR

BRT (0.6–0.8 Gy/h to a total dose of 50 Gy) after BCS for low-risk invasive carcinoma and low-risk ductal carcinoma in situ. An Intergroup phase III trial (National Surgical Adjuvant Breast and Bowel Project B-39/Radiation Therapy Oncology Group 0413) is currently comparing whole breast irradiation vs. PBI, performed either with MammoSite or 3D conformal ERT or multicatheter BRT (NSABP B-39, RTOG 0413 2006).

11.7 Mammosite

Interstitial BRT has traditionally been one modality of breast radiotherapy after conservative surgery. However, the difficulty in teaching and learning the technique by radiation oncologists and the use of multiple catheters that limited a widespread patient acceptance confined its use to a restricted number of cancer centers. In the early 2000s, the MammoSite breast BRT catheter (manufactured by Cytyc, Bedford, Mass) was developed to deliver accelerated PBI, either as a sole modality or as a boost dose. After clearance of the device by the US food and drug administration (FDA) for use in clinical practice in May 2002, it has been the most frequently employed method of PBI in the US. The device is a dual lumen spherical balloon catheter inflatable to 4–5 cm with a central lumen for the high-dose-rate Ir^{192} source. The catheter is a silicon balloon and shaft containing a small inflation channel and a larger central channel that allow the passage of the HDR source. Through an adapter, the device is connectable to any brand of commercially available HDR remote afterloading device. The applicator is inserted into the lumpectomy cavity at the time of surgery or up to 10 weeks afterward, inflated with saline and contrast material to fill the cavity, such that the surrounding tissue is stretched tightly around it. The treatment is delivered by a high dose rate source that travels from the afterloading device through the inner lumen into the center of the balloon to deliver the dose to the tissue surrounding the lumpectomy cavity (Fig. 11.3).

In order to test safety and performance, MammoSite was initially tested between 2000 and 2001 in a multiinstitution prospective phase I/II trial (Keisch et al. 2003) on 70 patients older than 45 years with a < 2 cm invasive ductal carcinoma. Fifty-four patients were implanted and 43 were finally eligible to receive BRT as the sole radiation modality after lumpectomy. A dose of 34 Gy was delivered in 10 fractions over 5 days prescribed to 1 cm from the applicator surface using Ir^{192}. Major reasons for not been implanted or treated were technical, such as inadequate skin spacing or suboptimal conformance of the surgical cavity to the applicator balloon. Treatment was well tolerated. The most common side effects related to device placement included mild erythema, drainage, pain, and bruising. No severe side effects related to implantation, BRT, or explantation occurred. Side effects related to RT were mild and cosmetic results good to excellent in 88% of the patients. The trial led to US Food and Drug Administration approval of the device in May 2002.

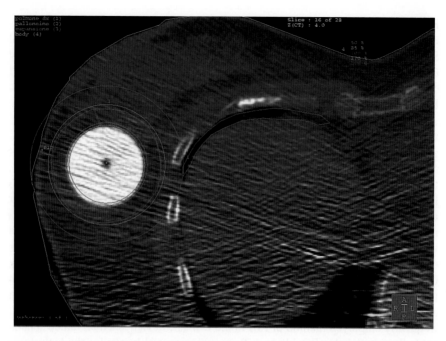

Fig. 11.3 Computed tomography imaging showing MammoSite balloon BRT applicator inserted into lumpectomy cavity and isodose distribution

Since the initial study of the MammoSite device, various new balloon diameters are available to better conform to different resection cavities. Furthermore, a few different versions of the original single dwell position spherical device have been developed. A number of patients have been already treated with a multiple dwell positions model produced in order to improve PTV coverage, reduce skin dose, and optimize implant with unfit balloon geometry. Also an elliptical balloon with multiple dwell positions has been produced to improve the filling of the sometimes irregularly shaped lumpectomy cavity.

The results of the FDA study at 4 years showed no local failure and an interesting correlation between cosmetic outcome and skin spacing of the balloon applicator. For most patients, cosmetic result was excellent/good for skin spacing ≥ 8 mm and decreased for spacing of 5–7 mm. Besides additional MammoSite clinical research ongoing in several institutions, the manufacturer initiated in 2002 a registry trial that closed in 2004. The preliminary data on 1,419 patients are confirming a similar relationship between skin spacing and cosmetic outcome. Over time, more patients are being implanted after lumpectomy, instead of at the time of lumpectomy to lower the explantation rate due to adverse pathology.

The most common acute side effects observed with the MammoSite are erythema and subsequent hyperpigmentation of the skin overlying the implant, seroma formation, and breast tenderness. They usually involve a small volume of tissue and resolve quickly. Very few complications requiring surgical intervention have been reported. Seroma requiring aspiration has been the most common (5–10% of the cases). Chronic toxicity includes fat necrosis, skin atrophy, telangiectasia, and fibrosis (Vicini et al. 2003a). Fat necrosis is most of the time asymptomatic (5% of cases) and less frequent compared to multicatheter BRT. In the great majority of cases, fat necrosis is self-limiting and does not require intervention. In few cases, fine needle aspiration of the necrotic collection and a few sessions of clinical care are sufficient to resolve symptoms. A less frequent side effect is the infection correlated to the indwelling catheter that is reported by different authors, with a variable rate of 5–16%. It has been observed that infection is related to the level of catheter site care and possibly reduced by the use of prophylactic antibiotics. Cuttino et al. reported a pooled analysis of a multiinstitutional experience on 483 patients with a median follow-up of 24 months. They observed a significant reduction in the rate of infection when the catheter was placed after lumpectomy and a reduced risk of severe acute skin reaction and telangiectasia with a skin spacing > than 6 mm (Cuttino et al. 2008). Furthermore, prophylactic antibiotics reduced the risk of acute skin reaction and the use of multiple dwell positions reduced the risk of severe hyperpigmentation. At present time, no series has sufficiently long follow-up to draw conclusions on local control, survival, late toxicity, and long-term cosmetic outcome. Vicini recently reported data on treatment efficacy in 1,440 patients treated with MammoSite for PBI at 97 institutions enrolled in the American Society of Breast Surgeons, Breast Brachytherapy Registry Trial. Dose delivered was 34 Gy in 3.4 Gy/fractions. At a median follow-up of 30.1 months, 23 patients (1.6%) developed ipsilateral breast tumor recurrence and 6 (0.4%) had axillary failure. A subset analysis of the first 400 consecutive enrolled cases with a median follow-up of 37.5 months showed that the actuarial rate of IBTR was 1.79%. The authors observe that efficacy and toxicity of the MammoSite treatment modality is comparable to other form of PBI with similar follow-up.

In conclusion, the overall procedure of placing the balloon catheter and treatment is relatively simple. The use of a hypofractionated schedule that reduces treatment time, coupled with the fact that patients find it less frightening than interstitial BRT, make the MammoSite a promising option for administering adjuvant irradiation after breast BCS.

11.8 3D Conformal Radiotherapy

3D CRT and intensity modulated radiotherapy (IMRT) have been introduced for accelerated partial breast irradiation (ABPI). The main advantage is the noninvasive nature of the procedure and the administration of treatment when final histopathologic parameters are known. Compared to conventional external radiotherapy, the high conformality of these external beam techniques allows a precise coverage of the lumpectomy site and an improvement of dose homogeneity within the target volume. This approach employs multiple (between 3 and 8) noncoplanar or mini-tangent photon treatment fields, eventually combined with an en face electron field

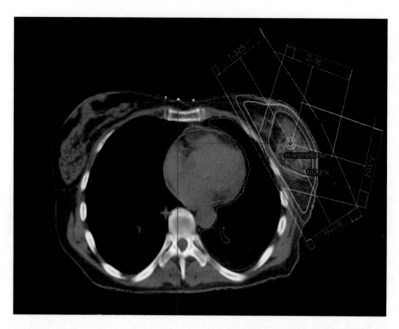

Fig. 11.4 Three dimensional conformal external beam (CRT) radiotherapy with noncoplanar photon beams

to provide a dose distribution conformed to target volume (Fig. 11.4). Selection of patients with small target, specific locations, and normal tissue dose limitations has been advocated in order to limit the increase of the integral dose received by surrounding normal structures. High-technology equipment including 3D computer-based planning and advanced linear accelerator units is essential for conformal external RT. The optimal planning target volume remains to be investigated, but generally an additional safety margin of 1–2 cm around the index quadrant is included. Surgical clips within the surgical bed help to better define the target volume. To improve geometric uncertainties of dose distribution within the breast which may result from breathing motions, respiratory-gated RT, the so called 4D-CRT, offers a significant potential for improvement. Two institutions have published phase I/II trials, one treating patients in prone position and the other in supine position. Formenti used 30 Gy in five fractions of 6 Gy each. After a follow-up of 18 months, toxicity was minimal and no recurrence was observed. In the RTOG study, treatment was performed twice daily in ten fractions of 3.85 Gy, up to a total dose of 38.5 Gy. A minimum 10 mm safety margin around the clinical target volume was required. Inclusion criteria were: stage I and II (T1N0-T2N1), tumor size ≤ 3 cm, unifocality, and negative surgical margins. Dose volume constraints in this study are strictly defined for lungs, heart, and uninvolved breast. Ideally < 50% of the whole breast should receive ≥ 50% of the dose (Formenti et al. 2004; Vicini et al. 2003b).

To further investigate this approach, the ongoing RTOG0413/NSABP B-39 phase III trial is randomly allocating patients after BCS to WBI vs. PBI, 3D-CRT being one of the three options.

11.9 Protons for Breast Irradiation

In recent years, an increasing number of radiation treatment facilities offer protons as treatment modality. Proton beam therapy is able to achieve optimal dose conformation due to a low to median entrance dose, followed by a unified high dose region (Bragg peak region) and a steep fall-off to zero dose behind the target. Such a conformal and homogeneous dose distribution can be particularly useful when critical organs such as lung and heart are just beside the target as in breast treatment. Studies on long-term toxicity of radiotherapy showed that the overall favorable effect of postoperative radiotherapy in the reduction of breast cancer mortality is tightened by this long-term toxicity that causes excess mortality due to cardiac and other vascular causes, and to lesser extent, to secondary malignancies, particularly pulmonary. This detrimental effect has been shown to decrease when patients treated more recently are considered, confirming the positive effect obtained by the increasing use in clinical practice of more sophisticated techniques able to better spare critical organs. Comparative treatment-planning studies investigated the ability of protons to achieve better dose conformation compared to conventional photons for both WBI and PBI. Lomax (Lomax 2008) compared standard photons/electrons, IMRT, and forward-planned proton treatment plans on a single patient with the intent to treat the involved breast, internal mammary, supraclavicular, and axillary nodes. Target coverage homogeneity was equally better with IMRT and proton plans compared with the standard plan. Furthermore, the most favorable lung and heart dose volume histogram (DVH) were generated with the proton plan. A dosimetric study comparing protons and photon-electron with a three dimensional conformal technique for accelerated partial breast irradiation (3D-CPBI) was conducted by Kozak et al. (2006) at the Massachusetts General Hospital. The comparison was made on 24 stage I breast cancer patients who received adjuvant proton 3D-CPBI with a dose of 32 cobalt gray equivalent (CGE) and had also a treatment plan generated using mixed modality photon-electron 3D-CPBI both optimized for PTV coverage and normal tissue sparing. Both techniques provided good PTV coverage and excellent dose homogeneity, but overall, proton ensured a statistically significant reduction of dose delivered to ipsilateral and contralateral lung and heart. The same group also reported preliminary clinical results on twenty breast cancer patients treated with a dose of 32 CGE proton 3D-CPBI in a phase I/II clinical trial. Breast cosmesis was rated good or excellent in 100% of cases both by the physician and the patients at 12 months follow-up. Acute skin toxicity was significant with moderate to severe color change in 79% of the patients and moderate to severe moist desquamation in 22%. No conclusive data on chronic toxicity were available.

Recently, Bush et al. (2007) reported on a new technique of proton partial breast irradiation in prone position using titanium surgical clips placed at the boundaries of the excision cavity to assist targeting and daily treatment set-ups. Twenty patients were treated with a multiple fields technique at a total dose of 40 CGE in ten daily fractions of 4 CGE. Ten consecutive CT data sets were used for treatment planning comparison between the proton plan and two methods of photon PBI. The use of the prone position reduced breast respiratory motion during CT acquisition and treatment delivery. DVH comparisons between the two modalities showed a higher volume of nontarget breast tissue and skin receiving significant dose with the two photons plans compared to protons.

Several new proton centers all over the world have recently opened or are in the construction phase. There is a growing capacity to treat more patients with a wide variety of malignancies where the sparing of adjacent critical structure is required, including breast cancer. Nevertheless, the enthusiasm generated by proton dose distribution should always first consider clinical data investigating substantial improvements in efficacy and safety of breast irradiation.

11.10   Summary

All techniques used for PBI, including BRT, MammoSite, intraoperative orthovoltage radiotherapy, electron intraoperative radiotherapy, and 3-D conformal or intensity-modulated external beam radiotherapy, have similar indications, but differ in the source of radiation as well as volume of breast treated. Eight randomized phase III trials were designed to investigate the role of PBI. The ELIOT trial has been closed and results are pending. The only completed phase III trial that published long-term results is the Hungarian trial that reported no significant difference between PBI and WBI in the 5-year actuarial rate of LR, overall, cancer-specific, and disease-free survival. The fact that the median age of the randomized patients was 59 with more than 70% being postmenopausal supports the efficacy of this treatment modality in elderly women. Other Phase II and III trials evaluating adjuvant peroperative modalities are actively recruiting patients in United States, Europe, United Kingdom, and Australia. Final results are pending and identification of patients appropriate for PBI remains under investigation. Long-term results from these trials will be necessary to ultimately demonstrate late effects, LR rate, and survival data with these approaches. Although still preliminary, the positive data released in studies on PBI of the recent past suggest that a change in treatment paradigm for early disease management can be reasonably expected in a short time. This implies that PBI could be proposed in selected patients based on individual clinical evaluation and informed consent. An attempt to identify eligible patients can be made considering the different distribution of risk factors in the current PBI trials. Patients with a significant risk of harboring microscopic disease within the breast located outside the index quadrant are not optimal candidates for PBI. Early experiences had to be very highly selective and two societies have pointed out very

Table 11.1 Median age of patients treated with PBI in phase I-II trials

Study	Median age (years)
RTOG 95-17 (Arthur et al. 2008)	62
William Beaumont Hospital (LDR/HDR) (Vicini et al. 2007)	65
ASBS Registry trial (Vicine et al. 2008)	65
William Beaumont Hospital (3D conformal) (Chen et al. 2008)	62
RTOG 0319 (Vicini et al. 2008)	61

strict selection criteria. The American Brachytherapy Society patients selection criteria include: ≥ 45 years of age, invasive ductal carcinoma only, tumor size $\leq$ 3 cm, negative resection margins (defined as no tumor on ink), and negative axillary nodal status. Although similar in concept, the patients selection criteria endorsed by the American Society of Breast Surgeons includes: ≥ 50 years of age, invasive ductal carcinoma or ductal carcinoma in situ, tumor size of ≤ 2 cm, negative resection margin (defined as at least 2 mm in all directions), and a negative axillary nodal status. The age criteria (≥ 45 and ≥ 50) was adopted by the two society because most women treated with PBI in reported experiences with > 5 years follow-up showing LR rate comparable to conventional treatment were postmenopausal having a median age of > 60 years. Table 11.1 reports the median age of patients treated with PBI in Phase I-II trials and single/multiinstitutional experience with longer follow-up. (Arthur et al. 2008; Vicini et al. 2007, 2008; Chen et al. 2008; Vicini et al. 2008) In reviewing the literature, many authors added other features into eligibility criteria in order to maintain a very prudent approach to PBI, as there is no presence of an EIC, no G3, and no vascular invasion, until more definitive data are available. More controversial is the role of lymph node involvement; some investigators consider PBI only for N0 patients, whereas others treat patients up to three positive nodes with this technique. Overall, the higher percentage of low-risk factors associated with a demonstrated lower risk of local relapse in postmenopausal breast cancer patients could justify the use of PBI in this age group. Nonetheless, even patients who would be treated outside clinical trials must receive PBI in centers with adequate expertise that can evaluate the best technical approach and within well-defined quality assurance protocols.

It is not unusual to see older patients decline BCS because receiving 6 weeks of RT would be too demanding. Numerous studies found that elderly patients tend to undergo mastectomy instead of BCS, because of a number of barriers to receiving the standard adjuvant RT (Lazovich et al. 1991; Newcomb et al. 1993; Nold et al. 2000). Older patients living far away from a radiation facility often find it difficult to bear the costs of relocating for the treatment or to find transportation to and from a radiation facility on a daily basis. PBI in elderly patients, by reducing the inconvenience of the conventional 6 weeks of daily RT to zero in the case of IORT or a maximum of a week for most of the other procedures, is expected to be more accepted, thereby increasing the rate of women undergoing BCS instead of mastectomy. PBI, by better targeting and tailoring postoperative radiotherapy, could farther reduce morbidity that will eliminate the fear for the dreaded side effects and, coupled with a less tiresome treatment, in the long term could also increase survival by motivating more elderly women to an earlier detection.

References

Arthur DW, Koo D, Zwicker RD et al (2003) Partial breast brachytherapy after lumpectomy: low-dose-rate and high-dose-rate experience. Int J Radiat Oncol Biol Phys 56:681–689

Arthur DW, Winter K, Kuske RR et al (2008) A phase II trial of brachytherapy alone after lumpectomy for select breast cancer: tumor control and survival outcomes of RTOG 95-17. Int J Radiat Oncol Biol Phys 72(2):467–473

Bartelink H, Horiot JC, Poortmans P et al (2001) Recurrence rates after treatment of breast cancer with standard radiotherapy with or without additional radiation. N Engl J Med 345:1378–1387

Bush DA, Slater JD, Garberoglio C et al (2007) A technique of partial breast irradiation utilizing proton beam radiotherapy: comparison with conformal x-ray therapy. Cancer J 13(2):114–118

Chen PY, Gustafson GS, Mitchell C et al (2008) Three-year clinical experience utilizing 3D-conformal radiation therapy to deliver accelerated partial breast irradiation (APBI). Int J Radiat Oncol Biol Phys 72(1):S3–S4

Clarke M, Collins R, Darby S et al (2005) Effects of radiotherapy and of differences in the extent of surgery for early breast cancer on local recurrence and 15-year survival: an overview of the randomised trials. Lancet 366:2087–2106

Cuttino LW, Keisch M, Jenrette JM et al (2008) Multi-institutional experience using the MammoSite radiation therapy system in the treatment of early-stage breast cancer: 2-year results. Int J Radiat Oncol Biol Phys 71(1):107–114

Formenti SC, Truong MT, Goldberg JD et al (2004) Prine accelerated partial breast irradiation after breast conserving surgery: preliminary clinical results and dose-volume histogram analysis. Int J Radiat Oncol Biol Phys 60(2):493–504

Holmes DR, Baum M, Joseph D (2007) The TARGIT trial: targeted intraoperative radiation therapy versus conventional postoperative whole-breast radiotherapy after breast-conserving surgery for the management of early-stage invasive breast cancer (a trial update). Am J Surg 194:507–510

Ivaldi GB, Leonardi MC, Orecchia R et al (2008) Preliminary results of electron intraoperative therapy boost and hypofractionated external beam radiotherapy after breast-conserving surgery in premenopausal women. Int J Radiat Oncol Biol Phys 72(2):485–493

Keisch M, Vicini F, Kuske RR et al (2003) Initial clinical experience with the MammoSite breast brachytherapy applicator in women with early stage breast cancer treated with breast-conserving therapy. Int J Radiat Oncol Biol Phys 55:289–293

Kozak KR, Smith BL, Adams J et al (2006) Accelerated partial-breast irradiation using proton beams: initial clinical experience. Int J Radiat Oncol Biol Phys 66:691–698

Lazovich DA, White E, Thomas DB et al (1991) Underutilization of breast-conserving surgery and radiation therapy among women with stage I or II breast cancer. JAMA. 266:3433–3438

Lomax AJ (2008) Intensity modulated proton therapy and its sensitivity to treatment uncertainties 2: the potential effects of inter-fraction and inter-field motions. Phys Med Biol 53(4):1043–1056

Luini A, Orecchia R, Gatti G et al (2005) The pilot trial on intraoperative radiotherapy with electrons (ELIOT): update on the results. Breast Cancer Res Treat 93:55–59

Mussari S, Sabino Della Sala W, Busana L et al (2006) Full-dose intraoperative radiotherapy with electrons in breast cancer. First report on late toxicity and cosmetic results from a single-institution experience. Strahlenther Onkol 182(10):589–595

Newcomb PA, Carbone PP (1993) Cancer treatment and age: patient perspectives. J Natl Cancer Inst 85:1580–1584

Nold RJ, Beamer RL, Helmer SD et al (2000) Factors influencing a woman's choice to undergo breast-conserving surgery versus modified radical mastectomy. Am J Surg 180:413–418

NSABP B-39, RTOG 0413 (2006) A Randomized Phase III Study of conventional whole breast irradiation versus partial breast irradiation for women with stage 0, I, or II breast cancer. Clin Adv Hematol Oncol 4:719–721.

Petit JY, Veronesi U, Rey P et al (2008) Nipple-sparing mastectomy: risk of nipple-areolar recurrences in a series of 579 cases. Breast Cancer Res Treat 114:97–101

Polgár C, Major T, Fodor J et al (2004) High-dose-rate brachytherapy alone versus whole breast radiotherapy with or without tumor bed boost after breast-conserving surgery: seven-year results of a comparative study. Int J Radiat Oncol Biol Phys 60:1173–1181

Polgár C, Lovey K, Major T et al (2006) Partial breast irradiation (PBI) versus whole breast irradiation (WBI) after breast conserving surgery for low risk breast cancer patients: 5-year results of a randomized study. Radiother Oncol 81:S148

Proulx GM, Stomper PC, Hurd T et al (2001) Breast-conserving therapy (BCT): radiatiating the entire breast may not be necessary. Breast J 7(4):275

Reitsamer R, Sedlmayer F, Kopp M et al (2006) The Salzburg concept of intraoperative radiotherapy for breast cancer: results and considerations. Int J Cancer 118:2882–2887

Strnad V, Ott O, Pötter R et al (2004) Interstitial brachytherapy alone after breast conserving surgery: interim results of a German-Austrian multicenter phase II trial. Brachytherapy 3(3):115–119

Vaidya JS, Baum M, Tobias JS et al (2001) Targeted inra-operative radiotherapy (TARGIT): an innovative method of treatment for early breast cancer. Ann Oncol 12:1075–1080

Veronesi U, Marubini E, Mariani L et al (2001) Radiotherapy after breast-conserving surgery in small breast carcinoma: long-term results of a randomized trial. Ann Oncol 12:997–1003

Veronesi U, Cascinelli N, Mariani L et al (2002) Twenty-year follow-up of a surgery with radical mastectomy for early breast cancer. N Engl J Med 16:1227–1232

Vicini F, Beitsch PD, Quiet CA et al (2008) Three-year analysis of treatment efficacy, cosmesis, and toxicity by the American Society of Breast Surgeons MammoSite Breast Brachytherapy Registry Trial in patients treated with accelerated partial breast irradiation (APBI). Cancer 112:758–766

Vicini FA, Kestin L, Chen P et al (2003a) Limited-field radiation therapy in the management of early stage breast cancer. J Natl Cancer Inst 95:1205–1210

Vicini FA, Remouchamps V, Wallace M et al (2003b) Ongoing clinical experience utilizing3D conformal external beam radiotherapy to deliver partial-breast irradiation in patients with early-stage breast cancer treated with breast-conserving therapy. Int J Radiat Oncol Biol Phys 57(5):1247–1253

Vicini FA, Antonucci JV, Wallace M et al (2007) Long-term efficacy and patterns of failure after accelerated partial breast irradiation: a molecular assay-based clonality evaluation. Int J Radiat Oncol Biol Phys 68(2):341–346

Vicini FA, Winter K, Straube W et al (2008) Initial efficacy results of RTOG 0319: three dimensional conformal radiation therapy (3D-CRT) confined to the region of the lumpectomy cavity for state I/II breast carcinoma. Int J Radiat Oncol Biol Phys 72(1):S3

Chapter 12
General and Local Anesthetics

Bernadette Th. Veering

12.1 Introduction

As the elderly population continues to increase and surgical techniques and management continue to improve, the number of elderly surgical patients will continue to grow.

An aging population carries profound implications for the practice of anesthesiology. Geriatric issues impact every aspect of anesthesiology. The preoperative evaluation of the geriatric patient is typically more complex than that of the younger patient because of the heterogeneity of this patient group and the greater number and complexity of comorbid conditions that usually accumulate with age. An understanding of general concepts of human aging and of organ function in older adults may contribute to adequate perioperative management of the elderly patient. One of the most important manifestations of aging is increased sensitivity to internal and external environmental stressful stimuli. With an acute disease or a surgical procedure, the elderly may be more prone to complications given their diminished reserve capacity and decreased ability to respond to the demand. Normal aging results in changes in cardiac, respiratory, and renal physiology. Because of physiologic heterogeneity, the response of the elderly patient to surgical stress is often unpredictable.

12.2 The Risk of Anesthesia in the Elderly

Aging per se is not a major factor in predicting the risk of anesthesia and operation. The overall physical status or disease state or both are better predictors of outcome (Dunlop et al. 1993) (Fig. 12.1). The American Society of Anesthesiologists (ASA)

B.Th. Veering (✉)
Department of Anesthesiology, Leiden University Medical Center, Leiden, The Netherlands
e-mail: b.th.veering@lumc.nl

M.W. Reed and R.A. Audisio (eds.), *Management of Breast Cancer in Older Women*,
DOI 10.1007/978-1-84800-265-4_12, © Springer-Verlag London Limited 2011

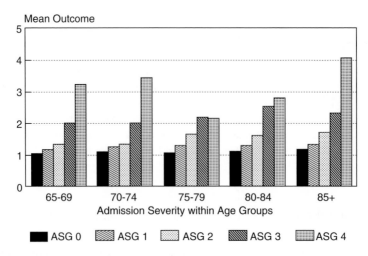

Fig. 12.1 Effect of admission severity (ASG) and age on outcome, showing that mean outcome increases with admission severity in each age group. Reprinted from Dunlop et al. (1993) with permission from Elsevier

physical status classification system, also known as the ASA score, has been a good predictor of risk of death following surgery in patients of 80 years of age and older (Table 12.1). Risk is directly related to the number and extent of coexisting preoperative diseases. Ischemic heart disease, diabetes mellitus, hypertension, chronic respiratory disease, and impaired renal function are the preoperative conditions most indicative of a higher risk of peri- and postoperative morbidity and mortality. Surgeries involving the abdominal and thoracic cavities and emergency cases have the highest mortality. The importance of the site as a major determinant of perioperative risk in the elderly applies equally to both emergency and elective surgery.

12.3   Body Composition, Pharmacokinetics, and Pharmacodynamics

Major changes occur in overall body composition as people become older. Total body water volume decreases because there is a loss of intracellular water with advancing age. There is a decrease in lean body mass as a proportion of total body mass and a relative increase in body fat with age, which is slightly higher in women than in men.

Aging affects both pharmacokinetics and pharmacodynamics (Vuyk 2003; Sadean and Glass 2003). Age-related changes in proportions of body water and fat may affect drug disposition. Water-soluble drugs may be expected to distribute into smaller apparent volumes, resulting in higher initial plasma concentrations following a bolus. Lipid-soluble drugs (inhalation agents, barbiturates, benzodiazepines) may demonstrate increased distribution volumes.

Albumin and α_1 [alpha$_1$]-acid glycoprotein (AAG) are the primary sites of plasma protein binding. Albumin concentrations decrease with age, while AAG concentrations do not change with age (Veering et al. 1990). The reduced concentration of albumin would be expected to result in reduced binding of acid drugs, for which albumin is the major binding protein.

Pharmacodynamic changes (concentration-response changes) reflect differences in pharmacological sensitivity, which are not directly related to pharmacokinetic changes. Changes in pharmacodynamics may lie at a number of points between the drug/receptor interaction and the final pharmacological effect (Vuyk 2003). The pharmacodynamics of anesthetic drugs in elderly patients have not been studied extensively. Despite the lack of pharmacodynamic information available, it is generally agreed that elderly patients require less anesthetic drugs, as they seem to be more sensitive to them.

12.4   Anesthetic Technique for Breast Cancer Surgery

Breast carcinoma surgery can be performed under local, general, or regional anesthesia.

12.5   Local Anesthesia

Local anesthesia was reported to be safe in 27 patients with poor preoperative medical condition undergoing simple mastectomy (Oakley et al. 1996). The limits of this technique include difficulties to perform axillary dissection and the potential systemic toxicity of high doses of local anesthetic agents.

12.6   General Anesthesia

The central nervous system (CNS) is the target organ for most anesthetic drugs and adjuvants. The precise neuro-anatomic basis for the age-related decline in anesthetic requirement is unknown. Reduced neuron quantity or quality, decrease in synaptic transmission, a reduction in the number of receptor sites, or a combination of these factors may contribute to the greater sensitivity of elderly patients to the depressant effects of anesthetics that act on the CNS.

Table 12.1   Physical status classification by the American society of anesthesiologists

Class I	Healthy patient, no medical problems
Class II	Mild systemic disease
Class III	Severe systemic disease, but not incapacitating
Class IV	Severe systemic disease that is a constant threat to life
Class V	Moribund, not expected to live 24 h irrespective of operation

Note that the age itself is not a parameter taken into account by the classification

Advanced age is clearly associated with a reduction in median effective dose requirements for all agents that act within the CNS, regardless of whether these drugs are administered via the oral, parenteral, or inhalational route (Table 12.2).

12.6.1   Inhalation Agents

This anesthetic sensitivity is manifested by a decreased minimum alveolar concentration (MAC) of the inhalation agents (Mapleson 1996). The MACs of the individual agents (halothane, isoflurane, desflurane, and sevoflurane) decrease by about 4% for each decade after 40. By the age of 80, inhaled anesthetic requirements are generally reduced by 30% compared with younger adults.

12.6.2   Induction Agents

The increased sensitivity of the aged brain to induction agents has been reported to be primarily due to pharmacokinetic differences which occur with aging (Vuyk 2003; Sadean and Glass 2003). The sleep-dose requirement of thiopental, etomidate, and propofol decreases linearly with age.

12.6.3   Opioids

Elderly patients may demonstrate increased sensitivity to opioids (Shafer 2000). Increased effects in the elderly may be explained by either pharmacodynamic or

Table 12.2 Recommendations for dosage adjustment consequence of altered pharmacokinetics and pharmacodynamics in the elderly

Class of drug	Dosage adjustment
Barbiturates	Modest reduction in bolus dose and infusion rates
Etomidate	Reduction of up to 50% in bolus dose
Propofol	Reduction of 30–50% in bolus dose and infusion rates
Benzodiazepines	Reduction of up to 75% in bolus dose and infusion rates
Opioids	Reduction of up to 50% in bolus dose and infusion rates
Nondepolarizing neuromuscular blocking agents	No reduction in bolus dose, but generally reduced infusion rates depending on the drug
Volatile agents	Reduction in inspired concentrations of 0.6% per decade
Local anesthetics	Small to moderate reduction in segmental dose

From Sadean and Glass (2003) With permission from Elsevier

pharmacokinetic differences. It was demonstrated by electroencephalography (EEG) that the most important difference is an increase in pharmacodynamic sensitivity in the elderly compared to the young. Changes in pharmacokinetics of opioids with increasing age do not play a major role.

12.6.4 Muscle Relaxants

The dosages of nondepolarizing agents do not decline in parallel with the age-related atrophy of skeletal muscle because the number of neuromuscular receptors does not decrease with aging. The required initial dose of muscle relaxants does not change in elderly patients. The pharmacodynamics of muscle relaxants is unchanged in the elderly. Aging is accompanied by decrease in hepatic and renal blood flow. Because the majority of nondepolarizing neuromuscular blocking agents are eliminated through hepatic and renal mechanisms, alterations in pharmacokinetics do occur. Their clearance is decreased and elimination half-life is increased, and as a consequence, the time to clinical recovery may be prolonged.

12.6.5 Benzodiazepines

Clinical experience suggests an increased sensitivity to benzodiazepine compounds. Jacobs et al. (1994) showed increased age-related intrinsic sensitivity to midazolam consistent with pharmacodynamic changes and independent of pharmacokinetic factors.

12.7 Regional Anesthesia

Thoracic epidural anesthesia and paravertebral blocks are both regional anesthetic techniques which are suitable for breast surgery.

Thoracic epidural anesthesia is a type of central neural blockade and paravertebral block is a type of a peripheral nerve blockade.

12.7.1 Age-Related Changes Relevant to Regional Anesthesia

Anatomical and physiological changes, associated with advancing age, may affect the nerve block characteristics and the pharmacokinetics following administration of local anesthetics (Veering 1998). A declining number of neurons, deterioration in myelin sheaths in the dorsal and ventral roots, changes in the anatomy of the spine, and intervertebral foramina may contribute to altered nerve block characteristics following a regional anesthetic procedure. Furthermore, the number of axons in peripheral nerves decreases with advancing age, and the conduction velocity diminishes, particularly in motor nerves. With increasing age, changes in the connective tissue ground substances may result in changes in local distribution, i.e., in the distribution rate of the local anesthetic from the site of injection (the epidural space) to the sites of action.

Age may affect peripheral nerve blocks because by the age of 90 years, one third of myelinated fibers disappear from peripheral nerves. By the age of 90 years, one third of the myelinated fibers disappear from peripheral nerves. In addition, conduction velocity, especially of the motor nerve, decreases with age (Dorfman and Bosley 1979).

The clearances of local anesthetic agents following epidural administration decrease with age, possibly resulting in increased accumulation of the local anesthetic solution with continuous epidural infusion or intermittent multiple administrations in the elderly (Veering et al. 1987; Simon et al. 2002).

12.7.2   Thoracic Epidural Anesthesia

Anatomically, the epidural space is a cylindrical space between the dura mater and the ligaments and periosteum lining the vertebral canal, extending from the foramen magnum to the sacrococcygeal membrane. Epidural anesthesia can produce profound anesthesia over a large area by blocking nerve pathways to, from, and most likely also within the neuraxis.

Thoracic epidural anesthesia is used mainly as an adjunct to general anesthesia (combined anesthesia) or as postoperative analgesic technique in patients undergoing breast cancer surgery. When a catheter is placed into the epidural space, a continuous infusion can be maintained for several days, if needed. The optimal level of placement of an epidural catheter depends on the dermatomal level at which the majority of the pain will be perceived. For breast surgery (occurring in the second to fifth intercostal space), the epidural can be placed anywhere between T2 and T4. High segmental thoracic epidural anesthesia extending to C5 appears to be feasible for breast surgery with axillary lymph node dissection. With patient-controlled epidural analgesia (PCEA), a patient has the ability to control postsurgical pain medications administered through the epidural catheter by way of intermittent boluses. PCEA technique can be used only in elderly patients who can participate in self-medication, which excludes those with cognitive dysfunction.

The physiological consequences of epidural anesthesia are almost completely due to sympathetic block affecting major organ systems (Veering and Cousins 2000). High thoracic epidural anesthesia from the first to fifth thoracic blocks the cardiac afferent and efferent sympathetic fibers with loss of chronotropic and inotropic drive to the myocardium.

12.7.2.1   Effect of Age

Performing epidural anesthesia may be more difficult in the elderly patients. It is often not easy to position the elderly patient appropriately because of the anatomical distortion that is to be found in many old people, particularly curvature or rotation of the spine. The inability of the elderly patient to flex the back as much as the younger one makes axial blockade hard.

The level of analgesia increases with advancing age after lumbar epidural administration of a given dose (fixed volume and concentration) of a local anesthetic solution (Veering et al. 1987; Simon et al. 2002) and following thoracic epidural administration of a fixed dose (Hirabayashi and Shimizu 1993) (Fig. 12.2). In older patients, lateral escape of the local anesthetic solution is minimal, due to the sclerotic intervertebral foramina.

12.7.2.2   Advantages of Thoracic Epidural Anesthesia

Thoracic epidural anesthesia covering the cardiac segments (T1–T4) improves myocardial function and is associated with an excellent attenuation of the perioperative stress response by a reversible blockade of sympathetic afferents and efferents (Waurick 2004).

Optimized pain control and early mobilization decrease the risk of pulmonary complications.

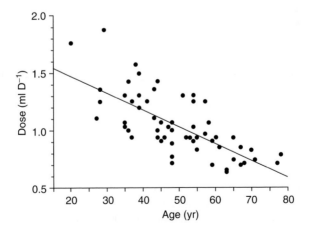

Fig. 12.2   Relationship between age and peridural dose requirement in thoracic epidural anesthesia. D > dermatome. Reproduced from Hirabayashi and Shimizu (1993) Used with permission

12.7.3   Potential Disadvantages of Thoracic Epidural Anesthesia

12.7.3.1   Risk

The most common complication of epidural anesthesia is accidental dural perfora-
tion (Tanaka et al. 1993). Spinal epidural hematoma formation is a rare but devastating complication after epidural anesthesia. An increased risk has been associated
with the use of anticoagulants and clotting disorders. National guidelines with the
establishment of recommended time interval between the administration of anticoagulants and epidural anesthesia or catheter withdrawal have aided in reducing the
incidence of this risk.

12.7.3.2   Hypotension

Hypotension is the most common cardiovascular disturbance associated with
epidural anesthesia, with a particularly frequent incidence in the elderly. It occurs
due to decreases in systemic vascular resistance and central venous pressure from
sympathetic block with vasodilatation and redistribution of central blood volume to
lower extremities and splanchnic beds (Veering and Cousins 2000). High levels of
analgesia and old age appeared to be the two main factors associated with the development of hypotension. A greater spread of analgesia with epidural ropivacaine in
elderly patients was accompanied by a higher incidence of hypotension and brady-
cardia (Simon et al. 2002). Marked hypotension is especially harmful to elderly
patients with limited cardiac reserve. Common strategies used to prevent or reduce
the incidence and severity of hypotension include IV fluid bolus and the use of
vasopressors.

12.7.3.3   Hypothermia

Both accidental and perioperative hypothermia (a decrease in core temperature)
are common in the elderly during general and epidural anesthesia (Frank et al.
1992). Because of age-related changes in temperature regulation, the elderly are
prone to hypothermia during surgery. Thus, low core temperature may not trigger
protective autonomic responses. Higher levels of analgesia are associated with
increased blocking of peripheral sympathetic and motor nerves which prevents
thermoregulatory vasoconstriction and shivering. The greater the proportion of
the body that is blocked, the more impairment of thermoregulatory function is to
be expected. Shivering is also a potentially greater problem in elderly patients,
who have a higher incidence of ischemic heart disease and may not be able to
tolerate the increased oxygen demands associated with the shivering state. The
time required for postoperative rewarming to recover normal body temperature
also appears to increase directly with advancing age. Controlling and monitoring

body temperature in older patients could decrease the risk of hypothermia and its complications.

12.7.3.4 Paravertebral Block

Thoracic paravertebral block (TPVB) is the technique of injecting local anesthetic adjacent to the thoracic vertebra close to where the spinal nerves emerge from the intervertebral foramina (Vila et al. 2007; Boezaart and Raw 2006). This results in ipsilateral somatic and sympathetic nerve blockade in multiple contiguous thoracic dermatomes above and below the site of injection. The quality at the dermatomal site of injection is very high. It is effective in treating acute and chronic pain of unilateral origin from the chest and abdomen. Bilateral use of TPVB has also been described.

Paravertebral blocks are a well-established option to provide anesthesia and postoperative analgesia during breast surgery (Greengrass et al. 1996). This block has the potential to offer long-lasting pain relief and fewer postoperative side effects when used for breast surgery.

Not only is acute pain better controlled, but the development of chronic mastectomy pain syndrome may be reduced by preoperative placement of paravertebral block. In addition, the other general related complications, such as postoperative nausea and vomiting (PONV), and prolonged sedation, are also reduced.

Continuous thoracic paravertebral block (TPVB) placed at 1 level has the obvious advantage of long-term analgesia into the postoperative period (Boezaart and Raw 2006). Pneumothorax after paravertebral catheter placement is a potential disadvantage of this technique; however, the incidence of pneumothorax after single-injection techniques is rare when the blocks are performed by experienced anesthesiologists.

No specific studies have been performed to investigate the effect of age on the clinical profile of paravertebral blocks.

12.8 Postoperative Pain Treatment

The management of postoperative pain in elderly patients can be a difficult task (Aubrun 2005). Older patients have coexisting diseases and concurrent medications, diminished functional status and physiological reserve, and age-related pharmacodynamic and pharmacokinetic changes. Pain assessment presents numerous problems arising from differences in reporting cognitive impairment and difficulties in measurement. The elderly are also at higher risk of adverse consequences from surgery and unrelieved or undertreated pain. Selection of analgesic therapy needs to balance the potential efficacy with the incidence of interactions, complications, or side effects in the postoperative period. Drug titration in the postanesthesia care unit should be encouraged together with analgesia on request in the wards.

Use of small intravenous boluses of morphine in the immediate postoperative period allows a rapid titration of the dose needed for adequate pain relief. Multimodal analgesia, using acetaminophen, nonsteroidal antiinflammatory drugs, or other nonopioid drugs, is the best way to decrease opioid consumption and thus opioid-related adverse events.

Patient controlled analgesia (PCA) devices are very effective means to provide postoperative analgesia in elderly patients. PCA is a method by which the patient controls the amount of pain medicine they receive. The person pushes a button and a device delivers a dose of an opioid into the bloodstream through a vein.

Using PCA, elderly patients self-administer less opioid than young patients, but report comparable pain relief and high satisfaction (Lavand'Homme and de Kock 1998). Morphine is the preferred drug for PCA because it is a well-known, efficient, and inexpensive agent.

Local anesthetic and lipid-soluble opioid at low concentration are often used in thoracic epidural analgesia for postoperative pain relief. A high success rate is dependent on sensory block covering the incision and the drains. Sophisticated analgesic methods like PCA, regional analgesia, and PCEA are not contraindicated in the elderly, but pain relief and side effects should be monitored.

12.9   Postoperative Nausea and Vomiting

Breast surgery performed under general anesthesia is associated with a high incidence of PONV. Between 60 and 80% of patients undergoing mastectomy (with axillary dissection) experience PONV. Pharmacological approaches have been investigated to reduce PONV after breast surgery. Traditional antiemetics (droperidol and metoclopramide) are frequently used for the prevention of PONV during the first 24 h after anesthesia. Antiserotonins (ondansetron, granisetron, tropisetron, dolasetron, and ramosetron) are highly effective for preventing PONV for 24 h postoperatively, compared with traditional antiemetics. Combinations of an antiserotonin (granisetron or dolasetron) and droperidol or dexamethasone are more effective than monotherapy with antiserotonins for preventing PONV after breast surgery (Layeeque et al. 2006).

12.10   Postoperative Cognitive Function

A proportion of mostly elderly orthopedic patients develop early postoperative cognitive dysfunction (POCD), confusion, and delirium, which are all nonspecific symptoms of CNS dysfunction (Newman et al. 2007). POCD is most frequently characterized by an impairment of memory and concentration and can be detected by neuropsychological testing. This postoperative mental condition may persist for several days to several weeks and can result in increased morbidity, delayed functional recovery, and prolonged hospital stay. The mechanism of early postoperative confusion following orthopedic surgery and other operations is probably multifactorial. In most cases recovery of cognitive function is prompt and complete within 1 week in elderly patients. Neither the choice of anesthetic technique nor the modality employed for the management of postoperative pain appears to be an important determinant of postoperative confusion in elderly patients. The factors that most likely explain the development of postoperative brain dysfunction are age, hospitalization, and extension and duration of surgery. The most important risk factors for POCD are increasing age, type of surgical procedure, duration of anesthesia, postoperative complications, and low level of education. Many scientific studies have focused on the comparison between regional and general anesthesia, but beyond the first week after surgery, no beneficial effect of regional anesthesia has been found (Rasmussen et al. 2003).

12.11   Conclusion

Age-associated change of the physiological systems results in impaired function and reserve, which affects most of the organs (there is of course variability of such decline between patients). The importance of this, when it comes to anesthesia, is that such a patient is less able to respond to perioperative stress and more likely to suffer from an adverse postoperative outcome. Complications can, however, be minimized by a combination of careful preoperative, intraoperative, and postoperative care, adapted to the needs of the elderly patient.

An understanding of the physiology of aging and an awareness of concomitant diseases, in combination with careful selection, monitoring, and preoperative assessment and care, can ensure a satisfactory outcome for the majority of these patients. Elderly patients are at greater risk of perioperative morbidity and mortality because of a high incidence of comorbidities. The importance of doing a thorough preoperative evaluation and identifying risk factors cannot be over emphasized in this frail and vulnerable group. Optimal anesthetic management of the elderly involves prior diagnoses and treatment of coexisting disease.

It should always be kept in mind that even if age-related trend of pharmacokinetics is true for many drugs, intersubject variability is usually large. The clinician, therefore, should titrate the lowest available dose against the desired effect in individual patients.

Older subjects are more sensitive to local anesthetic agents. Elderly are also at somewhat greater risk for arterial hypotension due to the sympatholytic consequences of acute peripheral autonomic blockade. Safe regional anesthesia in elderly patients requires reduced clinical doses for the same effect.

No single anesthetic technique has been found to be superior for the elderly, who are at increased risk for cardiopulmonary complications and deterioration of mental function after anesthesia and surgery.

A continuous evaluation of the clinical and often special pharmacological aspects of anesthesia in older patients remains necessary.

References

Aubrun F (2005) Management of postoperative analgesia in elderly patients. Reg Anesth Pain Med 30:363–379

Boezaart AP, Raw RM (2006) Continuous thoracic paravertebral block for major breast surgery. Reg Anesth Pain Med 31:470–476

Dorfman LJ, Bosley TM (1979) Age related changes in peripheral and central nerve conduction in man. Neurology 29:38–44

Dunlop WE, Rosenblood L, Lawrason L et al (1993) Effects of age and severity of illness on outcome and length of stay in geriatric surgical patients. Am J Surg 165:577–580

Frank SM, Beattie C, Christopherson R et al (1992) Epidural versus general anesthesia, ambient operating room temperature, and patient age as predictors of inadvertent hypothermia. Anesthesiology 77:252–257

Greengrass R, O'Brien F, Lyerly K et al (1996) Paravertebral block for breast cancer surgery. Can J Anaesth 43:858–861

Hirabayashi Y, Shimizu R (1993) Effect of age on extradural dose requirement in thoracic extradural anaesthesia. Br J Anaesth 71:445–446

Jacobs R, Reves JG, Marty J et al (1994) Ageing increases pharmacodynamic sensitivity to the hypnotic effect of midazolam. Anest Analg 80:143–148

Lavand'Homme P, de Kock M (1998) Practical guidelines on the postoperative use of patient-controlled analgesia in the elderly. Drugs Aging 13:9–16

Layeeque R, Siegel E, Kass R, Henry-Tillman RS et al (2006) Prevention of nausea and vomiting following breast surgery. Am J Surg 191:767–772

Mapleson WW (1996) Effect of age on MAC in humans: a meta-analysis. Br J Anaesth 76:179–185

Newman S, Stygall J, Hirani S, Shaefi S, Maze M (2007) Postoperative cognitive dysfunction after noncardiac surgery: a systematic review. Anesthesiology 106:572–590

Oakley N, Dennison AR, Shorthouse AJ (1996) A prospective audit of simple mastectomy under local anaesthesia. Eur J Surg Oncol 22:134–136

Rasmussen LS, Johnson T, Kuipers HM et al (2003) Does anaesthesia cause postoperative cognitive dysfunction? A randomised study of regional versus general anaesthesia in 438 elderly patients. Acta Anaesthesiol Scand 47:260–266

Shafer SL (2000) The pharmacology of anesthetic drugs in the elderly patients. Anesthesioly Clin of North Am 18:1–29

Sadean MR, Glass PSA (2003) Pharmacokinetics in the elderly. Best Pract Res Clin Anaesthesiol 17:191–205

Simon MJG, Veering BT, Stienstra R, van Kleef JW, Burm AGL (2002) The effects of age on the neural blockade and hemodynamic changes following epidural anesthesia with ropivacaine. Anesth Analg 94:1325–30

Tanaka K, Watanabe R, Harada T et al (1993) Extensive application of epidural anesthesia and analgesia in a university hospital: incidence of complications related to technique. Reg Anesth 18:34–38

Veering BT (1998) Pharmacological aspects of local anesthetics in the elderly. Acta Anaesth Belg 49:117–122

Veering BT, Cousins MJ (2000) Cardiovascular and pulmonary effects of epidural anaesthesia. Anaesth Intensive Care 28:620–635

Veering BT, Burm AGL, Van Kleef JW et al (1987) Epidural anesthesia with bupivacaine: effects of age on neural blockade and pharmacokinetics. Anesth Analg 66:589–94

Veering BT, Burm AGL, Souverijn JHM et al (1990) The effect of age on serum concentrations of albumin and α_1-acid glycoprotein. Br J clin Pharmac 29:201–206

Vila H Jr, Liu J, Kavasmanech D (2007) Paravertebral block: new benefits from an old procedure. Curr Opin Anaesthesiol 20:316–318

Vuyk J (2003) Pharmacodynamics in the elderly. Best Pract Res Clin Anaesthesiol 17:207–218

Waurick R (2004) Update in thoracic epidural anaesthesia. Best Pract Clin Anaesth 19:201–213

Chapter 13
The Surgical Management of Breast Cancer in Elderly Women

Malcolm W.R. Reed, Lynda Wyld, and Riccardo A. Audisio

13.1 Introduction

One third of all women diagnosed with breast cancer are over 70 years of age, equating to some 13,000 women in the UK annually. As the UK population ages, this number will increase. Whilst many of these older women will be fit for standard therapies, increasing age, frailty, and co-morbidity levels may render some women unfit for certain treatments. This chapter will deal with the role of surgery in these women. It has long been recognized that older women do not receive the same surgical and adjuvant treatments as younger women (Balasubramanian et al. 2003; Wyld et al. 2004; Lavelle et al. 2007; Mustacchi et al. 2003; Eaker et al. 2006; Louwman et al. 2005; BCCOM 2007). Chemotherapy is usually omitted, surgery may be omitted or minimized to be less onerous, (in particular axillary staging is less likely to be performed) and radiotherapy may be omitted after surgery. How these changes impact on local and systemic disease control has been largely studied in the context of observational studies with few good-quality randomized clinical trials having been performed. Rates of local control are inferior when surgery is omitted and there is some suggestion that systemic disease control rates are impaired in the elderly generally, although this is based on few good quality studies (Bouchardy et al. 2003). This is a difficult area to research as survival in this age group is heavily influenced by competing causes of death and the very heterogeneous nature of the population in terms of basal health status. Recent research has demonstrated that surgery, supported by modern anesthetic techniques (general, regional, and local), is well-tolerated, precluding fewer women (Wildiers et al. 2007). However, there are still women for whom extreme age, co-morbidity, and frailty render surgery more hazardous. This chapter will examine the evidence for the role of surgery in older women and suggest alternative strategies for those in whom the risks are raised. The evidence base for these modified strategies is poor,

M.W.R. Reed (✉)
Academic Unit of Surgical Oncology, University of Sheffield and Sheffield Teaching
Hospitals NHS Trust, Sheffield, England, UK
e-mail: m.w.reed@sheffield.ac.uk

M.W. Reed and R.A. Audisio (eds.), *Management of Breast Cancer in Older Women*,
DOI 10.1007/978-1-84800-265-4_13, © Springer-Verlag London Limited 2011

due to a lack of good-quality primary research in this age group and the inherent difficulties in studying disease processes, patient-related variance, and treatment variance in such a heterogeneous patient group.

13.2   Tumor Biology and Stage at Presentation

There are differences in tumor biology, which may make it acceptable to moderate the treatment of breast cancer in older women. The biology of the disease is less aggressive with higher rates of estrogen receptor positivity, reduced rates of HER-2 receptor expression, and a higher rate of favorable histological subtypes such as tubular and mucinous cancers. These features suggest a less aggressive disease course, a longer time to recurrence, and reduced rates of recurrence. However, these beneficial biological features may be offset by a later stage of presentation in the elderly. There is a slightly higher rate of locally advanced and metastatic disease, and the size of the primary cancer is larger. This is likely to be due to a combination of two factors: a lack of screening in the elderly and a lower level of breast awareness and self-examination. It is therefore not clear how these factors interact when examining outcome data and this complicates attempts at extrapolation of outcomes from studies in younger women.

13.3   Impact of Breast Cancer on Survival in Older Women

Increasing age is inevitably associated with a reduction in life expectancy partly due to the normal physiological decline in organ function (senescence) and the increasing incidence of co-morbid diseases. Consequently, overall survival for women with breast cancer is markedly influenced by age, with 73% of women aged 50 to 54 with breast cancer dying of the disease compared to only 29% of women of 85 and over (Diab et al. 2000). There are a number of computer-based algorithms that allow estimation of this interaction (http://www.adjuvantonline.com/index.jsp, http://www.cancermath.net/). Both of these tools, whilst very useful, do not allow for detailed assessment of co-morbidity, but can give useful guidance. As a result of this, breast cancer is proportionately less of a threat to an older woman's life than to a younger woman's, which is one of the justifications for the modified treatment regimes sometimes employed. For younger women, surgery is the mainstay of treatment, and until the 1980s was also the mainstay of treatment for all but the frailest elderly (Kesseler and Seton 1978; Hunt et al. 1980). In the 1980s, the concept of primary hormonal therapy with Tamoxifen was first suggested by researchers in Edinburgh (Preece et al. 1982). This idea rapidly gained popularity as several trials demonstrated that there was no survival disadvantage to omission of surgery in women over the age of 70 and the concept that breast cancer was a systemic disease held sway. Whilst local control rates were inferior, even long-term follow-up showed little detriment in overall survival with only one of the trials showing a slight but significant improvement in survival with surgery, although meta-analysis of all studies demonstrated only a small, nonsignificant trend for improved survival with surgery (Hind et al. 2007). The role of PET is discussed in more detail elsewhere in this book.

Breast cancer-specific mortality in this age group is difficult to determine from the literature. This is due to the fact that outcomes are rarely adjusted to reflect patient co-morbidity, there is widespread disease understaging in older women as many either have no surgery or limited surgery (often excluding axillary staging), and lastly, overall treatment is often substandard when compared to younger patients. All of these factors result in inaccurate or misleading comparisons with younger women's outcomes. Progress in this area can only be made either by the conduct of randomized controlled trials in this age group or detailed observational studies which accurately stratify patient outcomes according to age, disease stage, and health status.

13.4   Age and Surgical Treatment

Aging has significant effects on normal physiological processes (senescence) independent of any associated disease processes. For example, cardiac reserve is reduced due to a reduction in the number of myocytes, a reduction in the number of pacemaker cells, and a reduction in the maximal heart rate with age. Renal reserve is similarly reduced with a halving in the number of nephrons and in renal blood flow by age 70. As a result, tolerance to dehydration and fluid overload are poor. Cognitive function is also reduced, as is balance and coordination, all of which delay recovery or impair tolerance to anesthesia and surgery (Audisio et al. 1997; Ramesh et al. 2005).

However, despite this the operative mortality associated with surgery for breast cancer is negligible (0–0.3%) in most historic series. This reflects the fact that breast surgery is body-surface surgery and causes very little hemodynamic or pulmonary-function disturbance. In addition, most of the surgical procedures are of fairly short duration and patients are ambulatory immediately afterwards. In many cases, the surgery can also be performed under local or regional anesthesia, further reducing the risks. Morbidity is generally low, although lymphedema, chronic wound pain, and the psychological morbidity associated with the loss of a breast may cause some women considerable distress and should not be underestimated.

In addition to the above-mentioned senescent organ impairment, co-morbid diseases are increasingly common with age and may significantly impact on life expectancy and treatment tolerance (Satariano and Ragland 1994). For example, the prevalence of angina in 45–55 year olds is less than 1%, compared to almost 5% in people of 75 and over. Similarly the risk of significant cardiac arrhythmia increases from 0.6 to 4.2% between the ages 45 and 75. Rates of dementia increase from 0.9 to 40% between the ages of 65 and 90 years. These conditions impact significantly on both life expectancy and on the risks associated with anesthesia. As the number of co-morbid conditions increase, the relative risk of death from breast cancer is reduced. As mentioned above there are some computer-based algorithms that allow prediction of life expectancy and relative risk of death from breast cancer with age and co-morbidity (http://www.adjuvantonline.com/index.jsp, http://www.cancermath.net/). These are simple and easy to use and access but perhaps oversimplify the situation when making decisions about whether surgery is appropriate. Simply using the crude number of co-morbid conditions should not be considered as the only criteria for denying a surgical option as the nature and severity of each co-morbidity may have a widely varying impact (Read et al. 2004). A number of more complex and specific scoring systems have been developed to predict life expectancy and guide treatment decision-making in the elderly with cancer. One of the first to be developed was the Charlson Index, which considers both the number and severity of a defined selection of co-morbid diseases and can predict mortality with modest accuracy (Charlson et al. 1987). More recently, the Comprehensive Geriatric Assessment and the multidimensional assessment for cancer in the elderly (MACE) have been developed and validated. These include a detailed assessment of co-morbidity, functional status, cognitive function, and depression scores (Extermann et al. 2004; Gosney 2005). Measures of global functional ability have also been shown to be independently useful in predicting life expectancy. For example, the activities of daily living (ADL), the instrumental activities of daily living (IADL) and the mini mental state examination (MMSE) scores have all been shown to have prognostic value (Repetto et al. 2002; Inouye et al. 1998; Audisio et al. 2005; Pope et al. 2006; Fried et al. 2001).

Some of these tools are relatively time-consuming to administer and may require specialist interpretation. For this reason it has been proposed to utilize quick screening tools during clinical practice in order to provide a thorough assessment and identify frailty (PACE participants 2008).

13.4.1   Surgical treatment and disease control in older women with breast cancer

Until the 1980s when primary endocrine therapy was first proposed, all but the frailest elderly were treated with surgery for their breast cancer. A number of large series of surgical outcomes demonstrated that this was associated with a low morbidity and mortality. Primary endocrine therapy is similarly associated with a low mortality and morbidity with little to choose between the two strategies in older women based on comparative RCT data comparing the two (Hind et al. 2007). Seven randomized trials were performed. All these studies recruited women over the age of 70 with operable breast cancer who were fit for surgery under general anesthesia. Endocrine treatment was with tamoxifen although most of the studies did not assess the estrogen receptor status of the tumors as this was not widely accessible technology at the time. Three studies (Fentiman et al. 2003; Robertson et al. 1992; Gazet et al. 1994) compared surgery without adjuvant tamoxifen to tamoxifen alone. Four studies (Mustacchi et al. 2003; Fennessy et al. 2004; Capasso et al. 2000; Willsher et al. 1997) compared surgery with adjuvant tamoxifen to tamoxifen alone. Surgery included mastectomy or wide local excision with or without radiotherapy combined with axillary clearance or staging in most of the trials.

These studies demonstrated that endocrine therapy alone is inferior to surgery with adjuvant endocrine therapy for the local control of breast cancer in this group of patients. However, meta-analysis demonstrated no significant difference in overall survival between the two treatments. One of the trials showed a small but significant survival advantage for surgery at 13 years follow-up (Fennessy et al. 2004). Despite the lack of clear evidence of survival benefit for surgery, the clear advantage in local disease control suggests that PET should be reserved for women with a poor premorbid state likely to reduce life expectancy to 2–5 years.

Comparison of quality of life between these two treatment strategies has been poorly assessed in the trials with only one undertaking any assessment of this. This comparison showed that surgery was associated with impaired outcomes in the short term, (3 months), and that there is no difference at longer follow-up, (2 years). It is worth noting, however, that the tool used for this assessment was not a breast-cancer-specific QoL tool and it is likely to have been insufficiently sensitive to detect many of the life-domain issues that may be influenced by these treatments (Al-Ghazal et al. 2000; Fobair et al. 2006; Goldberg et al. 1992; Kornblith and Ligibel 2003; Ray 1977).

Another area of concern for the use of PET is the risk that some patients will not comply with their endocrine medication, which will be less of a problem if this medication is an adjuvant to surgery rather than the primary treatment. This may be a particular problem for patients on multiple medications as is commonly the case in the older population. There is good data in the geriatric literature that compliance with medication, especially for women on multiple medications, is poor in this age group.

Furthermore, patients on primary endocrine therapy may be called back more frequently for clinical review than patients who undergo surgery – this may have a negative impact on quality of life, although conversely patients may appreciate the close clinical review and the knowledge that the tumor is reducing in size (Husain et al. 2008; Repetto and Audisio 2006).

However, recent audits demonstrate the continued use of primary endocrine therapy in a substantial proportion of older, less fit patients with breast cancer in the UK (Wyld et al. 2004; Lavelle et al. 2007; BCCOM Report 2007; Wildiers et al. 2007). These studies, demonstrating the continued use of primary endocrine therapy in a substantial proportion of older women, are at variance with the results of a survey of UK breast surgeons, 98% of who state that age alone is not relevant in offering surgery for the treatment of breast cancer. However, 34% of respondents acknowledged that the patient's biological age is a significant factor although less than half utilize any form of assessment of fitness with only a very small minority using tools such as comprehensive geriatric assessment (Audisio et al. 2004). There is also a wide variation in rates of nonsurgical treatments amongst UK surgeons, as demonstrated by the BCCOM audit (2004), which found rates varying from 11 to 40% in women aged 70 and older treated without surgery BCCOM Report 2007.

These findings demonstrate that while surgeons in the UK are open to treating older patients with standard approaches, including surgery, they frequently fail to do so; this is predominantly due to concerns about the patient's fitness and overall life expectancy, as well as lack of familiarity with screening tools for frailty.

Less information is available on the rates of omission of surgery in other countries but recent publications indicate similar trends in other European countries (Eaker et al. 2006; Louwman et al. 2005). Little is known about patient attitudes and choices in relation to these different options. Recent small qualitative studies in the UK demonstrate that this group of patients generally do not show strong preferences and tend to defer decisions about treatments to their physicians with overall high levels of satisfaction with either surgery or primary endocrine therapy (Husain et al. 2008).

Until evidence from clinical trials is available the appropriate management of older patients with breast cancer should include adequate surgery and appropriate adjuvant therapies in all patients. In the subset of patients with a predicted limited life expectancy, due to extreme age or poor functional status, the surgical and adjuvant treatments may be modified or in some cases omitted.

13.5   Surgery to the Breast

There are two main surgical approaches to the treatment of primary breast cancer: mastectomy or wide local excision plus radiotherapy. Overall survival for these two approaches is equivalent, although there is a slightly higher rate of long-term local control for women who have mastectomy. The importance of local control on long-term overall survival outcomes has recently been highlighted by the overview analysis of the Early Breast Cancer Trialists' Collaborative Group. This demonstrated the importance of adequate local treatment in the management of primary operable breast cancer. They demonstrated that for both mastectomy and wide local excision treated patients, radiotherapy reduced the risk of local recurrence. Of great interest was their finding that there was a small but significant survival advantage at 15 years for patients treated with radiotherapy in addition to breast conserving surgery or mastectomy. The benefit in the mastectomy group was predominantly seen in patients with axillary node involvement whereas the survival benefit for patients treated by breast conservation was independent of nodal status. The EBCTCG concluded that "in the hypothetical absence of other causes of death, about one breast cancer death over the next 15 years would be avoided for every four local recurrences avoided." The implication of this for older women with breast cancer is that adequate local control of disease is important and may have a significant impact on survival in women with a life expectancy of between 10 and 15 years. Therefore, for a fit woman of 70 years with a predicted life expectancy of 15 years, treatment should follow standard guidelines based on evidence from trials recruiting younger women. However, in women of more advanced age or with associated co-morbidity where life expectancy may be restricted to less than 5 years it is reasonable to consider alternative approaches. Data from the PRIME trial will be of great value in establishing the importance of radiotherapy following wide local excision in older women. At present, follow-up data from this trial are only very short term, (1 year), but 5, 10, and 15-year survival and local control data will be extremely valuable in advising treatment strategies in these older women.

For any age group of women, the "absolute" indications for mastectomy include large primary tumors, (UICC TNM stage T3), and multifocal disease within more than one quadrant of the breast. In addition, for some women mastectomy may be mandated by a relatively large primary tumor in patients with small breasts, and in patients with an extensive in situ component to their invasive cancer. A further important indication for mastectomy is patient preference. A recent UK audit demonstrated that a significant proportion of patients with small tumors, suitable for breast conservation surgery prefer mastectomy if given a choice BCCOM Report 2007. In older women, primary tumor size is slightly larger than average, which may be one reason for the increased mastectomy rate and older women may be less concerned about the impact of mastectomy on body image and perhaps more anxious about the time and inconvenience that radiotherapy may entail. However, the loss of the breast is still a major cause of psychological distress for many older women. Surgeon and healthcare professional factors may also be important in guiding decision-making about choice of surgery for older women.

Another factor to consider in choice of surgery is whether it necessitates general anesthesia. Some frailer older women may be averse to general anesthesia and for some they may face increased risks. Wide local excision is almost always possible under local anesthetic, whereas for a larger-breasted woman mastectomy under local anesthetic may not be feasible due to the possibility of toxicity levels of the amount of local anesthetic required for adequate anesthesia. However, a series of cases of mastectomy under LA did demonstrate that LA mastectomy was feasible and rarely necessitated the use of harmful levels of local anesthetics (Oakley et al. 1996); however, there are no data on patient tolerance of the procedure or the pain associated with it. Axillary sampling is possible under local anesthetic, although isotope and blue dye guided sentinel node biopsy is now the most appropriate staging procedure. Axillary clearance is not amenable to LA.

For those patients whose tumors are too large for breast conservation or where the tumor is locally advanced and the tumor is ER positive, primary endocrine therapy may be utilized to downstage the tumor. In this neo-adjuvant setting, Letrozole has increased efficacy compared to Tamoxifen, (55 vs. 36% response rate) (Ellis and Ma 2007). Although, there are no data to support the use of neo-adjuvant chemotherapy in this patient group, it may be theoretically possible to use this technique for women with larger ER negative tumors but caution must be exercised in patient selection as toxicity levels are increased in this age group, especially with doxorubicin-based regimes where cardiac and other toxicities may be more significant.

13.6   Surgery to the Axilla

The staging and treatment of the axilla is important for two reasons. Firstly, where there is clear clinical or biopsy proven nodal disease, axillary clearance is indicated to prevent local progression and its attendant morbidity (pain, lymphedema, brachial plexus compression). Increasingly, preoperative axillary ultrasound and biopsy of suspicious nodes is gaining acceptance, and reducing the need for a two-stage surgical procedure in the axilla (sentinel lymph node biopsy followed by clearance). Routine axillary clearance has been superseded by less invasive approaches such as sentinel lymph node biopsy (Fleissig et al. 2006; Veronesi et al. 2003; Mansel et al. 2006). SLNB involves the injection of a radioisotope-labeled colloid and/or blue dye into the breast prior to surgery to localize the first lymph node in the breast drainage nodal chain. The radioactive and/or blue-colored sentinel nodes are identified using a handheld gamma probe and removed at surgery. The degree of axillary dissection is greatly reduced and the procedure is associated with a lower morbidity than standard axillary management (Fleissig et al. 2006). In most centers, standard postoperative histological assessment is performed on the nodes and axillary clearance performed as a second procedure. Some Units undertake peroperative frozen section, imprint cytology, or molecular biological assessment of nodal disease permitting immediate completion of the axillary dissection where axillary nodal metastases are identified. A number of studies have demonstrated the accuracy of SLNB, improved quality of life, and reduced arm morbidity associated with this approach (Fleissig et al. 2006; Veronesi et al. 2003; Mansel et al. 2006). In many ways the SLNB approach is ideally suited to older patients where the potential morbidity associated with more radical axillary surgery may have a greater impact on arm function. It is interesting to note, however, that axillary morbidity following both, standard axillary management or SLNB, is lower in older women than younger women (Fleissig et al. 2006).

Apart from ensuring local disease control, determining the extent of axillary nodal disease is important for estimating prognosis and selecting appropriate adjuvant therapies. Older women are much less likely to be offered adjuvant chemotherapy and therefore some would suggest axillary staging is less important. However, axillary positivity will also determine whether a woman is advised to have adjuvant chest wall or supra-clavicular fossa radiotherapy. Therefore, unless a woman is judged too frail to undergo these treatments, axillary staging should be undertaken.

13.7   Alternative Approaches in Patients with Restricted Life Expectancy

A small number of women will present with breast cancer who are extremely frail due to very advanced age or co-morbidity and for whom life expectancy will be predicted to be very short. Treatment tolerance for all but the simplest interventions will be reduced. For these women, their breast cancer is unlikely to have a major impact on life expectancy, which will be largely determined by their general health status. Similarly, the treatment of their cancer will have little impact and surgery may be an unnecessary imposition, especially if local control can be achieved with endocrine therapy. However, surgical treatment may still be appropriate in such patients to avoid the development of distressing symptoms, such as pain, ulceration, and bleeding due to local disease progression if the disease is estrogen receptor negative. Surgery may be performed under local, regional, or a carefully tailored general anesthetic. Axillary surgery may be omitted in the clinically uninvolved axilla or axillary clearance under a regional block or axillary radiotherapy offered for those with clinical axillary disease. In general terms, even in frail elderly patients, general anesthesia is a safe option with a mortality of less than 1%, although the morbidity may be higher. In such cases a formal anesthetic assessment should be performed prior to surgery by an experienced anesthetist who will recommend the most appropriate approach. This is extensively discussed in Chap. 11.

Omission of axillary surgery in these cases where the axilla is clinically uninvolved and surgery to the primary is only possible under LA, is acceptable and has little impact on overall survival. In women aged 75 or over studies indicate a local axillary progression rate of less than 10%, which, in the majority of cases, can be controlled with radiotherapy (Truong et al. 2002; Rudenstam et al. 2006).

Recently, a number of minimally invasive procedures have been proposed, i.e., percutaneous tumor excision, radio-frequency ablation, focused US ablation, interstitial laser ablation, and cryotherapy. These techniques may be associated with improved cosmetic results, reduced psychological morbidity, and short hospital stay; they require a close interaction with the X-ray department and might be suitable for frail individuals; although, they should be regarded as investigational until more data are available (Vlastos and Verkooijen 2007; Hamazoe et al. 1991; Jeffrey et al. 1999; Singletary et al. 2002).

For those frail elderly women with ER positive disease, primary endocrine therapy may be all that is required to control their disease for the remainder of their life. Disease control rates are high in the short to medium term and in some cases complete tumor resolution may occur. This is discussed in more detail elsewhere in this text.

13.8   Complications of Surgery

Breast cancer surgery is generally regarded as low-risk body-surface surgery and is associated with a very low mortality rate even amongst the elderly. However, morbidity rates can be quite high and include scar formation, wound pain, seroma formation, hematoma, infection, and skin necrosis following mastectomy. Axillary surgery is also associated with complications, including seroma and hematoma, infection, paraesthesia and neuropathic pain, mammary edema, shoulder stiffness, and rarely damage to the long thoracic nerve resulting in "winging" of scapula. The most significant complication of axillary node clearance is lymphedema which may occur in up to 38% of patients following a full axillary clearance (Kissin et al. 1986). Sentinel node biopsy and axillary sampling techniques are less likely to be associated with these complications but may still occur (Fleissig et al. 2006). The incidence of these complications following surgery is not significantly increased by patient age or co-morbidity (Houterman et al. 2004) and in particular the morbidity of axillary surgery may be lower in older women than in younger.

In addition to the physical morbidity of breast cancer surgery, there is also considerable psychological morbidity, especially for those women who undergo mastectomy. There is evidence that physical appearance is less significant in older than in younger women (Franzoi and Koehler 1998; King et al. 2000; Figueiredo et al. 2004).

Uniquely in this older population we have some data of the impact of surgery vs. no surgery in those women who have primary hormonal therapy. Whilst there is no difference in the long-term psychological outcomes between these two treatments, surgery has negative effects at 3 months postoperatively which disappear by 2 years (Fallowfield et al. 1994).

Little is known about the occurrence of postoperative delirium. This is a relatively frequent complication of general anesthesia in the elderly but is rarely studied. The detection of delirium and the early implementation of adequate management can resolve the condition in over 50% cases (Cole et al. 1996). Postoperative delirium independently associates to postoperative morbidity, mortality, length of hospital stay, and costs. An early discharge of elderly women to their usual environment may play a significant role to their psychiatric well-being. It is important to notice how the detection of depression at the diagnosis of cancer is linked to a longer hospital stay; this reinforces the value of utilizing the Comprehensive Geriatric Assessment instruments which also assesses depression.

13.9 Breast Reconstruction and Oncoplastic Surgical Techniques

Over the last 10 years there has been a substantial increase in the rates of breast reconstruction following mastectomy. This has been associated with an increase in the range of approaches available for breast conservation such as therapeutic mammoplasty and breast reshaping by volume displacement known as oncoplastic surgical approaches. These new techniques have had a substantial impact in the management of women with breast cancer but to date the evidence indicates that older women, particularly those over the age of 70 years of age, are not benefiting from breast reconstruction or oncoplastic approaches despite guidelines indicating how these techniques should be widely available. There are a number of potential reasons for this, including patient and health care professional factors, or the assumption that older patients may consider the physical impact of the surgical treatment of breast cancer less important than younger patients and have fewer concerns about their body image (Franzoi and Koehler 1998). However, body integrity is an important issue for some patients and some case series describe excellent results of breast reconstruction in older women. These report the results of techniques using autologous flaps (latissimus dorsi and Transverse Rectus Abdominis Myocutaneous, TRAM flaps) although in general simple implant-based approaches tend to be utilized more frequently in older women (Lipa et al. 2003; Alderman et al. 2003). In addition to patient factors the extremely low utilization of breast reconstruction in women over the age of 75 may indicate that surgeons also have reservations despite the lack of an evidence base. There is no doubt that reconstructive techniques, particularly those utilizing autologous myocutaneous flaps are more major surgical procedures which can be associated with an increased risk of side effects and complications such as flap necrosis. Studies in younger women indicate that these complications are more prevalent in patients with associated co-morbidity and it is this factor which is likely to be influencing surgeons and resulting in a failure to offer these options in the older population of women with breast cancer. Patients are also aware of these concerns and this may contribute to their decision not to seek breast reconstruction (Reaby 1998). The national mastectomy and reconstruction audit being conducted in the UK will provide comprehensive data on this topic within the near future.

13.10 A Surgical Strategy for Older Patients with Breast Cancer

Wherever feasible in women with an expectation of a reasonable life expectancy and where treatments are likely to be well-tolerated, older patients should be treated with standard surgical procedures applicable to younger patients. This should include the choice of breast conservation or mastectomy where appropriate and breast reconstruction or oncoplastic procedures should be included in the options available. The choice of surgical treatment should be decided in consultation with the patient after appropriate information has been made available. The inclusion of a geriatrician within the multidisciplinary team will assist in delivering tailored treatment. The axillary nodal status should be assessed in all suitable patients and nodal metastases should be confirmed by preoperative biopsy or sentinel lymph node biopsy techniques before proceeding to full axillary node clearance or radiotherapy for those patients with nodal disease.

In the subset of patients with an impaired life expectancy due to extreme age or frailty alternative approaches may be considered. These patients should be managed in consultation with specialist geriatricians and anesthetists in addition to surgeons and oncologists. Appropriate assessment tools such as CGA should be utilized and patient preferences carefully sought.

Patients with ER positive tumors may opt for surgery or primary endocrine therapy. In this group of frailer patients surgery may be performed under local or regional anesthesia if not fit for general anesthesia.

The difficult task with these patients is to avoid the onset of distressing symptoms while offering the largest chances of cure; a slight increase in overall survival does not justify any treatment modality that might significantly impair the patient's well-being. It is therefore essential to include patient preferences in the decision-making process and to undertake procedures which combine the minimum risk with the maximum achievable benefit in terms of avoiding morbidity either as a result of the surgical procedure or due to disease progression. In patients with proven axillary node disease complete clearance should be considered; radiotherapy to the axilla is an alternative for frail patients and primary endocrine therapy might be considered when the patient is not fit enough for a prolonged course of radiotherapy. In patients with a clinically node-negative axilla, a sentinel lymph node biopsy may be employed or axillary surgery omitted altogether, particularly for patients with estrogen receptor positive disease.

13.11   Summary

Older women are a very heterogeneous group in terms of their health status and likely treatment tolerances. For the frailer woman, for whom breast cancer may pose a reduced threat to life, and its treatment be associated with increased risk, tailored strategies to surgery may be needed. In some women surgery may be minimized or even avoided without detriment to breast cancer outcomes. The advice of specialist geriatricians and anesthetists will ensure treatment is optimized in each case.

References

Alderman AK, McMahon L Jr, Wilkins EG (2003) The national utilization of immediate and early delayed breast reconstruction and the effect of sociodemographic factors. Plast Reconstr Surg 111:695–703; discussion 704–705

Al-Ghazal SK, Fallowfield L, Blamey RW (2000) Comparison of psychological aspects and patient satisfaction following breast conserving surgery, simple mastectomy and breast reconstruction. Eur J Cancer 36:1938e43

Audisio RA, Veronesi P, Ferrario L, Cipolla C, Andreoni B, Aapro MS (1997) Elective surgery in gastrointestinal tumors in the aged. Ann Oncol 8(4):317–327

Audisio RA, Osman N, Audisio MM et al (2004) How do we manage breast cancer in the elderly patients? A survey among members of the British Association of Surgical Oncologists (BASO). Crit Rev Oncol Hematol 52:135–141

Audisio RA, Ramesh H, Longo WE et al (2005) Preoperative assessment of surgical risk in oncogeriatric patients. Oncologist 10:262–268

Balasubramanian SP, Murrow S, Holt S et al (2003) Audit of compliance to adjuvant chemotherapy and radiotherapy guidelines in breast cancer in a cancer network. Breast 12:136–141

BCCOM (2007) Breast Cancer Clinical Outcome Measures Report. http://www.wmpho.org.uk/wmciu/documents/BCCOM%20Year%20.3%20report.pdf

Breast Cancer Clinical Outcome Measures (BCCOM) Report 2007 http://www.wmpho.org.uk/wmciu/documents/BCCOM%20Year%203%20report.pdf

Bouchardy C, Rapiti E, Fioretta G et al (2003) Undertreatment strongly decreases prognosis of breast cancer in elderly women. J Clin Oncol 21:3580–3587

Capasso INF, Labonia V et al (2000) Survery + tamoxifen vs tamoxifen as treatment of stage I and II breast cancer in over to 70 years old women; Ten years follow-up. Ann Oncol 11(4):20

Charlson ME, Pompei P, Ales KL et al (1987) A new method of classifying prognostic comorbidity in longitudinal studies: development and validation. J Chronic Dis 40:373–383

Cole MG, Primeau F, McCusker J (1996) Effectiveness of interventions to prevent delirium in hospitalized patients: a systematic review. CMAJ 155:1263–1268

Diab SG, Elledge RM, Clark GM (2000) Tumor characteristics and clinical outcome of elderly women with breast cancer. J Natl Cancer Inst 92:550–556

Eaker S, Dickman PW, Bergkvist L et al (2006) Differences in management of older women influence breast cancer survival: results from a population-based database in Sweden. PLoS Med 3:e25

Ellis MJ, Ma C (2007) Letrozole in the neoadjuvant setting: the P024 trial. Breast Cancer Res Treat 105:33–43

Extermann M, Meyer J, McGinnis M et al (2004) A comprehensive geriatric intervention detects multiple problems in older breast cancer patients. Crit Rev Oncol Hematol 49:69–75

Fallowfield LJ, Hall A, Maguire P et al (1994) Psychological effects of being offered choice of surgery for breast cancer. BMJ 309:448

Fennessy M, Bates T, MacRae K et al (2004) Late follow-up of a randomized trial of surgery plus tamoxifen versus tamoxifen alone in women aged over 70 years with operable breast cancer. Br J Surg 91:699–704

Fentiman IS, van Zijl J, Karydas I et al (2003) Treatment of operable breast cancer in the elderly: a randomized clinical trial EORTC 10850 comparing modified radical mastectomy with tumorectomy plus tamoxifen. Eur J Cancer 39:300–308

Figueiredo MI, Cullen J, Hwang Y-T, Rowland JH, Mandelblatt JS (2004) Breast cancer treatment in older women: Does getting what you want improve your long term body image and mental health? J Clin Oncol 22(19):4002–4009

Fleissig A, Fallowfield LJ, Langridge CI et al (2006) Post-operative arm morbidity and quality of life. Results of the ALMANAC randomized trial comparing sentinel node biopsy with standard axillary treatment in the management of patients with early breast cancer. Breast Cancer Res Treat 95:279–293

Fobair P, Stewart SL, Chang S et al (2006) Body image and sexual problems in young women with breast cancer. Psychoncology 15:579e94

Franzoi SL, Koehler V (1998) Age and gender differences in body attitudes: a comparison of young and elderly adults. Int J Aging Hum Dev 47:1–10

Fried LP, Tangen CM, Walston J et al (2001) Frailty in older adults: evidence for a phenotype. J Gerontol A Biol Sci Med Sci 56(3):M146–M156

Gazet JC, Ford HT, Coombes RC et al (1994) Prospective randomized trial of tamoxifen vs surgery in elderly patients with breast cancer. Eur J Surg Oncol 20:207–214

Goldberg JA, Scott RN, Davidson PM et al (1992) Psychological morbidity in the first year after breast surgery. Eur J Surg Oncol 18:327e31

Gosney MA (2005) Clinical assessment of elderly people with cancer. Lancet Oncol 6:790–797

Hamazoe R, Maeta M, Murakami A et al (1991) Heating efficiency of radiofrequency capacitive hyperthermia for treatment of deep-seated tumors in the peritoneal cavity. J Surg Oncol 48:176–179

Hind D, Wyld L, Reed MW (2007) Surgery, with or without tamoxifen, vs tamoxifen alone for older women with operable breast cancer: Cochrane Review. Br J Cancer 96:1025–1029

Houterman S, Janssen-Heijnen ML, Verheij CD et al (2004) Comorbidity has negligible impact on treatment and complications but influences survival in breast cancer patients. Br J Cancer 90:2332–2337

Hunt KE, Fry DE, Bland KI (1980) Breast carcinoma in the elderly patient: an assessment of operative risk, morbidity and mortality. Am J Surg 140:339–342

Husain LS, Collins K, Reed M et al (2008) Choices in cancer treatment: a qualitative study of the older women's (>70 years) perspective. Psychoncology 17:410–416

Inouye SK, Peduzzi PN, Robison JT et al (1998) Importance of functional measures in predicting mortality among older hospitalized patients. JAMA 279:1187–1193

Jeffrey SS, Birdwell RL, Ikeda DM et al (1999) Radiofrequency ablation of breast cancer: First report of an emerging technology. Arch Surg 134:1064–1068

Kesseler HJ, Seton JZ (1978) The treatment of operable breast cancer in the elderly female. Am J Surg 135:664–666

King MT, Kenny P, Shiell A, Hall J, Boyages J (2000) Quality of life 3 months and 1 year after first treatment for early stage breast cancer: Influence of treatment and patient characteristics. Qual Life Res 9:789–800

Kissin MW, Querci della Rovere G, Easton D et al (1986) Risk of lymphedema following the treatment of breast cancer. Br J Surg 73:580–584

Kornblith AB, Ligibel J (2003) Psychosocial and sexual functioning of survivors of breast cancer. Semin Oncol 30:799e813

Lavelle K, Todd C, Moran A et al (2007) Non-standard management of breast cancer increases with age in the UK: a population based cohort of women > or >65 years. Br J Cancer 96:1197–1203

Lipa JE, Youssef AA, Kuerer HM et al (2003) Breast reconstruction in older women: advantages of autogenous tissue. Plast Reconstr Surg 111:1110–1121

Louwman WJ, Janssen-Heijnen ML, Houterman S et al (2005) Less extensive treatment and inferior prognosis for breast cancer patient with comorbidity: a population-based study. Eur J Cancer 41:779–785

Mansel RE, Fallowfield L, Kissin M et al (2006) Randomized multicenter trial of sentinel node biopsy versus standard axillary treatment in operable breast cancer: the ALMANAC Trial. J Natl Cancer Inst 98:599–609

Mustacchi G, Ceccherini R, Milani S et al (2003) Tamoxifen alone versus adjuvant tamoxifen for operable breast cancer of the elderly: long-term results of the phase III randomized controlled multicenter GRETA trial. Ann Oncol 14:414–420

Oakley N, Dennison AR, Shorthouse AJ (1996) A prospective audit of simple mastectomy under local anesthesia. Eur J Surg Oncol 22:134–136

PACE participants (2008) Shall we operate? Preoperative assessment in elderly cancer patients (PACE) can help – a SIOG surgical task force prospective study. Crit Rev Oncol Hematol 65(2):156–163

Pope D, Ramesh H, Gennari R, Corsini G, Maffezzini M, Hoekstra HJ, Mobarak D, Sunouchi K, Stotter A, West C, Audisio RA (2006) Pre-operative assessment of cancer in the elderly (PACE): a comprehensive assessment of underlying characteristics of elderly cancer patients prior to elective surgery. Surg Oncol 15(4):189–197

Preece PE, Wood RA, Mackie CR et al (1982) Tamoxifen as initial sole treatment of localised breast cancer in elderly women: a pilot study. Br Med J (Clin Res Ed) 284:869–870

Ramesh HSJ, Pope D, Gennari R, Audisio RA (2005) Optimising Surgical Management of Elderly Cancer Patients. World J Surg Oncol 3:17

Ray C (1977) Psychological implications of mastectomy. Br J Soc Clin Psychol 16:373e7

Reaby LL (1998) Reasons why women who have mastectomy decide to have or not to have breast reconstruction. Plast Reconstr Surg 101:1810–1818

Read WL, Tierney RM, Page NC, Costas I, Govindan R, Spitznagel EL, Piccirillo JF (2004) Differential prognostic impact of comorbidity. J Clin Oncol 22(15):3099–3103

Repetto L, Audisio RA (2006) Elderly patients have become the leading drug consumers: it's high time to properly evaluate new drugs within the real targeted population. J Clin Oncol 24(35):e62–e63

Repetto L, Fratino L, Audisio RA et al (2002) Comprehensive geriatric assessment adds information to Eastern Cooperative Oncology Group performance status in elderly cancer patients: an Italian Group for Geriatric Oncology Study. J Clin Oncol 20:494–502

Robertson JF, Ellis IO, Elston CW, Blamey RW (1992) Mastectomy or tamoxifen as initial therapy for operable breast cancer in elderly patients: 5-year follow-up. Eur J Cancer 28A(4–5):908–910

Rudenstam CM, Zahrieh D, Forbes JF et al (2006) Randomized trial comparing axillary clearance versus no axillary clearance in older patients with breast cancer: first results of International Breast Cancer Study Group Trial 10–93. J Clin Oncol 24:337–344

Satariano WA, Ragland DR (1994) The effect of comorbidity on 3-year survival of women with primary breast cancer. Ann Intern Med 120:104–110

Singletary SE, Fornage BD, Sneige N et al (2002) Radiofrequency ablation of early-stage invasive breast tumors: An overview. Cancer J 8:177–180

Truong PT, Bernstein V, Wai E et al (2002) Age-related variations in the use of axillary dissection: a survival analysis of 8038 women with T1-ST2 breast cancer. Int J Radiat Oncol Biol Phys 54:794–803

Veronesi U, Paganelli G, Viale G et al (2003) A randomized comparison of sentinel-node biopsy with routine axillary dissection in breast cancer. N Engl J Med 349:546–553

Vlastos G, Verkooijen HM (2007) Minimally invasive approaches for diagnosis and treatment of early-stage breast cancer. Oncologist 12(1):1–10

Wildiers H, Kunkler I, Biganzoli L et al (2007) Management of breast cancer in elderly individuals: recommendations of the International Society of Geriatric Oncology. Lancet Oncol 8:1101–1115

Willsher PC RJ, Jackson L, Al-Hilaly M, Blamey RW (1997) Investigation of primary tamoxifen therapy for elderly patients with operable breast cancer. The Breast 6:150–154

Wyld L, Garg DK, Kumar ID et al (2004) Stage and treatment variation with age in postmenopausal women with breast cancer: compliance with guidelines. Br J Cancer 90:1486–1491

Chapter 14
Breast Reconstruction

Marcus J.D. Wagstaff, Malcolm W.R. Reed, and Christopher M. Caddy

14.1 Introduction

Surgeons are invited to discuss breast reconstruction with all breast cancer patients (Improving Outcomes in Breast Cancer – Manual Update 2002). In practice, this counseling and decision-making process is not solely surgeon- and patient-based, but is frequently complemented by the breast care nurse and other members of the multidisciplinary team. The intention is that this recommendation should apply equally to the older patient as to the younger. This chapter presents what is relevant to this older group of patients and how this may affect our practice. For the purposes of this chapter, and keeping in line with the literature discussed below, older or elderly patients are defined as those over 60 years of age.

The literature specifically relating to issues regarding breast reconstruction in the elderly patient is sparse. Previous studies have addressed changes in body image, patient preferences, technical aspects and risks of surgery, and outcomes, but no prospective study has been undertaken to follow a group of patients through the journey with comparison to their younger counterparts. Randomized controlled trials are difficult in this group where patients make an active choice whether to have a reconstruction and, if so, the type of reconstruction.

In the absence of specific trials in the elderly, clinicians and patients have had to rely on data and experience accrued from treating younger patients. There are, however, significant changes associated with increasing age, including psychological, psychosocial, and medical (co-morbid) conditions. In this chapter, we review the standard approaches to breast reconstruction in younger patients with the considerations necessary when applying these to the population of older women with breast cancer.

M.J.D. Wagstaff (✉)
Department of Reconstruction Plastic and Burns Surgery, University of Sheffield and Sheffield Teaching Hospitals NHS Trust, Sheffield, England, UK
e-mail: wagstaff@doctors.org.uk

M.W. Reed and R.A. Audisio (eds.), *Management of Breast Cancer in Older Women*, 213
DOI 10.1007/978-1-84800-265-4_14, © Springer-Verlag London Limited 2011

14.2 An Overview of Breast Reconstruction

The aims of unilateral breast reconstruction following mastectomy are to achieve symmetry with the contralateral breast, particularly to restore cleavage, and to improve the quality of life for the patient following breast cancer treatment. Volume match in a bra, and color and contour symmetry out of a bra, can avoid the need for an external prosthesis, with a greater choice of clothing, restoration of femininity, and a feeling of wholeness. These are patient-reported goals outlined in a qualitative study of younger Australian patients (Reaby 1998).

The combination of plastic and oncological surgery principles has led to the development of techniques to improve the cosmetic outcome following breast conserving surgery or mastectomy, known as oncoplastic surgery (Rainsbury 2007). Following breast conserving surgery, smaller (<20% of estimated total breast volume) defects can be reconstructed using volume displacement techniques utilizing local parenchymal or dermoglandular flaps. Larger partial mastectomy defects can be filled with volume replacement techniques such as local perforator or muscle flap transposition. Specific outcomes in older patients have yet to be reported for oncoplastic procedures following breast conserving surgery and therefore these techniques are not discussed in detail here. However, these techniques are applicable to older patients as described in another chapter in this text. For the purposes of this chapter, breast reconstruction relates to the surgical re-creation of the whole breast following mastectomy.

The texture of the reconstruction and its symmetry with the contralateral breast is dependent on the technique selected and applied for each individual patient. This presents the patient and the surgeon with choices, four of which predominate. What follows is a brief description of these techniques for the purposes of subsequent discussion with regard to the older patient. Detailed and varied descriptions of these techniques and their outcomes are described in other texts (Spear 2006).

1. Implant-based reconstruction – An expanding breast implant is sited under the pectoralis major muscle, and expanded over time using saline injected percutaneously via a subcutaneous filler port (Fig. 14.1). This may be a one-stage reconstruction using a prosthesis with a removable or permanent port or a two-stage procedure with a temporary expander implant, requiring subsequent replacement with a permanent reconstruction implant.
2. Pedicled latissimus dorsi (LD) based reconstruction with implant – The LD muscle and an overlying skin island are mobilized and transposed from the back of the patient about its insertion on the upper humerus, passed through a subcutaneous tunnel below the axilla, and inset to the breast site (Fig. 14.2). It is inset over an expander or breast implant to complement the volume.
3. Pedicled autologous (utilizing solely the patients own tissue) reconstruction – The LD muscle and skin paddle can be harvested, with surrounding fat and fascia to provide enough tissue volume so that an implant is not required (autologous or "extended" LD). Alternatively, skin and fat of the lower abdomen can be raised with the rectus abdominis muscle, passed under a skin bridge and inset

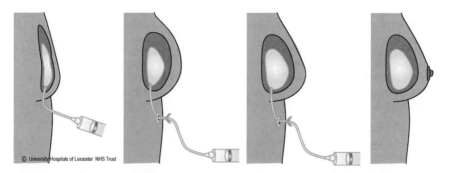

Fig. 14.1 Serial percutaneous breast implant expansion using saline injected into a subcutaneous filler port. Medical Illustration, University Hospitals of Leicester NHS Trust. Used with permission

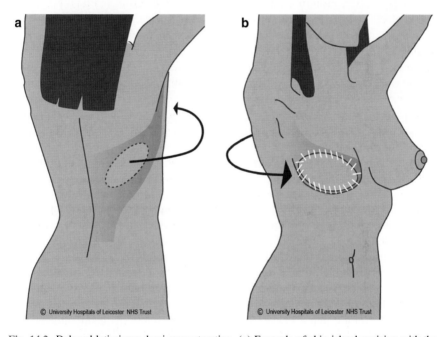

Fig. 14.2 Delayed latissimus dorsi reconstruction. (a) Example of skin island excision with the underlying latissimus dorsi (LD) muscle in situ prior to elevation and transposition under the axillary skin into (b) the breast defect commonly overlying a prosthetic expander or implant. Medical Illustration, University Hospitals of Leicester NHS Trust. Used with permission

into the chest, the pedicled transverse rectus abdominis musculocutaneous (TRAM) flap (Fig. 14.3). The abdominal wall defect is repaired with a synthetic mesh and the skin wound is closed with a hip-to-hip scar, similar to that seen following an abdominoplasty procedure.

4. Free flap tissue transfer – Most commonly taken from the lower abdomen, fat and skin, with or without muscle, are moved and inset into the breast defect by

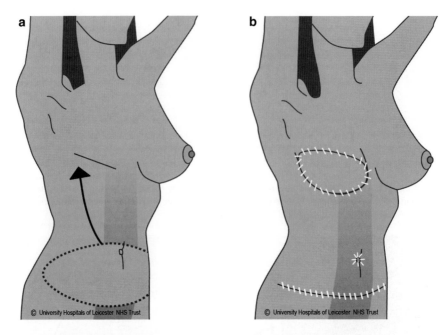

Fig. 14.3 Delayed abdominal flap reconstruction. (**a**) Planned skin island excision with underlying rectus abdominis muscle prior to pedicled TRAM or free microsurgical TRAM or DIEP transfer into (**b**) a right mastectomy defect with closure of the abdominal wound and repositioning of the umbilical stalk, similar to an abdominoplasty. Medical Illustration, University Hospitals of Leicester NHS Trust. Used with permission

dividing the supplying blood vessels at their origins and reconnecting them using microvascular surgery (microsurgery) to blood vessels in the chest or axilla. The free TRAM and a variety of muscle-sparing variants, including the deep inferior epigastric perforator flap (DIEP), are examples of this. Alternative free flaps of different size with different donor sites can also be harvested, for example, from the buttock (superior or inferior gluteal artery perforator flap – SGAP/IGAP), inner thigh (transverse upper gracilis flap – TUG), and the back (thoracodorsal artery perforator flap – TDAP), but these are much less frequently utilized than LD or TRAM flap procedures.

As you descend this list, operations increase in complexity and duration, with specific complications for each procedure; however, in patients with larger, more ptotic breasts, the greater use of autologous tissue improves symmetry with the contralateral breast. Greater volume reconstruction is achievable with the free TRAM and DIEP flaps (Fig. 14.4). Implant-based reconstructions may offer limited ptosis and techniques are described to enhance this; however, long-term results can be less satisfactory than with autologous tissue reconstruction, with many requiring subsequent revision or replacement. They can, however, fill a bra and offer visible upper-pole fullness of the breast and cleavage, along with decreased initial operative time, inpatient stay, and risk of complications (Fig. 14.5). Use of

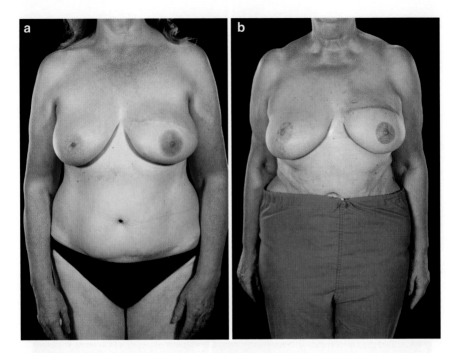

Fig. 14.4 Delayed free TRAM flap reconstruction. These cases exemplify the natural appearance and ptosis achievable by autologous tissue transfer. (**a**) Right reconstruction in a 60 year old with subsequent adjustment by liposuction. She is wearing a prosthetic nipple-areola complex. The abdominal scar is also visible. (**b**) 64-year-old patient who has also undergone nipple-areola reconstruction and contralateral symmetrizing mastopexy

an LD with an implant creates some natural-appearing ptosis outside a bra and this may be enough to achieve symmetry with a contralateral breast of smaller volume (Fig. 14.6).

Breast reconstruction can be immediate, i.e. performed at the time of mastectomy, or delayed – performed at a later date once the mastectomy wound has healed and any adjuvant therapy completed. The principal advantage of immediate reconstruction is the opportunity to preserve the breast skin envelope, including the nipple-areola complex in some cases, and the inframammary fold resulting in an esthetically superior reconstruction (Kroll et al. 1995). Although immediate reconstruction has been shown to improve the psychological recovery from breast cancer (Atisha et al. 2008), the patient awakes with a new breast and a comparison may be drawn with its predecessor in contrast to delayed reconstruction when the comparison with a mastectomy scar may be more satisfactory.

A major concern of immediate reconstruction is the possible effects of subsequent radiotherapy if this is required. It is known that breast implants underlying irradiated skin and muscle are approximately 30% more likely to demonstrate palpable capsular contracture due to fibrosis around the implant, than nonirradiated implants, although patient satisfaction may remain high up to 6 years postoperatively

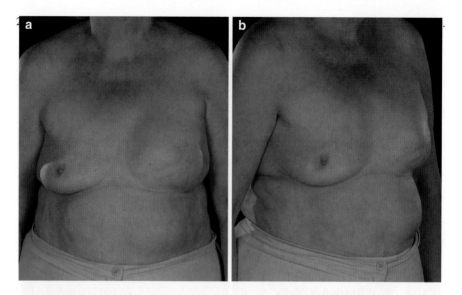

Fig. 14.5 Right delayed-implant-based reconstruction in a 60-year-old patient. Submuscular expansion was performed with a one-stage expander prosthesis achieving adequate volume but limited ptosis. The contralateral breast had undergone wide local excision and radiotherapy 11 years previously

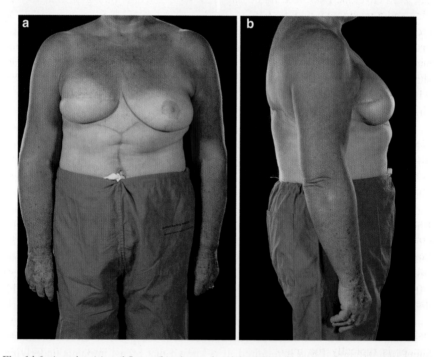

Fig. 14.6 Antorior (a) and Later (b) views of a right delayed LD and tissue expander breast reconstruction with contralateral breast reduction for symmetrization performed on a 62-year-old patient. The lateral view demonstrates ptosis achievable with this technique, and also the transverse donor scar on the back. Abdominal scarring is secondary to a recent unrelated "fleur-de-lys" abdominoplasty

(Cordeiro et al. 2004). Autologous tissue better withstands radiotherapy exposure following immediate reconstruction, but results are unpredictable and it is difficult to advise the patient of the outcome. Alternatively, delayed autologous reconstruction imports new skin and soft tissue with its own blood supply into the previously irradiated field. Recent protocols have been described using breast implants, placed at mastectomy, to fill and preserve the skin envelope for the period of adjuvant chemotherapy, then deflated for the duration of the radiotherapy. Reconstruction is subsequently completed with implants or autologous tissue (Kronowitz et al. 2004). This "delayed-immediate" reconstruction protocol has as yet, not been widely adopted.

Irradiated chest skin becomes less pliable and therefore difficult to stretch. Therefore, following delayed reconstruction with breast expander implants, tissue expansion to match the contralateral breast may be problematic and be associated with an increased risk of implant extrusion or an unsatisfactory cosmetic result. Irradiation is considered by many to be an absolute contraindication to delayed reconstruction with expanding implants without associated autologous tissue transfer.

Surgery to the contralateral breast is often necessary to achieve symmetry. Reduction or augmentation with implants may be necessary for volume mismatch. The skin envelope may need tightening in order to elevate the nipple-areola complex and a mastopexy may be required to adjust any ptosis when compared to the reconstructed side. This may be performed at the time of the initial reconstruction or at a later date, when swelling has resolved and the resulting changes in volume and ptosis have plate out, in order to better guide design of the contralateral breast shape and volume. However, many patients prefer to avoid surgery to their otherwise normal breast and consideration is given to this when discussing the initial choice of reconstructive procedure.

Following breast reconstruction, further adjustments may be desirable to complete the process such as liposuction or fat transfer to adjust volume and contour discrepancies, nipple reconstruction, and tattooing of the nipple-areola complex. However, many patients may be satisfied with a prosthetic nipple and accepting of modest volume and contour differences.

The above descriptions and pathways are principally concerned with technical issues such as symmetry, esthetics, revision rates, and risk rather than patient outcomes with regard to satisfaction, body image, and social or cultural context. The best looking reconstruction in a surgeon's eyes amounts to little if the patient is not satisfied, or if the reconstruction has not met with the patient's expectations. Conversely, an inferior esthetic result may be regarded as perfectly satisfactory by the patient.

Breast reconstruction is a complex process, requiring careful consideration of risks and benefits by both the surgeon and patient. Adequate treatment of the breast cancer is typically the major priority and this must be balanced with realistic expectations of the cosmetic result. The pathway can involve several procedures, sometimes over years, and therefore a realistic prediction of esthetic outcomes, the degree of risk, donor site morbidity, and disruption to normal life of each procedure need to be discussed with the patient with care and clarity at the outset. Once the information has been understood, the patient's wishes are paramount in choosing the most appropriate approach. Multiple visits to the clinic or additional consultations with a breast care nurse or clinical nurse specialist with experience in this area may be required before a mutually confident decision can be made.

14.3   The Aging Breast

Structural changes in the aging breast have been investigated both radiologically and using morphometric analysis. Objective measurements confirm that the central and lateral positions of the inframammary fold, nipple-areola complex, and inferior-most pole of the breast descend with increasing age, with increasing diameter of the areola (Brown et al. 1999). This is due to both skin and parenchymal changes. Aging skin changes are influenced by intrinsic factors with decreased elasticity and thinning of the dermis – compounded by estrogen withdrawal at the menopause; alongside extrinsic factors, including the effect of gravity, sun exposure, and cigarette smoking (Hall and Phillips 2005). The parenchyma regresses following the menopause as the glandular epithelium involutes by apoptosis, secondary to estrogen and progesterone withdrawal, leaving behind islands of ductal tissue and the stroma is replaced by fatty tissue. Decreased epithelial-to-stromal proportion causes decreased density of the breast tissue, which may be compounded by estrogen antagonists such as tamoxifen (Abramson et al. 2007). This decreased density further contributes to ptosis. This ptosis is subjectively obvious but can be difficult to recreate using solely implant based reconstructions. Autologous tissue transfer, either with a LD musculocutaneous flap, free or pedicled TRAM flap reconstruction, or one of the alternative free tissue transfer techniques offers a soft, immediately ptotic, natural-feeling breast with improved symmetry. In comparison with immediate implant reconstruction, immediate or delayed TRAM flap symmetry persists in the long-term, and ages under the same influence with the patient (Clough et al. 2001a, b). When considering the purely esthetic perspective in older patients, the most appropriate choice may be an autologous tissue reconstruction to match the contralateral breast and offer a reconstruction with a good prospect of a long-term acceptable cosmetic outcome.

14.4   Demographics of Breast Reconstruction in the Elderly

In the United Kingdom, 80% of new patients diagnosed with breast cancer are aged 50 or over. The highest numbers of cases arise between the ages 50 and 64 (Office for National Statistics 2004). There has also been a decline in breast cancer mortality since 1989 in all age groups (Office for National Statistics 2005). It is clear, therefore, that within any practice encompassing either immediate or delayed reconstruction, older patients potentially form a significant part of the eligible patient group. In reality, patients who elect for breast conservation surgery, primary endocrine therapy, conservative management for advanced disease, or who simply decide against breast reconstruction will limit this practice.

Many studies demonstrate that older patients are less likely to undergo breast reconstruction. Three studies from the United States and one from Australia report the proportions of older women who undergo breast reconstruction after mastectomy (Reaby 1998; August et al. 1994; Lipa et al. 2003; Alderman et al. 2003; Joslyn 2005). The earlier series from Ann Arbor, Michigan reported that 7% of women older than 60 years underwent reconstruction compared to 38% of younger women (August et al. 1994).The oldest patient in this series was only 68. Comparable results were reported in 2003 by Lipa et al. who reviewed 13 years of their practice in Texas in the largest single retrospective series to date. In this series, 84 patients over 65 years of age underwent postmastectomy breast reconstruction. They reported an 8.5% reconstruction rate vs. 41.4% in patients less than 65 years (oldest patient 79) (Lipa et al. 2003).

Reaby reported regarding the demographics of patients in her qualitative study on the reasons why these women elect to undergo breast reconstruction. They noted that Australian patients who had undergone reconstruction ($n=31$) had a younger mean age (49.5 years) than those that had not ($n=64$, mean age >63 years)[2]. Other studies reported odds ratios of a patient undergoing reconstruction decreasing significantly with rising age in groups of women up to 65 and 75 years and older, respectively (Alderman et al. 2003; Joslyn 2005). From a series in the United Kingdom of 125 patients with locally advanced breast cancer questioned prior to neo-adjuvant chemotherapy, those patients interested in breast reconstruction had a younger mean age (47 years) than those who were not (55 years) (Keith et al. 2003). Possible reasons for these differences between age groups are discussed below. The ongoing National Mastectomy and Breast Reconstruction audit will address these issues in a large cohort of patients and also report on variations in patient subgroups such as socioeconomic status and ethnicity, along with regional variations in provision and uptake of reconstructive options.

14.5 The Surgeon's Perspective

A surgeons' perception of the risk that the older patient may not benefit with regard to body image and quality of life may be poorly founded and may depend on the individual surgeon's experience with the available techniques. Prior to the publication of guidelines by the National Institute of Clinical Excellence in 2002 on reconstructive practice in the United Kingdom, the age of breast surgeon was shown to influence reconstructive practice, with less patients being offered immediate reconstruction when the surgeon was between 51 and 60 years old (Callaghan et al. 2002). Younger surgeons were more likely to perform breast reconstruction. Although this study only looks at consultations with patients younger than 65 years, with no investigation into older women, it does confirm that surgeon experience may affect the choices offered to patients.

In the United States, it has recently been shown that one-third of general surgeons studied discuss breast reconstructive options with patients choosing between mastectomy and breast conserving surgery for the treatment of breast cancer. Of these surgeons, these discussions are more likely to take place with younger (mean age 56 years, against 61 not discussed), more educated patients with larger tumors (Alderman et al. 2008). This additional information was shown to affect the subsequent decision with patients more willing to consider mastectomy, which then affected the choice of surgical pathway.

Another study also demonstrates that in the United States, socioeconomic status also affects the surgeon's likelihood of discussing and offering reconstruction after mastectomy, demonstrating access to care is variable for patient groups with non-clinical, financial, and linguistic barriers (Greenberg et al. 2008). This study found that from their cohort of 626 patients, the more educated, younger, Caucasian group of women were more likely to have reconstruction discussed and subsequently performed ($n=253$). Indeed, Morrow and her colleagues demonstrated that age younger than 50 years was the greatest single predictor for a breast reconstruction (odds ratio 4.3) (Morrow et al. 2001). No single study has questioned the surgeons' clinical preconceptions of breast reconstruction in older women; however, these can be subdivided into those of concerns relating to co-morbidity and risk, benefit attributable to the expected esthetic outcome, and the perceptions of the patients' self-esteem and body image.

14.6 The Patient's Perspective

Handel et al. questioned patients who had elected not to undergo reconstruction following mastectomy and found that 40% cited age as a deciding factor (Handel et al. 1990). Other issues included concern about complications, uncertainty about outcome, and fear about the effect of reconstruction on future cancer recurrence. Reaby's qualitative study of patients in Australia who elected not to undergo reconstruction described their reasons as not being essential for physical or emotional well-being, not having enough information about the procedure, and not wanting anything unnatural in the body (Reaby 1998). The two main issues that emerged were a fear of complications and perception of being too old for the procedure.

Patients' perceptions of consultations regarding breast cancer do not appear to change significantly with age, nor does their ability to engage in the decision-making process. Indeed, Bowman and colleagues in Canada showed that 100% of patients older than 60 years, who had undergone reconstruction, felt in retrospect that immediate reconstruction should have been discussed with them at their first consult; the actual proportion where this happened was 16% (Bowman et al. 2006). In a recent multivariate analysis of the influence of age in breast surgery decision-making in the United States, when a choice was available, mastectomy rates were not significantly different in all age groups up to the age of 79 (Bleicher et al. 2008). Decisions were felt to have been surgeon-based, patient-based, and shared in comparable proportions between all age groups, as was confidence in the decisions made. The younger patients were, however, better informed regarding breast cancer.

14.7   Body Image

In a study of 1957 patients in the United States using a self-report questionnaire, those who have undergone breast conserving surgery for their primary cancer have greater self-esteem, better body image, and feelings of sexual attractiveness than those who have had a mastectomy (Rowland et al. 2000). Women who have undergone a mastectomy and reconstruction (immediate or delayed within 5 years of diagnosis) have a more negative view of the effect of cancer treatment on their sex life than those who undergo mastectomy alone. This may not be surprising as the group which chooses reconstruction is more likely to have concerns about the impact of mastectomy on their sexuality. However, these groups differed in age with the mastectomy-alone group being a mean age 10 years older than those undergoing reconstruction, suggesting that older patients are more able to accept the loss of a breast, or place a lower importance in body image issues. The groups are also confounded by other demographic differences: the reconstructive group is younger, more educated, and more affluent than the mastectomy-alone group. Because of this it is unwise to draw general conclusions regarding the older patient and body image.

One must be cautious in assuming that older women experience fewer concerns relating to body image than younger patients. This is a generalization that has been studied in healthy individuals using self-reporting methods, in particular by Franzoi and Koehler (1998). Older women (mean age 73.6 years) expressed greater satisfaction with their weight, but held less positive attitudes toward visible aging changes in the face. This acceptance of change in the body contour may be secondary to a cultural shift with age where thinness is less a defining standard of attractiveness than in younger women. Attitudes toward the breast however, appear similar between age groups. In older and younger women with breast cancer, body image concerns were also similar between the different age groups within a longitudinal cohort of 563 patients in the United States (Figueiredo et al. 2004). When considering breast cancer surgery, 31% of women older than 67 report physical appearance (body image) as an important factor, however only 7.5% of patients underwent reconstruction. Of those who had breast conservation, body image was better at 2 years than those undergoing mastectomy alone. Those who preferred breast conservation but eventually had a mastectomy had the poorest body image results, demonstrating that treatment discordant with the patient's preferences resulted in poorer body image results and reduced mental health scores.

14.8   Procedure Rates

The few retrospective studies published on breast reconstruction practice in older women have studied the numbers of reconstructive procedures and complication rates following mastectomy (August et al. 1994; Lipa et al. 2003; Bowman et al. 2006; Girotto et al. 2003). Up to 1994 in a retrospective review of 11 years' practice in Michigan, August et al. reported that younger patients ($n=224$ less than 60 years) were undergoing more implant-based reconstructions, with the older group ($n=18$ up to 68 years) undergoing proportionally higher numbers of autologous reconstructions (August et al. 1994). Analysis of data regarding 10,406 patients drawn from the National Cancer Institute's Surveillance, Epidemiology and End Results program (SEER) in 2003 covering the United States, showed that women older than 65 or younger than 35 were more likely to have implant-based reconstruction, with patients of the intervening years being more likely to undergo autologous reconstruction (Lipa et al. 2003). Furthermore, in looking at their own experience in Baltimore over 4 years with 316 patients, 24 of whom were older than 65, Girotto et al. found that older patients were less likely than younger patients to complete the reconstructive process, such as having nipple-areola reconstruction (Girotto et al. 2003). In this study and in Lipa et al.'s review in the over 65 age group in Texas, the reconstructions performed were, 30–50% implant-based, 11–29% LD based, and 39–40% free or pedicled (TRAM) flap (Lipa et al. 2003; Girotto et al. 2003).

14.9   Risks

The health of the elderly patient cohort is improving (Ramesh et al. 2005), although patients with preexisting co-morbidity or self-reported poor physical health have a greater incidence of medical complications following breast reconstruction (Lipa et al. 2003; Bowman et al. 2006). TRAM flap donor site complications were noted in patients with higher body mass index (BMI), current smokers, and higher American Society of Anaesthesiologists Classification of Physical Status (ASA). The translation of co-morbidity into contraindication when considering each reconstructive option can be difficult; however, older age alone should not be a factor in choosing the method of reconstruction. Individual patients with co-morbid conditions must be optimized prior to surgery both medically and with regard to patient-controlled risk factors such as smoking cessation and decrease in BMI.

Implant-based reconstruction, whether one stage, two stage, immediate, or delayed, may appear to be a simpler option for the older patient. The anesthetic time is shorter than for autologous-tissue-based reconstructions, and there is no donor site to develop complications. Lipa et al. report that the trade-off appears to be a higher breast-site complication rate, reported at 79% in their series (Lipa et al.

2003). These include hematoma, capsular contracture, seroma, infection, and implant removal and/or revision rate, with implant failure rates requiring removal at 41% which they compare with previously reported figures of 21% across the age groups (Kroll and Baldwin 1992). Their LD failure rates at 4.2%, and TRAM flap failure rates at 1.7% in patients older than 65, were comparable with previously published figures across all age groups from the same center (Kroll and Baldwin 1992). These implant/expander complication rates were greater in proportion to the combined donor and breast-site complications of the other patient groups. These are in contrast to August et al. who reported that complication rates in older women who have had immediate or delayed prosthetic reconstruction is less than in the younger population, however their age threshold was 60 with only 18 patients in the older group (August et al. 1994). Bowman's group in British Columbia noted in their series of 75 patients with an age range of 60–77 years, that the majority of patients over the age of 60 were satisfied with their reconstruction regardless of whether or not they suffered a complication (Bowman et al. 2006).

An increased risk of failure rate of microvascular surgery with increasing age appears to be a misconception. This technique allows the single-stage reconstruction of autologous tissue in TRAM and other free flap reconstructions. Experience of microvascular surgery and free tissue transfer in the elderly has been reviewed in several centers (Malata et al. 1996; Serletti et al. 2000; Coskunfirat et al. 2005; Ozkan et al. 2005). Malata and his colleagues looked specifically at their head and neck free flap survival rate in 49 cases, which including three successfully salvaged cases, was 95% in patients aged 70–83 years (Malata et al. 1996). Success rates of 97% were reported in free flaps to multiple sites including the breast by Serletti et al., who concluded along with Coskunfirat et al. who published similar results, that ASA status and length of operation were more important predictors of morbidity than age (Serletti et al. 2000; Coskunfirat et al. 2005). Ozkan et al., who published a 98.3% flap success rate in 55 free tissue transfers to the head, neck, lower limb, and one breast reconstruction, remark that ASA increases with increasing age but, again, age alone should not be a consideration in older patients (Ozkan et al. 2005). These papers demonstrate an increasing success rate over 10 years in elderly patients, reflecting the evolution of anesthetic and surgical experience, materials, and techniques alongside perioperative monitoring and care.

14.10   Outcomes

Only two studies of breast reconstruction in the elderly give details of patient-reported outcomes. In their retrospective series of Canadian patients, Bowman and colleagues report that 70% of a cohort of 75 patients aged older than 60 who underwent breast reconstruction over the previous 8 years self-reported satisfaction with the result as good or excellent – regardless of the type of reconstruction (Bowman et al. 2006). Almost 90% of patients said they would undergo the same treatment again. Low satisfaction correlated with depression as lower mental health scores assessed by the short form-12 questionnaire, although whether this is cause or effect is unknown.

Using the self-reporting short form 36 (SF-36), a frequently used tool designed to assess quality of life, Girotto and his colleagues retrospectively assessed their reconstructive outcomes in their patient group comparing 24 patients aged 65 and older with 292 younger patients (Girotto et al. 2003). They found that in the areas related to mental health, the older patients scored higher (better outcome) than age-matched controls and younger patients (less than 55 years) who had completed reconstruction. The physical function scores were higher in the older patient cohort than age-matched controls, but not better than the younger patient population. It may be that the self-selecting group of older patients electing for reconstruction are those who function better physically than the age-matched general population, but without preoperative prospective data this cannot be confirmed. Complication rates were similar between the older and younger groups. Although the SF-36 scores comparing autologous transfer with implant reconstruction in older patients showed similar scores for mental and general physical health, emotional limitation, and vitality, significantly lower scores (worse outcomes) were noted in physical pain and physical role limitation in the implant reconstructed group. No study to date uses independent observer reporting of symmetry, or esthetic outcomes in the older patient. In their experience therefore, older patients demonstrated benefit emotionally and psychologically from breast reconstruction, at least to the same degree as younger patients and within this group autologous reconstruction appeared to offer a better physical recovery than implant-based reconstruction. This may be a reflection of effective patient counseling and selection, which needs to be investigated with prospective studies.

14.11   Summary and Approach to the Older Patient

After consideration of the oncological treatment plan, and any anticipated adjuvant therapy, the context of the individual is as relevant in the older patient as the younger. Socioeconomic and cultural contexts will affect the desire of the patient to seek reconstruction, regardless of age. Currently, fewer elderly patients undergo reconstruction and may not complete the process. These patients may come to the consultation with fears about the risks of reconstruction, co- morbidity, and lack of importance of body image. It is not, however, reasonable to assume that older patients as a whole do not wish to be considered and counseled for reconstruction. In general older patients are able and wish to be involved in the decision-making process, including consideration of reconstructive options. Body image concerns persist into old age and need to be respected. These fears and issues of self-esteem need to be addressed so that the patient and surgeon can come to an agreed plan.

Each patient needs to be assessed for anesthetic risk, older patients may have higher co-morbidity and ASA scores, and this may affect morbidity in breast reconstruction.

In microsurgical centers, there are no increased failure rates of microanastomosis in the elderly with low ASA scores and therefore physiologically healthy patients are candidates for the longer operations such as free flap reconstruction. Uncovering any risks at the earliest opportunity enables planning for anesthetic and surgery, and physiological optimization of the patient.

With regards to esthetic outcomes, implant reconstructions have higher failure rates in older patients than younger, and yet these are the reconstructions performed in the majority of older patients. If the patients' chest has been irradiated then importing of unirradiated tissue from elsewhere offers an improved result. The aging, ptotic breast may be better matched with an autologous reconstruction such as a free or pedicled TRAM flap if larger volumes are required and there is enough abdominal tissue to harvest, or, if less volume is required, an autologous LD, LD with implant or smaller free flap reconstruction may be considered. Such a reconstruction offers longevity of symmetry, with ultimately lower numbers of revision operations. The patient's attitude to surgery to the contralateral breast should be ascertained at an early stage as this may affect the ultimate choice of reconstruction. Elderly patients should therefore be assessed with the full range of reconstructive options in mind, and a tailor-made plan designed for each individual.

It is therefore best to approach the consultation with an open mind and to discuss openly the patients' fears, body image concerns, and expectations. Starting with the full range of options, the more complex procedures such as free tissue transfer may be withdrawn due to medical contraindications such as high ASA status, smoking, hypertension, and diabetes mellitus which may increase the systemic risks of prolonged duration of surgery or wound healing at the donor site. Previous abdominal scars may preclude a TRAM flap reconstruction. Poor mobility or use of walking aids make harvesting of an abdominal core stabilizing muscle with a TRAM flap, or shoulder muscle with an LD transfer, unwise. Rehabilitation from these procedures is considerable, and older patients living alone or caring for dependents may find this too involved for their social circumstances. Implant-based reconstructions require less operative time, decreased in-patient stay, no donor site, and quicker recovery time. However, they may offer poor symmetry to the aging contralateral breast, with worsening long-term esthetic outcomes, a significant failure or revision rate and longer-term increased physical pain and limitation of physical function compared to autologous reconstruction. Patient information aids such as leaflets, a DVD, photographs of good and poor results, discussions with previous patient volunteers, and further discussions with breast care nurses can all help in the decision-making process. Multiple consultations can be offered to address questions or concerns and further reassure and reinforce the patients' decisions.

The majority of older patients are capable of engaging in these discussions and benefit from doing so. The appropriate choice of whether or not to undergo reconstruction, with the arguments for and against each option with the context centered on them as an individual, can be effectively discussed as a two-way process. A suitable pathway can then be mutually agreed.

Further prospective long-term studies would be useful to comparing body-image concerns, mental health, and social context between age groups both prior to and after surgery, looking at those who choose different types of reconstruction and those who elect not to have reconstruction, and their reasons. Risks, complications, failure rates, and outcomes, with regard to patient satisfaction and independent evaluation of esthetics in the long term could help guide future practice.

Acknowledgments The authors would like to thank the medical illustration department of University Hospitals of Leicester NHS Trust for their preparation of the illustrations, and Rachel Berry, Breast Practice Specialist Nurse at Sheffield Teaching Hospitals NHS Trust for helping with preparation of the photographs.

References

Abramson RG, Mavi A, Cermik T et al (2007) Age-related structural and functional changes in the breast: multimodality correlation with digital mammography, computed tomography, magnetic resonance imaging, and positron emission tomography. Semin Nucl Med 37:146–153

Alderman AK, McMahon L, Wilkins EG (2003) The national utilization of immediate and early delayed breast reconstruction and the effect of sociodemographic factors. Plast Reconstr Surg 111:695–703

Alderman AK, Hawley ST, Waljee J, Mujahid M, Morrow M, Katz JK (2008) Understanding the impact of breast reconstruction on the surgical decision-making process for breast cancer. Cancer 112:489–494

Atisha D, Alderman AK, Lowery JC, Kuhn LE, Davis J, Wilkins EG (2008) Prospective analysis of long-term psychosocial outcomes in breast reconstruction: two-year postoperative results from the Michigan breast reconstruction outcomes study. Ann Surg 247(6):1016–1028

August DA, Wilkins E, Rea T (1994) Breast reconstruction in older women. Surgery 115:663–668

Bleicher RJ, Abrahamse P, Hawley ST, Katz SJ, Morrow M (2008) The influence of age on the breast surgery decision-making process. Ann Surg Oncol 15:854–862

Bowman CC, Lennox PA, Clugston PA, Courtemanche DJ (2006) Breast reconstruction in older women: should age be an exclusion criterion? Plast Reconstr Surg 118:16–22

Brown TPL, Ringrose C, Hyland RE, Cole AA, Brotherston TM (1999) A method of assessing femal breast morphometry and its clinical application. Brit J Plast Surg 52:355–359

Callaghan CJ, Couto E, Kerin MJ, Rainsbury RM, George WD, Purushotham AD (2002) Breast reconstruction in the United Kingdom and Ireland. Brit J Surg 89:335–340

Clough KB, O'Donoghue JM, Fitoussi AD, Nos C, Falcou M-C (2001a) Prospective evaluation of late cosmetic results following breast reconstruction: I. Implant reconstruction. Plast Reconstr Surg 107:1702–1709

Clough KB, O'Donoghue JM, Fitoussi AD, Vlastos G, Falcou M-C (2001b) Prospective evaluation of late cosmetic results following breast reconstruction: II. TRAM flap reconstruction. Plast Reconstr Surg 107:1710–1715

Cordeiro PG, Pusic AL, Disa JJ, McCormick B, VanZee K (2004) Irradiation after immediate tissue expander/implant breast reconstruction: outcomes, complications, aesthetic results, and satisfaction among 156 patients. Plast Reconstr Surg 113:877–881

Coskunfirat OK, Chen H, Spanio S, Tang Y (2005) The safety of microvascular free tissue transfer in the elderly population. Plast Reconstr Surg 115:771–775

Figueiredo MI, Cullen J, Hwang Y, Rowland JH, Mandelblatt JS (2004) Breast cancer treatment in older women: does getting what you want improve your long-term body image and mental health? J Clin Oncol 22:4002–4009

Franzoi SL, Koehler V (1998) Age and gender differences in body attitudes: a comparison of young and elderly patients. Int J Ageing Hum Dev 47:1–10

Girotto JA, Schreiber J, Nahabedian MY (2003) Breast reconstruction in the elderly: preserving excellent quality of life. Ann Plast Surg 50:572–578

Greenberg CC, Schneider EC, Lipsitz SR et al (2008) Do variations in provider discussions explain socioeconomic disparities in postmastectomy breast reconstruction? J Am Coll Surg 206:605–615

Hall G, Phillips TJ (2005) Estrogen and skin: the effects of estrogen, menopause, and hormone replacement therapy on the skin. J Am Acad Dermatol 53:555–568

Handel N, Silverstein MJ, Waisman E, Waisman JR (1990) Reasons why mastectomy patients do not have breast reconstruction. Plast Reconstr Surg 86:1118–1122

Improving Outcomes In Breast Cancer – Manual Update (2002) National institute for clinical excellence. At: <http://www.nice.org.uk/nicemedia/pdf/Improving_outcomes_breastcancer_manual.pdf> Accessed 12 Jun 2008.

Joslyn SA (2005) Patterns of care for immediate and early delayed breast reconstruction following mastectomy. Plast Reconstr Surg 115:1289–1296

Keith DJW, Walker MB, Walker LG et al (2003) Women who wish breast reconstruction: characteristics, fears, and hopes. Plast Reconstr Surg 111:1051–1056

Kroll SS, Baldwin B (1992) A comparison of outcomes using three different methods of breast reconstruction. Plast Reconstr Surg 90:455–462

Kroll SS, Coffey JA, Winn RJ, Schusterman MA (1995) A comparison of factors affecting aesthetic outcomes of TRAM flap breast reconstructions. Plast Reconstr Surg 96:860–864

Kronowitz SJ, Hunt KK, Kuerer HM et al (2004) Delayed-immediate breast reconstruction. Plast Reconstr Surg 113:1617–1627

Lipa JE, Youssef AA, Kuerer HM, Robb GL, Chang DW (2003) Breast reconstruction in older women: advantages of autogenous tissue. Plast Reconstr Surg 111:1110–1121

Malata CM, Cooter R, Batchelor AGG, Simpson KH, Browning FSC, Kay SPJ (1996) Microvascular free-tissue transfers in elderly patients: the Leeds experience. Plast Reconstr Surg 98:1234–1241

Morrow M, Scott SK, Menck HR, Mustoe TA, Winchester DP (2001) Factors influencing the use of breast reconstruction postmastectomy: a national cancer database study. J Am Coll Surg 192:1–8

Office for National Statistics, Cancer Statistics registrations: Registrations of cancer diagnosed in 2004, England. Series MB1 n0.35. 2007. http://www.statistics.gov.uk/downloads/theme_health/MB1_35/MB1_No%2035_2004.pdf Accessed 12 Jun 2008

Office for National Statistics, Mortality Statistics: Cause. England and Wales 2005. Series DH2 n0.32. 2006. http://www.statistics.gov.uk/downloads/theme_health/Dh2_32/DH2_N032_2005.pdf Accessed 12 Jun 2008.

Ozkan O, Ozegentas HE, Islamoglu K, Boztug N, Bigat Z, Dikici MB (2005) Experiences with microsurgical tissue transfers in elderly patients. Microsurgery 25:390–395

Rainsbury RM (2007) Surgery insight: oncoplastic breast-conserving reconstruction-indications, benefit, choices and outcomes. Natl Clin Pract Oncol 4:657–664

Ramesh HSJ, Pope D, Gennari R, Audisio RA (2005) Optimising surgical management of elderly cancer patients. World J Surg Oncol 3:17–31

Reaby LL (1998) Reasons why women who have mastectomy decide to have or not to have breast reconstruction. Plast Reconstr Surg 101:1810–1818

Rowland JH, Desmond KA, Meyerowitz BE, Belin TR, Wyatt GE, Ganz PA (2000) Role of breast reconstructive surgery in physical and emotional outcomes among breast survivors. J Natl Cancer Inst 92:1422–1429

Serletti JM, Higgins JP, Moran S, Orlando GS (2000) Factors affecting outcome in free-tissue transfer in the elderly. Plast Reconstr Surg 106:66–70

Spear SL (ed) (2006) Surgery of the breast: principles and art 2nd edition. Lippincott Williams and Wilkins, Philadelphia, PA

Chapter 15
Adjuvant Endocrine Therapy

Laura Biganzoli

The major threat of breast cancer is that of distant metastasis. An adjuvant treatment is given with the aim to reduce the risk of tumor relapse and death. An adjuvant endocrine therapy represents a treatment option to be offered to patients with estrogen-receptor (ER) and/or progesterone-receptor (PgR)-positive early breast cancer. The value of this treatment is influenced by the extent of receptor expression (patients with a greater percentage of cells that are ER- or PgR-positive derive greater benefit) and the quality of receptor expression (patients with both ER- and PgR-positive tumors derive greater benefits than patients with tumors that are ER-positive and PgR-negative or ER-negative and PgR-positive). Anyhow, as recently confirmed by the St Gallen Panelists, an adjuvant endocrine treatment should be proposed to patients with highly endocrine-responsive tumors (high expression of both ER and PgR in a majority of tumor cells) as well as to patients with incompletely endocrine-responsive breast cancer (low expression of ER and/ or PgR) (Goldhirsch et al. 2007). Therefore, the majority of elderly patients are potential candidates for an adjuvant endocrine treatment since the number of tumors with ERs progressively increases with aging, with less than 20% of breast cancer cases being ER-negative in patients aged 65 years or more. Let us discuss the available options.

15.1 Tamoxifen: Efficacy and Safety Data

Tamoxifen, a selective ER modulator, has represented for several years the most commonly used hormonal therapy for endocrine sensitive early breast cancers. Data from the Oxford Overview clearly show that 20 mg/die is the recommended

L. Biganzoli (✉)
Department of Oncology, Hospital of Prato—Instituto Toscano Tumori, Prato, Italy
e-mail: lbiganzoli@usl4.toscana.it

M.W. Reed and R.A. Audisio (eds.), *Management of Breast Cancer in Older Women*, 231
DOI 10.1007/978-1-84800-265-4_15, © Springer-Verlag London Limited 2011

dose being as effective as 30–40 mg/die and that the optimal treatment duration is 5 years, even if benefit is observed with 1–2 years of treatment (Early Breast Cancer Trialists' Collaborative Group 2005). The administration of 5 years of tamoxifen vs. no treatment almost halves the annual recurrence rate (recurrence rate ratio 0.59 [SE 0·03]) and reduces the breast cancer mortality rate by a third (death rate ratio 0.69 [SE 0·04]). This translates in an absolute 15-year gain of 11.8 and 9.2% in terms of recurrence and breast cancer mortality, respectively (Early Breast Cancer Trialists' Collaborative Group 2005). This benefit is irrespective of patients age. In particular, the reduction in recurrence is substantial, and highly significant, both for women younger than 40 years of age and for those older than 70.

In terms of tolerability, treatment with tamoxifen is associated with an increased risk of endometrial cancer and thromboembolic events such as deep venous thrombosis, pulmonary embolism, and cerebrovascular accidents. This does not translate in a significant excess of deaths from any particular cause (Early Breast Cancer Trialists' Collaborative Group 2005). A nonsignificant excess mortality of about 0.2% from uterine cancer and tromboembolic disease is reported in women treated with 5 years of tamoxifen. Due to the low number of events, it is not possible to assess the dependence of risk on age, or on other factors. Overall mortality from vascular disease is nonsignificantly lower with tamoxifen than with control, since a nonsignificant excess of stroke and thromboembolic disease are outweighed by a nonsignificant deficit in other vascular mortality, mainly heart disease. This apparent reduction is compatible with a real protective effect against heart disease, perhaps from the favorable lipid changes produced by tamoxifen.

Coming back on the impact of age on the risk of thromboembolic events among tamoxifen users, Ragaz et al. calculated that the relative risk of mortality for thromboembolic events was 1.5 at the age of 50, but it dramatically increased to 17.5 at the age of 80 (Ragaz and Coldman 1998). However, also in this specific age group, this negative outcome was outweighed by a protective cardiac effect of tamoxifen. There is evidence that the risk of thromboembolic events is related to the duration of the treatment (doubled from 2 to 5 years) (Sacco et al. 2003). In the context of the International Breast Cancer Study Group (IBCSG) Trial IV favorable long-term effects were observed with 1 year of tamoxifen plus low-doses of prednisone in an elderly population (ages 66–80 years) of patients with node-positive breast cancer (Crivellari et al. 2003). Ragaz and IBCSG findings open the issue of the optimal duration of hormonal treatment in elderly patients. Aging has been shown to be related to alterations in the metabolism of tamoxifen, resulting in higher levels of tamoxifen and its metabolites in elderly women, but whether this leads to altered efficacy or side effects is unknown. A lower dose of tamoxifen might prove to be as useful and potentially less toxic than standard doses (Decensi et al. 2003). However, based on the available data, 20 mg/die for 5 years remains the standard treatment to be proposed to elderly women who are candidates to receive adjuvant tamoxifen.

15.2 Aromatase Inhibitors

The role of tamoxifen in postmenopausal women has been challenged in the last few years by the aromatase inhibitors (AIs). AIs are a class of endocrine agents that act by interfering with aromatization, a process that converts androgens to estrogens. The most studied AIs are anastrozole, exemestane, and letrozole. They are respectively given at the daily dose of 1, 25 and 2.5 mg. Based on the evidence of a favorable therapeutic index of the AIs in comparison to tamoxifen in advanced breast cancer, clinical trials have been conducted to evaluate the role of the AIs in the adjuvant setting. These trials can be grouped, according to the modality of introduction of the AI in the treatment program, as: (1) Upfront adjuvant therapy trials, in which there is a head-to-head comparison between tamoxifen and the AI; (2) switching trials, in which 5 years of therapy with tamoxifen is compared with tamoxifen for 2–3 years followed by AI for a global duration of 5 years; (3) extended adjuvant trials, evaluating the benefit of an AI after 5 years of tamoxifen. Study design and results of published trials are summarized in Table 15.1 and will be discussed in this chapter.

15.2.1 Efficacy Data

15.2.1.1 Upfront Trials

In the The Arimidex & Alone or in Combination (ATAC) trial a total of 9,366 post-menopausal patients who were eligible to receive adjuvant endocrine therapy were randomized to receive tamoxifen, anastrozole, or a combination of tamoxifen plus anastrozole for 5 years (The ATAC Trialists' Group 2002). Patients median age was 64 years. While results with the combination were not significantly different from those with tamoxifen alone, at a median follow-up of 100 months (range 0–126), single-agent anastrozole significantly prolonged disease-free survival (DFS), time to recurrence (TTR), time to distant recurrence (TDR), and controlateral breast cancer rate (CLBC) (HR 0.68; $p=0.020$) over tamoxifen (The ATAC Trialists' Group 2008). No difference was observed in terms of overall survival (OS) between the two agents. Similar results were obtained when the efficacy analysis was limited to the hormone-receptor positive population (84%, $n=5216$). Recently, Buzdar presented the results of an analysis that looked at the causes of death in the ATAC study population and aimed to examine the relationship between prognostic factors and competing causes of death (Buzdar and Cuzick 2008). After a median of 100 months of follow-up (mean age at this analysis 72 years), 10.2% of women enrolled in the trial had died following recurrence, and 8.8% had died without recurrence. Death from breast cancer was strongly related to nodal status, with node-positive patients having a twofold greater chance of death than nodes-negative women. Older age and a history of smoking were important predictors of non-breast cancer death.

Table 15.1 Trials evaluating the role of aromatase inhibitors (AIs) in the adjuvant setting

Study (No. patients)	Study design	Follow-up months	Endpoints				overall survival (OS)
Upfront adjuvant therapy							
ATAC (The ATAC Trialists' Group 2008) (n=6241)	5 y A 5 y T	100	DFS TTR	HR 0.90; p=0.025 HR 0.81; p=0.0004	TDR	HR 0.86; p=0.022	HR 1.0; p=0.99
Breast International Group (BIG) 1–98 (Coates et al. 2007) (n=4922)	5 y L 5 y T	51	DFS TTR	HR 0.82; p=0.007 HR 0.78; p=0.004	DDFS TDR	HR 0.87; p=0.07 HR 0.81; p=0.03	HR 0.91; p=0.35
Switching trials							
Intergroup Exemestane Study (IES) Coombes et al. 2007 (n=4724)	2–3y E 2–3y T	55.7	DFS	HR 0.75; p=0.0001	TDR	HR 0.83; p=0.03	HR 0.85; p=0.07
ABCSG8/Italian tamoxifen anastrozole (ITA)/ARN095 Jonat et al. 2006 (n=4600)	2–3y T 2–3y A 2–3y T	30	DFS	HR 0.59; p<0.0001	DDFS	HR 0.61; p=0.002	HR 0.71; p=0.04
Extended adjuvant therapy							
MA 17 Goss et al. 2005 (n=5187)	5y T 5 y L placebo 5y T	30	DFS	HR 0.58; p<0.001	DDFS	HR 0.60; p<0.002	HR 0.82; p=0.3

ABCSG 6a (Jakesz et al. 2007) (n=856)	5y T±AG	3 y A	62.3	DFS	HR 0.62; p=0.031			OS	NS
	5y T±AG	NT							
NSABP B-33 (Mamounas et al. 2008) (n=1598)	5y T	5y E	30	DFS	HR 0.68; p=0.07	RFS	HR 0.44; p=0.004	OS	NS
	5y T	placebo							

A anastrozole; T tamoxifen; L letrozole; E exemestane; NS not significant; HR hazard ratio; y years; AG aminoglutethimide; DFS disease-free survival; TDR time to distant recurrence; OS overall survival; TTR time to recurrence; DDFS distant disease-free survival; RFS relapse-free survival Modified from Biganzoli et al. (2007), with permission

The Breast International Group (BIG) 1–98 study is a randomized, phase 3, double-blind trial that compared 5 years of treatment with various adjuvant endocrine therapy regimens in postmenopausal women with hormone-receptor-positive breast cancer: letrozole, letrozole followed by tamoxifen, tamoxifen, and tamoxifen followed by letrozole. A total of 4,922 were randomized in the upfront comparison of tamoxifen vs. letrozole (Coates et al. 2007). Patients median age was 61 years, range 38–90. At a median follow-up of 51 months patients on letrozole presented a longer DFS, TTR, and TDR than patients on tamoxifen. No difference in terms of OS was observed between the two treatment arms, with a total of 194 and 211 events reported with letrozole and tamoxifen, respectively. Overall 2.2% of the patients died without recurrence.

In both the ATAC and BIG 1–98 trials subgroup analysis based on baseline and treatment characteristics (i.e., nodal status, tumor size, receptor status, age, prior treatments) favored the AIs in terms of DFS for all subsets (The ATAC Trialists' Group 2008; Buzdar and Cuzick 2008; Coates et al. 2007).

15.2.1.2 Switching Trials

In the intergroup exemestane study (IES) 4,724 postmenopausal women with ER-positive or ER-unknown breast cancer, who were disease-free on 2–3 years of tamoxifen, were randomly assigned to switch to exemestane or continue tamoxifen for the remainder of 5 years of treatment (Coombes et al. 2007). Patients' median age was 64 years. At a median follow-up of 55.7 months patients who switched to exemestane presented an advantage in terms of DFS and TDR. Adjusting for potential confounders related to baseline and treatment characteristics, i.e., nodal status, hormonal status, age, previous chemotherapy, and previous tamoxifen duration, did not substantially affect the estimates of treatment effect (DFS adjusted 0.75 [0.65–0.86, $p=0.0001$]). No difference in terms of OS was observed between the two treatment groups according to an intent-to-treat (ITT) analysis. A small advantage in terms of OS was observed in favor of exemestane when 122 patients originally reported as ER unknown and later found to be ER-negative were excluded from the efficacy analysis (HR 0.83, $p=0.05$). Overall 483 deaths were reported; 317 events had known breast-cancer cause or followed a breast-cancer relapse with an additional 23 patients dying of unknown cause and considered likely to be deaths due to breast cancer.

Three clinical trials, the Arimidex-Nolvadex (Arno 95), the Austrian Breast and Colorectal Cancer Study Group (ABCSG 8), and the Italian tamoxifen anastrozole (ITA) studies, have randomized postmenopausal women with hormone-sensitive early breast cancer to receive anastrozole after 2–3 years of tamoxifen or to continue to take tamoxifen up to 5 years of treatment. It should be noted that while the ITA and ARNO 95 are two classical switching trials, in ABCSG 8 patients were randomized from the outset with a pure sequencing strategy. A meta-analysis of these three clinical trials, including a total of 4,600 eligible patients, was published in 2006. Median patient age was 63 years. After a median follow-up of 30 months, a significant reduction in the DFS hazard rate and in the risk of death was observed in patients treated with anastrozole (Jonat et al. 2006). The advantage in term of OS in favor of the incorporation of

the AI in the treatment program has been recently confirmed in a separate analysis of
the ARNO trial. Among 979 postmenopausal patients aged ≤75 years, at a median
follow-up of 30.1 switching to anastrozole resulted in a statistically significant
improvement in DFS, with a 34% reduction in the relative risk of disease recurrence
or death (HR 0.66, $p=0.049$) and in OS, with a 47% improvement (HR 0.53, $p=0.45$),
compared with patients who continued with tamoxifen (Kaufmann et al. 2007). After
adjustment for potential prognostic factors (age, tumor size and grade, lymph-node
status, and type of primary surgery), switching to adjuvant anastrozole still resulted in
a statistically significant improvement in DFS and OS.

15.2.1.3   Extended Adjuvant Trials

The NCIC CTG MA.17 study targeted postmenopausal women with primary breast
cancer who had completed approximately 5 years of adjuvant tamoxifen therapy
(Goss et al. 2003). A total of 5,187 patients were randomized to receive (double-
blind) either letrozole or placebo for 5 years. Patients median age was 62 years,
25% of the patients were aged ≥ 70 years. The study was interrupted and unblinded
after the first interim analysis due to the clear advantage in terms of DFS with
letrozole. At a median follow-up of 30 months extended therapy with letrozole
resulted in prolonged DFS and DDFS (Goss et al. 2005). A subgroup analysis
showed also an advantage in terms of OS among node-positive patients (HR 0.61;
$p>0.04$). After the unblinding, patients in the placebo arm were offered letrozole.
At an intent to treat analysis performed after a median follow up of 54 month,
patients originally randomized to receive letrozole did better than patients originally randomized to placebo in terms of DFS (4y DFS HR$=0.64; p = 0.00002$) and
DDFS (4y DDFS HR$=0.76; p=0.041$) despite 73% of the patients on placebo
crossed to letrozole after unblinding (Ingle et al. 2006).

In the study ABCSG-6a, a total of 456 postmenopausal women who had
received, in the context of trial ABCSG6, either 5 years of tamoxifen or tamoxifen
plus aminoglutethimide for a 2-year period followed by 3 years of tamoxifen alone,
were re-randomized to switch to anastrozole or no treatment for a further 3 years
(Jakesz et al. 2007). Patients' median age was 61.8 years. At a median follow-up of
60 months, significantly fewer patients in the AI group experimented disease recurrence compared with the no-treatment group.

The National Surgical Adjuvant Breast and Bowel Project B-33 Trial, aimed to
randomize 3,000 postmenopausal patients who were disease-free after 5 years of
tamoxifen to 5 years of exemestane or 5 years of placebo (Mamounas et al. 2008).
Due to the results of MA.17, the study was discontinued with 1,598 randomized.
At that point treatment assignment was unblinded, and exemestane was offered to
patients in the placebo arm. On unblinding, 72% of the patients in the exemestane
group chose to continue exemestane while 44% of the patients on placebo switched
to exemestane. With 30 months of median follow-up, original exemestane assignment resulted in a borderline statistically significant improvement in 4-year DFS
and in a statistically significant improvement in 4-year RFS.

Briefly, all the above-discussed trials showed that AIs were superior to tamoxifen in reducing the risk of tumor relapse and some initial evidence of benefit in terms of OS was observed with the switching strategy. Based on the early results of these trials, the Panel of the American Society of Clinical Oncology technology assessment on the use of AIs as adjuvant therapy for postmenopausal women with hormone-receptor-positive breast cancer concluded that the optimal adjuvant hormonal therapy, in this subgroup of patients, should include an AI (Winer et al. 2005).

15.3   From The "Postmenopausal" to the Elderly Population

Can the results observed in the general "postmenopausal" population be transferred to older women? Except for the ABCSG8 and ARNO 95 trials, there was no age limit for study entry; patients' median age was between 61 and 64 years. No impact of age on DFS was observed in the upfront or switching trials. Results for the ATAC, BIG 1–98, IES, and combined analysis of the ABCSG8/ARNO95 trials are given in Table 15.2. A detailed analysis was performed by Crivellari et al. to explore potential differences in efficacy in elderly women receiving adjuvant tamoxifen or letrozole in the BIG 1–98 trial (Crivellari et al. 2008). The report included 4,922 patients with a median follow-up of 40.4 months. Subpopulation treatment effect pattern plot (STEPP) analysis was used to examine the patterns of differences in DFS according to age. The authors found that letrozole was superior to tamoxifen across the age spectrum and not significantly influenced by age (interaction of age and treatment, $p = 0.84$). Apparently, as already shown for tamoxifen, older patients derive the same benefit from AI than younger patients.

Regarding the extended adjuvant strategy, per age subgroup analysis data for DFS are summarized in Table 15.2. In particular, Muss and colleagues divided patients randomized in MA. 17 in three age-groups: younger than 60 (<60), 61–69, and 70 years old and older (70+) (Muss et al. 2008). There was no significant difference in DFS (4-year outcome = 92.4, 91.4, and 92.5% for women aged <60, 60–69, and 70+, respectively) and DDFS (4-year outcome = 96.0, 94.3, and 95.0% for women aged <60, 60–69, and 70+, respectively) between the three age groups. As expected, the OS was significantly different between these three age groups due to an increased risk of non-breast-cancer-related death with increasing age (4-year outcome = 97.4, 96.2, and 90.6% for women aged <60, 60–69, and 70+, respectively). The results remained the same after adjusting for other potential prognostic factors such as letrozole or placebo treatment, duration of prior tamoxifen, nodal status, and prior chemotherapy. Letrozole significantly improved both DFS and DDFS only in women younger than 60 years. However, the interaction between age and treatment was not statistically significant for any of these three outcomes ($P = 0.36, 0.77$, and 0.98 for DFS, DDFS, and OS, respectively), indicating no evidence of a heterogeneous effect of letrozole among age groups. MA.17 showed an OS advantage for all node-positive patients. In this age-directed subset analysis, only node-positive patients aged 70+ had significant improvement in OS.

Table 15.2 Per age subgroup analysis for disease-free survival in AIs adjuvant trials

Study	Follow-up	Age group	n	HR	95% CI	p
ATAC	100 months	<65	5137	0.76	0.63–0.91	NR
		65+	4229	0.77	0.63–0.93	NR
BIG 1–98	51 months	<65	3127	0.82	0.67–0.99	0.04
		65+	1795	0.82	0.67–1.01	0.06
IES	55.7 months	<60	1523	0.82	0.63–1.06	NR
		60–69	2021	0.70	0.56–0.87	NR
		70+	1180	0.81	0.63–1.04	NR
ABCSG8/ ARN095	28 months	<60	1265	0.63	0.40–1.00	0.05
		60+	1959	0.58	0.39–0.87	0.007
MA.17	4-year outcome	<60	2152	0.46	0.30–0.70	0.0004
		60–69	1694	0.68	0.44–1.04	0.078
		70+	1323	0.67	0.41–1.11	0.12
ABCSG 6a	62.3 months	<60	147	0.60	0.21–1.72	0.336
		60+	705	0.63	0.39–1.03	0.064
NSABP B-33	4-year outcome	<60	777	0.53	NR	0.06
		60+	785	0.80	NR	0.43

NR not reported
Modified from Biganzoli et al. (2007), with permission

15.4   Strategy: Upfront or Sequence?

An unresolved question is whether it is more beneficial for the patient to receive an AI upfront or to start with tamoxifen and then shift to an AI. In fact, data deriving from switching trials are not directly relevant to a prospective treatment strategy of commencing with tamoxifen with the intention of changing to an AI after two or more years. A clear answer to this dilemma will emerge from two trials, the BIG 1–98 and the tamoxifen exemestane adjuvant multinational (TEAM), which investigate upfront AI vs. AI after tamoxifen.

Using mathematical models with data coming from the aforementioned trials led Cuzick et al. to assert that early treatment with an AI is superior to sequencing after 2 years of tamoxifen (Cuzick et al. 2006). Punglia et al. reached the opposite conclusion when applying simulations on the basis of data from the same trials, namely that sequential therapy is preferable to an AI- alone treatment (Punglia et al. 2005). Mauriac et al. examined prognostic factors of an early relapse among patients in the BIG 1–98 trial to aid in treatment choices (Mauriac et al. 2007). Analyses included all 7,707 eligible patients treated on BIG 1–98. The median follow-up was 2 years, and the primary endpoint was breast-cancer relapse. Cox proportional hazards regression was used to identify prognostic factors. Two hundred and eighty-five patients (3.7%) had an early relapse (3.1% on letrozole, 4.4% on tamoxifen). Predictive factors for early relapse were node positivity ($P<0.001$), absence of both receptors being positive ($P<0.001$), high tumor grade ($P<0.001$), HER-2 overexpression/amplification ($P<0.001$), large tumor size ($P=0.001$), treatment with tamoxifen ($P=0.002$), and vascular invasion ($P=0.02$). After controlling for predictors of high risk, the authors found that letrozole significantly reduced the risk of early relapse compared with tamoxifen. Despite the lack of significant interaction between endocrine treatment and the prognostic factors of early relapse, multivariate analyses indicated that the beneficial effect of letrozole vs. tamoxifen may be qualitatively greater for patients with poor prognosis (four or more positive nodes, tumors >2 cm, or with vascular invasion) than for patients without poor prognosis (i.e., those with intermediate risk). For patients with intermediate risk of early relapse (less than four positive nodes, tumors ≤2 cm, and without vascular invasion), tamoxifen may be as effective as letrozole, and therefore sequential therapy may represent a good option, with toxicity profiles playing a greater role in therapy choice.

15.5   Side Effects

Aging is associated with an increased incidence and prevalence of co-morbidities and the presence of specific illnesses might drive the choice between tamoxifen and AIs in this population. Therefore safety issues are extremely important in older patients. The long-term safety profile of tamoxifen is well-known. In comparison with AIs, tamoxifen is associated with a higher risk of endometrial cancer and thromboembolic events. In comparison with tamoxifen, AIs are associated with a higher risk of musculoskeletal disorders. Among the side effects described with AIs, osteoporosis, bone fracture, and cardiac events are particularly worrisome for older patients.

Variation in bone mineral densitometry (BMD), incidence of osteoporosis, and bone fracture in patients treated in AIs adjuvant trials, are described in Table 15.3. Briefly, the introduction of AIs in the adjuvant setting was associated with an increased incidence of osteopenia and osteoporosis. With the exception of the extended strategy, therapy with AIs was also associated with a significant increase in clinical fracture. Data from IES and BIG 1–8 suggest that there is no significant effect of age on the risk of fracture (Crivellari et al. 2008; Coleman et al. 2007).

A higher incidence of cardiovascular events (CV), with AIs has been reported in some adjuvant trials. Detailed information is available for the ATAC, BIG 1–98, IES, and MA.17 trials (Table 15.4). In the ATAC trial, apart from a nonstatistically significant difference in angina, the occurrence of other ischemic CV events was similar between tamoxifen and anastrozole (The Arimidex & Alone or in Combination (ATAC) Trialists' Group 2006). In the BIG 1–98 trial, although the overall incidence of cardiac adverse events did not differ significantly between the two treatments, a trend for higher grade (3–5) cardiac events on letrozole compared with tamoxifen was seen (Coates et al. 2007). In particular, double the number of cardiac deaths was reported with letrozole vs. tamoxifen. Looking at the overall incidence of cardiac events, Crivellari et al. found that after adjusting for risk factors, a significant difference favoring tamoxifen was observed in the older age cohort (65–74 years) but not in the elderly cohort (≥75 years) (Crivellari et al. 2008). Regarding ischemic heart events, after adjusting for risk factors, a significant difference in time to first grade 3–5 ischemic heart event favoring tamoxifen was observed in the older age cohort (65–74 years), but not in the younger cohort (<65 years), or elderly cohort (≥75 years). On the basis of Cox model analysis, history of hypertension represented a statistically significant risk factor for both cardiac and ischemic heart events. Prior cardiac and ischemic heart events represented risk factors for respectively cardiac and ischemic heart events during treatment. In the IES trial, there was a trend for higher incidence in myocardial infarctions (MI) on exemestane. Of note, the effects of treatment on the risk of MI seemed largely restricted to patients with a history of hypertension. Seventy-one percent of patients on exemestane who had MI had hypertension at baseline compared with 32% of the corresponding patients on tamoxifen (Coombes et al. 2007). Apart from the BIG 1–98 trial, that showed that patients on letrozole experimented more CV events other than ischemia and cardiac failure and more severe cardiac events, no significant differences in terms of CV events were observed in all the other adjuvant trials. Extremely interesting are the data from the MA.17 trial, in which the AI was compared with placebo. The fact that no difference in terms of CV events was reported in this trial, suggests that the cardioprotective effect of tamoxifen may be the principle driving factor for difference in cardiac toxicity observed in all adjuvant trials when an AI is compared to tamoxifen. A longer follow-up will probably better clarify the safety profile of letrozole. For the time being conclusions regarding the relationship between AIs and cardiac risk are limited by the modest number of events reported.

Table 15.3 Bone toxicities from published adjuvant trials

Events	ATAC			BIG 1-98			ABSG8/ARNO 95			ITA		IES		
%	A	T	p	L	T	p	A	T	p	T	p	E	T	p
Bone fracture	11.0	7.7	<0.0001	8.6	5.8	<0.001	2	1	0.015	1.3	0.6	4.3	3.1	0.03
Osteopor-osis												7.3	5.5	0.01
BMD changes -lumbar spine	from baseline to 5 yrs −8.1		<0.0001									at 24 months −4.0		

Events	MA.17			ABCSG6a				NSABP- B33		
%	L	P	p	A	P	E	p	A	P	p
Bone fracture	5.3	4.6	0.25	0.8			1.1	1.0		0.33
Osteoporosis	8.1	6.0	0.003							
P	A	P		P	E	p	p	P		p
BMD changes at 24 months -lumbar spine	−5.4		0.008							

Empty blanks = data not reported *A* anastrozole; *T* tamoxifen; *L* letrozole; *E* exemestane; *BMD* bone mineral densitometry
Modified from Biganzoli et al. (2007), with permission

Table 15.4 Details on cardiovascular events (CV) from ATAC, BIG 1–98, IES and MA.17 trials

Adverse Events	ATAC			BIG 1–98			IES			MA.17		
	A	T	P	L	T	P	E	T	P	L	P	P
	No. (%)	No. (%)		No. (%)	No. (%)		No. (%)	No. (%)		No. (%)	No. (%)	
All patients	3,092	3,094		2,448	2,447		2,320	2,338		2,572	2,577	
Cardiovascular events[a,b,c]	127 (4)	104 (3)	0.1	134 (5.5)	122 (5.0)	0.48[h]	382 (16.5)	350 (15.0)	0.16	149 (5.8)	144 (5.6)	0.76
Ischemic events				54 (2.2)	41 (1.7)	0.21	185 (8.0)	162 (6.9)	0.17			
Myocardial infarction	37 (1)	34 (1)	0.7				31 (1.3)	19 (0.8)	0.08	9 (0.3)	11 (0.4)	
Angina[g]	71 (2)	51 (2)	0.07							31 (1.2)	23 (0.9)	
Cardiac failure				24 (1)	14 (0.6)	0.14						
Cerebrovascular events	62 (2)	88 (3)	0.03	34 (1.4)	35 (1.4)	0.9				17 (0.7)	15 (0.6)	
Thromboembolic events[d]	87 (3)	140 (5)	0.0004	50 (2)	94 (3.8)	<0.001	28 (1.2)	54 (2.3)	0.004	11 (0.4)	6 (0.2)	
Other CV events[e]				19 (0.8)	6 (0.2)	0.014						
Deaths due to CV events[f]	49 (2)	46 (1)										
Deaths due to cardiac events				11	5		14	13				
Deaths due to vascular events							17	11				
Deaths due to CBV events	14 (<1)	22 (1)										

Empty blanks = data not reported A anastrozole; T tamoxifen; L letrozole; E exemestane; CV cardiovascular; CBV cerebrovascular

[a] BIG 1–98: included ONLY cardiac events

[b] IES CV excluded venous tromboembolic events

[c] MA.17: CV included tromboembolic and cerebrovascular events

[d] ATAC and IES: venous thromboembolic events

[e] included cardiovascular disorders not otherwise specified, aneurysm, aortic aneurysm rupture, aortic dilation, aortic stenosis, arteriosclerosis, atherosclerosis (obliterans), femoral arterial stenosis, hypertensive angiopathy, iliac artery stenosis, and intermittent claudication

(continued)

Table 15.4 (continued)

[f]included myocardial infarction, myocardial ischemia, arteriosclerosis, coronary-artery disorder, coronary thrombosis, peripheral vascular disorder, heart arrest, arrhythmia, atrial flutter, cardiomyopathy, congestive heart failure, embolus, heart failure, sudden death, left-heart failure, lung edema, mesenteric occlusion, occlusion, hypertension, hypotension, hemorrhage, and vascular anomaly

[g]MA.17: angina = new or worsening angina

[h]Fisher's exact p<. 001 for incidence of grade 3–5 cardiac events

From Biganzoli et al. (2007), with permission

15.6   Treatment Options for Elderly Patients

A primary issue is whether or not endocrine therapy is necessary in all elderly patients with hormone-receptor-positive early breast cancer. For women with minimum risk disease, treatment decisions should be based on a risk–benefit analysis that takes into account the low relapse rate within the first 10 years, the potential reduction in ipsilateral and CLBC relapse, the patient's life expectancy, and treatment-related adverse events. Older patients who have small (<1 cm) node-negative tumors or have serious co-morbidity with an estimated survival less than 10 years are unlikely to derive any survival benefit from tamoxifen or other endocrine treatments (Fig. 15.1). No adjuvant treatment could be an option in these patients.

For patients who are considered candidates to endocrine therapy, a patient-profile–based approach should be considered to maximize the therapeutic index of the treatment. From the safety point of view, when hormonal therapy is proposed to a new patient, all risk factors for cardiovascular disease and for osteoporosis should be evaluated. Thus, in the presence of co-morbidities such as osteoporosis with preexisting bone fractures or cardiac diseases tamoxifen may be preferred, whereas, on the contrary, an increased risk for or a prior history of thromboembolic disease might favor the choice of an AI. Based on efficacy data, upfront AIs should be considered for patients at risk of an early relapse, i.e., patients with node-positive (i.e., 4+) and/or large tumors. Tamoxifen remains a valuable option for early breast cancers at low risk of relapse, i.e., T<1 cm, grade 1, low proliferative index.

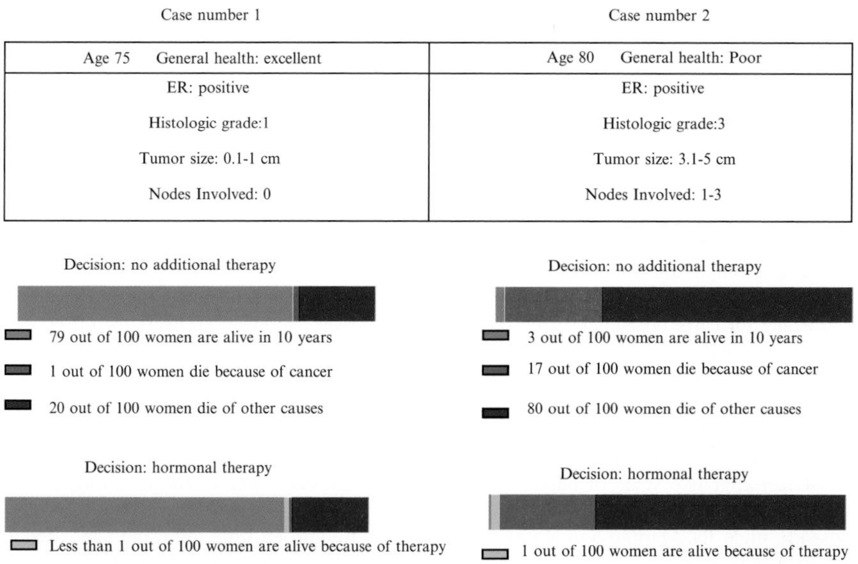

Case number 1	Case number 2
Age 75 General health: excellent	Age 80 General health: Poor
ER: positive	ER: positive
Histologic grade:1	Histologic grade:3
Tumor size: 0.1-1 cm	Tumor size: 3.1-5 cm
Nodes Involved: 0	Nodes Involved: 1-3

Decision: no additional therapy

- 79 out of 100 women are alive in 10 years
- 1 out of 100 women die because of cancer
- 20 out of 100 women die of other causes

Decision: hormonal therapy

- Less than 1 out of 100 women are alive because of therapy

Decision: no additional therapy

- 3 out of 100 women are alive in 10 years
- 17 out of 100 women die because of cancer
- 80 out of 100 women die of other causes

Decision: hormonal therapy

- 1 out of 100 women are alive because of therapy

Fig. 15.1 Expected effect of endocrine therapy on survival according to Adjuvant!Online www.adjuvantonline.com

In-between patients might be good candidates for sequential treatment. An extended adjuvant treatment with an AI found its rationale on evidences of a relatively constant risk of tumor relapse for ER-positive tumors over time. Individualized estimates of the risk of relapse and death after 5 years of tamoxifen based on standard pathologic prognostic markers suggest that extended adjuvant treatment could be avoided in women at low-risk of relapse (Kennecke et al. 2007). A subgroup analysis of the MA.17 trial showed that this "prolonged" approach is effective in healthy 70+ women with high-risk breast cancer.

References

Biganzoli L, Licitra S, Claudino W et al (2007) Clinical decisionmaking in Breast Cancer: TAM and aromatase inhibitors for older patients—a jungle? Eur J Cancer 43:2270–2278

Buzdar AU, J Cuzick (2008) Is overall survival an appropriate endpoint in early Breast cancer studies? Data from the ATAC study at 100-month median follow-up. J Clin Oncol 26 : 19s (abstract 552)

Coates AS, Keshaviah A, Thurlimann B et al (2007) Five years of letrozole compared with tamoxifen as initial therapy for postmenopausal women with endocrine-responsive early breast cancer: update of study BIG 1–98. J Clin Oncol 25:486–492

Coleman RE, Banks LM, Girgis SI et al (2007) Skeletal effects of exemestane on bone-mineral density, bone biomarkers, and fracture incidence in postmenopausal women with early breast cancer participating in the Intergroup Exemestane Study (IES): a randomized controlled study. Lancet 8:119–127

Coombes RC, Kilburn LS, Snowdon CF et al (2007) Survival and safety of exemestane versus tamoxifen after 2–3 years' tamoxifen treatment (Intergroup Exemestane Study): a randomized controlled trial. Lancet 369:559–5570

Crivellari D, Price K, Gelber RD et al (2003) Adjuvant endocrine therapy compared with no systemic therapy for elderly women (age 66–80 with early breast cancer: 21-year results of International Breast Cancer Study Group Trial IV. J Clin Oncol 21:4517–4523

Crivellari D, Sun Z, Coates AS et al (2008) Letrozole Compared With Tamoxifen for Elderly Patients With Endocrine-Responsive Early Breast Cancer: The BIG 1–98 Trial. J Clin Oncol. 26:1972–1979

Cuzick J, Sasieni P, Howell A (2006) Should aromatase inhibitors be used as initial adjuvant treatment or sequenced after tamoxifen? Br J Cancer 94:460–464

Decensi A, Robertson C, Viale G et al (2003) A randomized trial of low-dose tamoxifen on breast cancer proliferation and blood estrogenic biomarkers. J Natl Cancer Inst 95:779–790

Early Breast Cancer Trialists' Collaborative Group (2005) Effects of chemotherapy and hormonal therapy for early breast cancer on recurrence and 15-year survival: an overview of the randomised trials. Lancet 365:1687–1717

Goldhirsch A, Wood WC, Gelber RD et al (2007) Progress and promise: highlights of the international expert consensus on the primary therapy of elderly breast cancer 2007. Ann Oncol 18:1133–1144

Goss PE, Ingle JN, Martino S et al (2003) A randomised trial of letrozole in postmenopausal women after five years of tamoxifen therapy for early-stage breast cancer. N Engl J Med 349:1793–1802

Goss PE, Ingle JN, Martino S et al (2005) Randomised trial of letrozole following tamoxifen as adjuvant therapy in receptor-positive breast cancer: update findings from NCIC CTG MA.17. J Natl Cancer Inst 97:1262–1271

Ingle J, Du T, Shepherd L, Palmer M, Pater J, Goss P (2006) NCI CTG MA.17: Intent to treat analysis (ITT) of randomized patients after a median follow-up of 54 months. J Clin Oncol 24: (15S), abstract 549

Jakesz R, Greil R, Gnant M et al (2007) Extended adjuvant therapy with anastrozole among post-menopausal breast cancer patients : results from the randomized Austrian Breast and Colorectal Cancer Study Group Trial 6a. J Natl Cancer Inst 99:1845–1853

Jonat W, Gnant M, Boccardo F et al (2006) Effectiveness of switching from adjuavant tamoxifen to anastrozole in postmenopausal women with hormone-sensitive early stage breast cancer: a meta-analysis. Lancet 7:991–996

Kaufmann M, Jonat W, Hilfrich J et al (2007) Improved Overall survival in postmenopausal women with early breast cancer after nastrozole initiated after 2 years of treatment with tamox-ifen compared with continued tamoxifen: the ARNO 95 study. J Clin Oncol 25:2664–2670

Kennecke HF, Olivotto IA, Speers C et al (2007) Late risk of relapse and mortality among post-menopausal women with estrogen responsive early breast cancer after 5 years of tamoxifen. Ann Oncol 18:45–51

Mamounas EP, Jeong J-H, Wickerham DL et al (2008) Benefit from exemestane as extended adjuvant therapy after 5 years of adjuvant tamoxifen: intention-o-treat analysis of the National Surgical Adjuvant Breast and Bowel Projet B-33 Trial. J Clin Oncol 26:1965–1971

Mauriac L, Keshaviah A, Debled M et al (2007) Predictors of early relapse in postmenopausal women with hormone receptor-positive breast cancer in the BIG 1–98 trial. Ann Oncol 18:859–867

Muss HB, Tu D, Ingle JN et al (2008) Efficacy, Toxicity, and Quality of Life in Older Women With Early-Stage Breast Cancer Treated With Letrozole or Placebo After 5 Years of Tamoxifen: NCIC CTG Intergroup Trial MA.17. J Clin Oncol 26:1956–1964

Punglia RS, Kuntz KM, Winer EP et al (2005) Optimizing adjuvant endocrine therapy in post-menopausal women with early-stage breast cancer: a decision analysis. J Clin Oncol 23:5178–5187

Ragaz J, Coldman A (1998) Survival impact of adjuvant tamoxifen on competing causes of mor-tality in breast cancer survivors, with analysis of mortality from controlateral breast cancer, cardiovascular events, endometrial cancer and throemboembolic episodes. J Clin Oncol 16:2018–2024

Sacco M, Valentini M, Belfiglio M et al (2003) Randomized trial of 2 versus 5 years of adjuvant tamoxifen for women aged 50 years or older with early breast cancer: Italian Interdisciplinary Group for Cancer Evaluation study of adjuvant treatment in breast cancer. J Clin Oncol 21:2276–2281

The Arimidex Tamoxifen, Alone or in Combination (ATAC) Trialists' Group (2006) Comprehensive side-effect profile of anastrozole and tamoxifen as adjuvant treatment for early-stage breast cancer: long-term safety analysis of the ATAC trial. Lancet Oncol 7:633–643

The ATAC Trialists' Group (2002) Anastrozol alone or in combination with tamoxifen versus tamoxifen alone for adjuvant treatment of postmenopausal women with early breast cancer: first results of the ATAC randomised trial. Lancet 359:2131–2139

The ATAC Trialists' Group (2008) Effect of anastrozole and tamoxifen as adjuvant treatment for early-stage breast cancer: 100-month analysis of the ATAC trial. Lacet Oncol 9:45–53

Winer EP, Hudis C, Burstein HJ et al (2005) American Society of Clinical Oncology technology assessment on the use of aromatase inhibitors as adjuvant therapy for postmenopausal women with hormone receptor-positive breast cancer: status report 2004. J Clin Oncol 23:619–629

Chapter 16
Adjuvant Chemotherapy

Sumanta Kumar Pal, Nilesh Vora, and Arti Hurria

16.1 Introduction

Age constitutes the greatest risk factor for breast cancer – the median age at the time of diagnosis is 61, and the median age at the time of death from breast cancer is 69 (Ries et al. 2008). In patients with non-metastatic disease, adjuvant chemotherapy to decrease the risk of relapse and mortality remains a consideration regardless of age. Although substantial evidence supports the use of adjuvant chemotherapy in postmenopausal women, limited data specifically address the risks and benefits of adjuvant chemotherapy for patients over the age of 65, and even less data are available for those over 75.

Unique therapeutic considerations arise with older adults. With increasing age, breast cancers exhibit a distinct biology (i.e., increased hormone sensitivity, attenuated HER2 expression, lower tumor grade, and decreased proliferative indices). These biological characteristics help define the potential benefits from various treatment options designed to decrease the risk of relapse (Diab et al. 2000). For example, with hormone receptor positive tumors, the benefit of chemotherapy or trastuzumab (for HER2-positive tumors) in addition to endocrine therapy needs to be quantified. Additionally, the risks of adjuvant chemotherapy also vary by age. Medical co-morbidities and age-related changes in physiology increase the possibility of chemotherapy toxicity in older adults. These risks need to be weighed against potential benefits (Hurria et al. 2006a; Wildiers et al. 2007). In this chapter, we describe previous and ongoing efforts to define and optimize the role of adjuvant chemotherapy in the older adult.

A. Hurria (✉)
Department of Medical Oncology and Experimental Therapeutics,
City of Hope Comprehensive Cancer Center, Duarte, CA, USA

M.W. Reed and R.A. Audisio (eds.), *Management of Breast Cancer in Older Women*,
DOI 10.1007/978-1-84800-265-4_16, © Springer-Verlag London Limited 2011

16.2   Benefits of Chemotherapy

16.2.1   Prospective Trials in Older Adults

Data from prospective trials specifically addressing adjuvant breast cancer therapy in an older population are limited. Two available studies compare (1) adjuvant chemotherapy compared with endocrine therapy alone, and (2) polychemotherapy vs. single-agent chemotherapy.

The French Adjuvant Study Group 08 trial (FASG 08) randomized patients aged ≥65 years with node-positive, operable breast cancer to receive tamoxifen with or without epirubicin-based chemotherapy (Fargeot et al. 2004). Tamoxifen dose was 30 mg orally every day for 3 years, while epirubicin was given at 30 mg intravenously on days 1, 8, and 15 of a 28-day cycle for a total of 6 cycles. Both groups received radiotherapy following the completion of chemotherapy, if it was applicable. A total of 338 patients were enrolled in the study, with 318 patients ultimately included in the efficacy analysis. At a median follow-up of 72 months, 84 patients experienced recurrence: 46 (30%) in the tamoxifen-only arm and 38 (23%) in the combination-therapy arm (Fig. 16.1). Upon multivariate analysis, an increased relative risk of relapse (1.93; 95% CI, 1.70–2.17) was observed in patients receiving tamoxifen alone compared with epirubicin and tamoxifen. However, no difference was observed in overall survival (OS) related to disease progression (79% for tamoxifen alone vs. 80% with combination therapy; $P=0.41$). Comparison of hazard ratio for recurrence suggested a benefit from chemotherapy, principally in the estrogen receptor (ER) negative population ($P=0.01$). With respect to toxicity, no cases of congestive heart failure (CHF) occurred among 160 patients treated with epirubicin-based chemotherapy. Additionally, only eight cases of left ventricular ejection fraction (LVEF) declines were recorded, all of which were transient and controlled with medical management. These data reflect a benefit with single-agent chemotherapy and endocrine therapy over endocrine therapy alone in the older adult with node-positive breast cancer, as well as the safety of such therapy. As anticipated, this benefit is more pronounced among patients with ER-negative disease.

While the FASG 08 trial offers a comparison of chemotherapy with or without endocrine therapy, the Cancer and Leukemia Group B (CALGB) 49907 trial represents a comparison of distinct cytotoxic regimens (Table 16.1) (Muss et al. 2009). Eligibility criteria included an age of ≥65, non-metastatic breast cancer with tumors ≥1 cm, adequate organ functions, and estimated survival >5 years. Patients with Eastern Cooperative Oncology Group (ECOG) performance status >2 were excluded. Six hundred and thirty-three patients were randomized to receive either (1) capecitabine for 6 cycles, or (2) standard combination therapy consisting of cyclophosphamide, methotrexate, and fluorouracil (CMF) for 6 cycles, or doxorubicin and cyclophosphamide (AC) for 4 cycles. With a median follow-up of 2.4 years, analysis of RFS using a Cox proportional hazards model showed that patients receiving capecitabine had twice the relapse risk of standard therapy

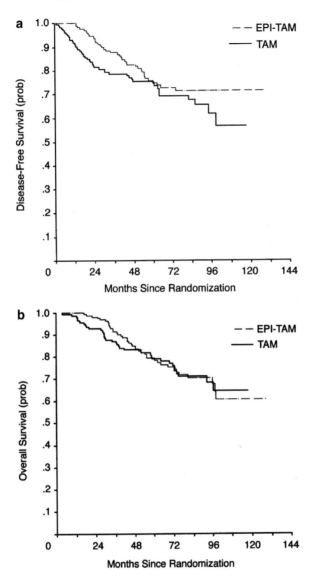

Fig. 16.1 Kaplan–Meier curves delineating DFS and OS from FACS 08, comparing tamoxifen alone for 3 years to tamoxifen for 3 years with epirubicin-based chemotherapy for 6 cycles (*DFS* disease-free survival; *OS* overall survival; *EPI* epirubicin; *TAM* tamoxifen). From Fargeot et al. (2004). Reprinted with permission from the American Society of Clinical Oncology (ASCO)

(hazard ratio [HR] 2.09, $P<0.001$). Similar findings were noted with respect to OS (HR 1.85, $P=0.02$). Among patients randomized to receive CMF or AC chemotherapy, 52 and 54% experienced grade 3 or 4 hematologic toxicity, respectively. In contrast, only 2% of patients receiving capecitabine experienced these toxic effects. Non-hematologic grade 3 or 4 toxicity was most common among patients receiving

Table 16.1 Summary of prospective trials including older patients with breast cancer

	Trials	
Trial design	FASG 08	CALGB 49907
Comparison	Tamoxifen alone × 3 years vs. tamoxifen × 3 years with epirubicin-based chemotherapy × 6 cycles	Capecitabine × 6 cycles vs. AC × 4 cycles or CMF × 4 cycles
Patient characteristics	Age ≥65 with node-positive, operable breast cancer	Age ≥65 with non-metastatic breast cancer, estimated survival >5 years
Number of participants	338	633
Median follow-up, years	6	2.4
HR for recurrence	1.93[a]	2.09[b]
95% CI	1.7–2.2	1.4–3.2

[a]Favoring chemotherapy and tamoxifen vs. tamoxifen alone
[b]Favoring AC or CMF chemotherapy vs. capecitabine alone
FASG French Adjuvant Study Group; *CALGB* Cancer and Leukemia Group B; *HR* hazard radio; *CI* confidence interval

CMF (41% CMF, 25% AC, 33% capecitabine). Notably, only two drug-related deaths occurred in the trial; both were in the capecitabine arm (one death from colitis, and another from infection).

Taken together, the results of the trials indicate that polychemotherapy is associated with improved relapse-free and OS compared with single-agent therapy. However, polychemotherapy is also associated with an increased risk of hematologic and non-hematologic toxicity, although the two treatment-related deaths occurred among patients receiving single-agent capecitabine.

16.2.2   Retrospective Data

The Early Breast Cancer Trialists' Collaborative Group (EBCTCG) meta-analysis incorporates data from randomized trials completed prior to 1995 (Early Breast Cancer Trialists Collaborative Group 2005). Over 150,000 women from 200 randomized trials were included in the meta-analysis, featuring studies that had >20 years of follow-up. Data in postmenopausal women indicate that polychemotherapy decreased the risk of recurrence and mortality from breast cancer; however, an age-related decrease in the benefit from polychemotherapy was also observed. These findings must be interpreted cautiously, given that women >70 years of age represented only 5% of the population assessed in this meta-analysis. In broader terms, this statistic reflects the poor representation of older adults in randomized trials.

Two separate studies utilizing data from the surveillance, epidemiology, and end results (SEER) database identify a potential benefit from chemotherapy in patients with ER-negative, lymph-node positive disease (Elkin et al. 2006; Giordano et al. 2006a). The first study assessed patients age ≥65 with hormone-receptor-negative, non-metastatic breast cancer diagnosed between 1992 and 1999. Associated data regarding chemotherapy use were obtained using Medicare claims linked to the SEER record (Elkin et al. 2006). Among 5,081 women in the analysis, 1,711 (34%) had received adjuvant chemotherapy. The study assessed predictors of chemotherapy receipt, including clinical and sociodemographic variables. This study showed that receipt of adjuvant chemotherapy was associated with a 15% reduction in mortality. Controlling for all other variables, age was a strong predictor of adjuvant chemotherapy use, with women age 70–74 being 44% less likely to receive chemotherapy compared with women age 66–69. The OS benefit was most pronounced in patients with lymph-node-positive disease and in patients with lymph-node-negative disease who were most likely to receive chemotherapy based on clinical and sociodemographic variables.

A second SEER database evaluation included patients with both hormone-receptor-negative and hormone-receptor-positive disease (Giordano et al. 2006a). Using otherwise similar criteria (age ≥65, stage I to III breast cancer, and diagnosis between 1991 and 1999), 41,390 patients were identified. A total of 4,500 (11%) received adjuvant chemotherapy, and again, a trend toward decreased chemotherapy use was observed with increasing patient age. Comparable to the previous study, women between the ages of 75 and 79 were 4 times less likely to receive chemotherapy than women between the ages of 65 and 69. In the analysis of survival benefit, a significant interaction was observed between hormone receptor status and chemotherapy use. Accordingly, analyses were stratified by ER status. Receipt of chemotherapy was not associated with a survival benefit in patients with ER-positive disease regardless of lymph-node status, nor was a benefit identified in patients with ER-negative, lymph-node-negative disease. Importantly, however, a survival benefit was elicited in patients with ER-negative, lymph-node-positive disease, mirroring results from the previous study. This subgroup may be of interest in shaping further trials of adjuvant therapy in the older adult.

Further insight into age-related benefits from chemotherapy regimens can be obtained from a combined report of 4 CALGB trials that evaluated the benefit of regimens that contained "more" chemotherapy (the experimental arm) vs. "less" chemotherapy (the standard arm) (Table 16.2) (Muss et al. 2005). The treatment arm that contained "more" chemotherapy typically built upon standard treatment at the time and was considered more toxic because it delivered higher doses or additional chemotherapy than the standard arm. Two trials included CMF-based therapy and two trials contained anthracycline-based chemotherapy. Among a total of 6,487 patients with lymph-node-positive breast cancer treated in these trials, 542 patients (8%) were ≥65 years of age and 159 patients (2%) were ≥70 years. An important finding from this study was that both younger and older cohorts obtained similar benefits in decreasing the risk of recurrence and mortality from the arm that contained "more" vs. "less" chemotherapy. On multivariate analysis, smaller tumor size, fewer positive lymph nodes, enrollment in the treatment arm that delivered "more chemotherapy," and tamoxifen use were significantly related to improvements

Table 16.2 Summary of CALGB trials comparing "less" and "more" chemotherapy ($N=6,487$)

Trial	CALGB 7581	CALGB 8082[a]	CALGB 8541	CALGB 9344
Regimen (more chemotherapy)	CMF+VP	CMF+VP; VATH	High-dose CAF	AC+T
Regimen (less chemotherapy)	CMF+MER	CMF+VP	Mid-/low- dose CAF	AC
Number of patients treated	884	933	1,549	3,121
Age≥65, N (%)	85 (10)	128 (14)	148 (10)	181 (6)

[a]Excluding patients aged 70 or older

AC doxorubicin and cyclophosphamide; *AC+T* doxorubicin and cyclophosphamide followed by paclitaxel; *CAF* cyclophosphamide, doxorubicin, and fluorouracil; *CMF* cyclophosphamide, methotrexate, and fluorouracil; *CMF+VP* CMF+vincristine and prednisone; *CMF+MER* CMF+the methanol extraction residue of bacillus Calmette-Guerin; *VATH* vinblastine, doxorubicin, thiotepa, and fluoxymesterone (halotestin)

in disease-free survival (DFS) and OS ($P<0.001$). Although age was not related to DFS, OS was significantly worse among patients age≥65, primarily because of deaths other than breast cancer.

Recently, interest has been directed toward substituting non-anthracycline regimens for an anthracycline regimen in order to minimize cardiac toxicity. This effort is particularly pertinent for older adults who may have preexisting cardiac co-morbidities. US Oncology Trial 9735 represents one such effort, comparing adjuvant docetaxel and cyclophosphamide (TC) to AC in patients with low-risk breast cancer (Jones et al. 2006). A significant disease-free and OS benefit with TC was observed, and an update of these data suggested similar efficacy in older as well as younger patients (Jones et al. 2008). Assessment of toxicity showed numerically higher rates of febrile neutropenia with TC, but greater incidence of anemia with AC in older patients. Additionally, fewer long-term toxicities (cardiac and hematologic) were observed with TC (Dominguez-Ventura et al. 2007).

16.3 Risks of Adjuvant Therapy

Several large studies have demonstrated that older adults are at increased toxicity risk from adjuvant chemotherapy. An extensive review of the International Breast Cancer Study Group (IBCSG) experience, including IBCSG trials I through IX, assessed CMF-related mortality in the context of these trials (Colleoni et al. 1999). In 6,926 patients, a total of 17 deaths (68%) were observed during CMF therapy. Of these, 3 deaths (0.08%) occurred in 3,653 patients age ≤50, 7 (0.26%) among 2,728 patients between age 51 and 64, and 7 (1.28%) among 545 patients age≥65 ($P<0.0001$). Notably, increased age was associated with a higher risk of treatment-related mortality. Seven of the CMF-related deaths were attributed to sepsis or toxic effects related to therapy, and these occurred among patients age 54–74 (median 63).

Table 16.3 Summary of treatment and toxicity data in CALGB trials 8541, 9344, and 9741 ($N=6,642$)

Toxicity/treatment course	Age		
	≤50 (%)	51–64 (%)	≥65 (%)
Grade 4 hematologic toxicity	17	17	18
Grade 3 or 4 non-hematologic toxicity	20	19	17
Treatment discontinued[a]	2	4	6
Overall treatment-related death	0.2	0.4	1.5
Cardiac[b]	0.03	0.2	1.1
AML[c]	0.11	0.08	0.4

[a]Toxicity-related
[b,c]Denotes treatment-related deaths related to cardiac dysfunction and AML

A similar correlation between age- and treatment-related toxicity was observed from a meta-analysis of 3 CALGB trials (Table 16.3). This study utilized data from two previously mentioned CALGB trials, including anthracycline therapy (CALGB 8541 and 9344), and additionally includes data from CALGB 9741, a trial of doxorubicin, cyclophosphamide, and paclitaxel every 2 weeks compared with every 3 weeks (Muss et al. 2007). Toxicity data were available for most of the 6,642 patients enrolled in these trials, and a total of 458 patients (7%) were age ≥65. Toxic deaths attributable to therapy occurred in 1.5% of patients age ≥65, 4% of patients age 51–64, and 19% of patients age <50. In addition, multivariate analysis demonstrated that older patients were more likely to have grade 4 hematologic toxicity, discontinue treatment because of toxicity, or die from acute myelogenous leukemia (AML), or myelodysplastic syndrome (MDS). Both these data and the IBCSG experience underscore the need to carefully assess the potential risks associated with adjuvant therapy in the older adult, and counter the assumption that risk profiles established from chemotherapeutic regimens are generalizable across all ages.

A separately reported assessment of IBCSG VII provides additional insight into both efficacy and toxicity related to adjuvant chemotherapy in the older adult. This trial randomized postmenopausal women to 1 of 4 treatment groups including tamoxifen alone or tamoxifen with 1 of 3 schedules of CMF chemotherapy (Crivellari et al. 2000). The 3 schedules included early CMF (3 consecutive cycles initiated on the same day as tamoxifen), delayed CMF (3 cycles administered at months 9, 12, and 15 of tamoxifen therapy), or a combination of early and delayed CMF. No upper age limit was included in the trial, and subgroup analysis suggested a significantly higher rate of hematologic toxicity ($P=0.0002$) and mucosal toxicity ($P=0.004$) in patients age ≥65. In addition, older patients were less likely to receive the protocol-specified CMF dose (48% vs. 65%, $P=0.0008$). Interestingly, while the addition of CMF to tamoxifen led to an overall improvement in 5-year (DFS; HR 0.78, 95% CI, 62%-97%, $P=0.03$), no such improvement was observed in older patients ($P=0.99$). It is important to note that interpretations of subset analyses by age are complicated by the limited representation of older patients and the lack of information regarding the health status of the older adults included in the trial. On the other hand, this study demonstrates that older adults tolerated less of the protocol-specified therapy than younger adults, highlighting a potential reason for the age-related decreased benefit from adjuvant chemotherapy.

A separate institutional review provides further insight regarding the utility of adjuvant CMF in older patients (De Maio et al. 2005). This study selected a total of 180 patients age >60 who had received adjuvant CMF therapy between March 1991 and 2002. Within this population, 100 patients were identified between the ages of 60-65, and 80 patients age ≥65, forming 2 comparator groups. With respect to toxicity, more severe and frequent events occurred in the older subset, including leucopenia, neutropenia, nausea, cardiac toxicity, and thrombophlebitis. Accordingly, poor compliance (defined as 1 of the following events: <6 cycles received, >1 day #8 chemotherapy omission, dose reduction in >25% of cycles, need for G-CSF or treatment interruption because of toxicity or refusal) occurred more frequently among older patients – 58% vs. 46%, $P=0.02$. Despite the data related to compliance and toxicity, DFS did not appear to be markedly different between the 2 groups, with 5-year DFS in 42% and 43% of older and younger patients, respectively ($P=0.84$), although interpretation of these results is limited by the small sample size.

16.3.1 Specific Toxicities from Adjuvant Therapy

16.3.1.1 Cardiac Toxicity

Several studies have assessed toxicity considerations that may be of particular importance in the older adult (Fig. 16.2). The risk of cardiac toxicity with anthracycline therapy in cancer patients is well-documented (Gianni et al. 2008). In the older adult, this risk is compounded by the presence of cardiovascular co-morbidities (Thomas and Rich 2007). An analysis of the SEER-Medicare database focused on the incidence of CHF in the older population (Giordano et al. 2006b). Patients age 66–90 who were diagnosed with breast cancer were included in this analysis. In this observational study, 34,261 patients were assessed: 28,640 received no chemotherapy, 3,253 received non-anthracycline chemotherapy, and 2,728 received anthracycline-based chemotherapy. Consistent with previous findings, women who received anthracycline-based chemotherapy were younger and had lower co-morbidity scores. Additionally, these patients generally had more advanced disease. The adjusted hazard ratio (HR) for the development of CHF with anthracycline therapy was 1.45 (95% CI, 1.19–1.76) vs. non-anthracycline chemotherapy. No statistically significant difference in the rates of CHF was determined among patients age 66–70 compared with patients age 71–90. However, given the retrospective nature of the study, selection biases cannot be excluded; i.e., the older patients may have been healthier at baseline, leading to the utilization of chemotherapy.

Beyond chemotherapy alone, several large randomized trials have led to the acceptance of chemotherapy in combination with trastuzumab for HER2-positive breast cancer. Data emerging from these studies also indicate an increased risk of

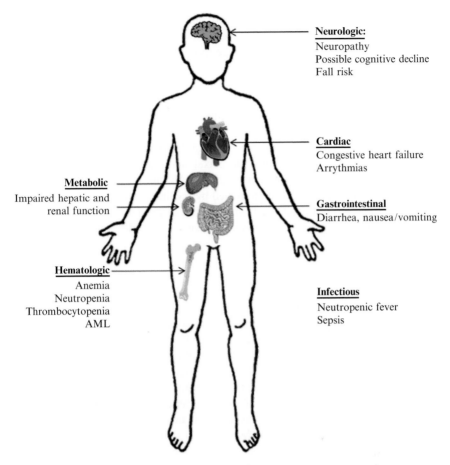

Neurologic:
Neuropathy
Possible cognitive decline
Fall risk

Cardiac
Congestive heart failure
Arrythmias

Metabolic
Impaired hepatic and
renal function

Gastrointestinal
Diarrhea, nausea/vomiting

Hematologic
Anemia
Neutropenia
Thrombocytopenia
AML

Infectious
Neutropenic fever
Sepsis

Fig. 16.2 Toxicity considerations in the older patient. From Fargeot et al. (2004). Reprinted with permission from the ASCO

cardiac toxicity with trastuzumab/chemotherapy combinations, in particular those that are anthracycline-based.

The North Central Cancer Treatment Group (NCCTG) N9831 and National Surgical Adjuvant Breast and Bowel Project (NSABP) B-31 trials randomized patients to either anthracycline-based chemotherapy alone or in combination with trastuzumab (Romond et al. 2005). A combined analysis at a median follow-up of 2 years demonstrated a 52% reduction in the risk of recurrence and a 33% reduction in the risk of death with the addition of trastuzumab. Notably, of 3,351 patients enrolled in the trial, only 535 patients (16%) were ≥60 years of age. Serious cardiac adverse events, including New York Heart Association (NYHA) class III or IV heart failure or death from cardiac causes, was more pronounced in the trastuzumab-containing arm in both studies (an absolute increase of 3.3% and 2.9% in NSABP B-31 and NCCTG N9831, respectively). Among patients enrolled in

NSABP B-31, older age (defined as age >50) and a post-AC left ventricular ejection fraction of 50–54% were significant predictors of CHF (Tan-Chiu et al. 2005). Similarly, data from NCCTG N9831 suggested older age (defined as age >50) was significantly associated with the risk of any cardiac event. Other risk factors included left ventricular ejection fraction (<55% but above lower limit of normal) at the time of registration for the study and the use of antihypertensive medication (either prior or current use) (Perez et al. 2008). Given these data, alternatives to the combined anthracycline and trastuzumab regimens in these trials may be desirable.

Breast Cancer International Research Group (BCIRG) trial 006 assesses a non-anthracycline regimen (specifically, docetaxel, and carboplatin) in combination with trastuzumab (TCH) (Slamon et al. 2007). An interim efficacy analysis suggested equivalence of TCH to AC followed by paclitaxel and trastuzumab. Subset analyses by age are not available from this trial at present; ultimately, however, TCH may represent a less cardiotoxic alternative for older adults with HER2-positive breast cancer.

16.3.1.2   Neurologic Toxicity

Concerns have recently emerged as to the impact of cancer therapy on cognitive function; however, few studies have focused specifically on the impact of cancer therapy on the cognitive function of older adults or those with preexisting cognitive problems. A pilot study recently reported serial cognitive function assessments in 28 women (mean age 71 years) receiving adjuvant chemotherapy for non-metastatic breast cancer (Hurria et al. 2006b). Cognitive scores were assessed at baseline and 6 months after adjuvant chemotherapy. Of 28 evaluable patients, 7 patients (25%) experienced a 1 SD decline in 2 or more neuropsychological domains from prior to and after receiving chemotherapy. The older patient's perception of the impact of adjuvant chemotherapy on memory was evaluated in a cohort of 45 patients with a mean age of 70 years (Hurria et al. 2006c). In this cohort of 45 patients, with a mean age of 70 years, approximately half the patients perceived a decline in memory from before chemotherapy to after receiving chemotherapy. These patients perceived that the ability to learn new information seemed most affected by adjuvant chemotherapy.

16.3.1.3   Hematologic Toxicity

Bone marrow reserve decreases with increasing age, placing older adults at increased risk for hematologic toxicity. Data from a prospective analysis indicate increasing rates of chemotherapy-induced neutropenia with advancing age (Dees et al. 2000). This study included 44 women with early stage breast cancer, and assessed pharmacokinetic variables during receipt of an initial cycle of AC chemotherapy. Laboratory values and other physiologic parameters were monitored through the course of 4 cycles of AC. Although there were no age-related differences in the pharmacokinetics of AC, an age-related decrease in the nadir ANC was seen.

Based on this and other studies, American Society of Clinical Oncology (ASCO) practice guidelines for the use of white blood cell growth factors recognizes age >65 as a risk factor for febrile neutropenia (Smith et al. 2006). Similarly, guidelines from the National Comprehensive Cancer Network (NCCN) recognize age as a risk factor that may compromise the ability to deliver full-dose chemotherapy (Crawford et al. 2007). Early initiation of white blood cell growth factors in older adults can decrease the risk of fever and neutropenia, making it possible to maintain the chemotherapy dose and schedule.

16.3.1.4 Secondary Acute Myelogenous Leukemia (AML)

Older adults who receive adjuvant chemotherapy are at an increased risk of developing AML. This was demonstrated in an observational study from the SEER-Medicare linked database. Women age $\geq$66 with a diagnosis of non-metastatic breast cancer were included in this analysis (Patt et al. 2007). The risk of AML was stratified based on receipt or nonreceipt of chemotherapy. A diagnosis of AML beyond the time of diagnosis with breast cancer was used as the primary endpoint. Of 64,715 patients reviewed in the study, 10,130 received adjuvant chemotherapy. Patients who received adjuvant chemotherapy had an increased risk of AML (HR1.53, 95% CI, 1.14–2.06) compared with patients who did not receive chemotherapy. This increased risk was independent of the type of chemotherapy received. For example, in a multivariate analysis, anthracycline therapy did not significantly increase the risk of AML (5-year cumulative hazard, 1.2% vs. 0.9%, $P=0.21$). Age >80, however, was noted to be a significant predictor of AML in patients who received adjuvant chemotherapy vs. those who did not (HR 3.35, 95% CI, 1.54–7.30).

16.4 Factors Influencing Adjuvant Therapy Decisions

Older adults of the same chronological age present with a heterogeneous pool of health states and co-morbid conditions. Results from a recent physician survey support the finding that both patient age and health status guide therapeutic decision-making (Hurria et al. 2008). The study participants comprised 150 oncologists and 155 primary care providers with geriatric expertise who were presented with case scenarios of hypothetical patients of varying ages (70, 75, 80, and 85) with a 4 cm, lymph-node-positive, ER-positive, HER2-negative-tumor, and health states good, average, and poor. The results demonstrated that both oncologists and geriatricians were less likely to recommend adjuvant therapy as the patient's age increased or health status declined ($P<0.0001$). This study highlights the need to incorporate health status and age in prospective studies of older adults with breast cancer, as well as to develop evidence-based guidelines that take these factors into account. A geriatric assessment (which includes an evaluation of an individual's functional status, co-morbid medications and concomitant medications, social support, nutritional, psychological, and cognitive status) can provide a better understanding of an individual's health status, "functional age," and life expectancy. Additional research is needed to identify those items in a geriatric assessment which are most predictive of the risk of toxicity to adjuvant chemotherapy in older adults. This calls for collaboration between the fields of geriatrics and oncology.

16.5 Conclusions and Future Directions

Limited prospective data are available to guide decisions regarding adjuvant breast cancer chemotherapy in the older adult, though further trials are either anticipated or ongoing (Table 16.4). As a result, most knowledge to date is derived from retrospective data, subset analyses by age, and observational studies.

A further understanding of breast cancer in the older adult depends upon several factors. First, as with patients of all ages, further efforts are needed to characterize the molecular pathogenesis of breast cancer in order to select those patients who are likely to derive the greatest benefit from chemotherapy. Second, clinical assessment of older patients with breast cancer must reflect the current understanding of age-related toxicities and incorporate novel metrics to assess global health status. As outlined previously, existing studies suggest that older patients experience higher rates of neutropenia and cardiac toxicity, among other adverse effects. Nonetheless, several large studies also suggest that older patients may derive as much benefit from adjuvant treatment as younger patients, even in the face of increased toxicity. Therefore, general breast cancer treatment guidelines pertain as much to an older adult as a younger adult (Gridelli et al. 2007; Harbeck and Jakesz 2007). Recently published recommendations from the International Society of Geriatric Oncology (SIOG) may further aid in the management of adjuvant chemotherapy decisions (Wildiers et al. 2007). In addition, a geriatric assessment can provide a more thorough understanding of the patient's health status in order to weigh the risks and benefits of therapy. Ultimately, understanding the patient's preferences for adjuvant treatment is an integral part of the treatment decision.

Table 16.4 Currently active, randomized, prospective clinical trials focused on older adults with breast cancer

Trial	Anticipated accrual	Cooperative group/ sponsor	Description
Elderly breast cancer-docetaxel adjuvant therapy (ELDA)	300	Clinical Trials Unit, National Cancer Institute of Naples	Patients age 65–80 will be randomized to docetaxel alone or CMF as adjuvant therapy.
Ibandronate with or without capecitabine in elderly patients with breast cancer (ICE)	1,500	German Breast Group (GBG)	Ibandronate alone will be compared to ibandronate with capecitabine in patients age ≥65.

In the future, utilizing the breast cancer's genotypic data to quantify the risk of relapse as well as the benefits to be derived from chemotherapy, in combination with information from a geriatric assessment and an understanding of the patient's preferences, will allow oncologists to optimize and tailor adjuvant therapy for the older adult with breast cancer. Ultimately, additional prospective studies are needed to accomplish these goals.

Acknowledgment of Research Support Dr. Hurria's efforts are supported by K23 AG026749-01 (Paul Beeson Career Development Award in Aging Research) and American Society of Clinical Oncology-Association of Specialty Professors-Junior Development Award in Geriatric Oncology.

References

Colleoni M, Price KN, Castiglione-Gertsch M et al. (1999) Mortality during adjuvant treatment of early breast cancer with cyclophosphamide, methotrexate, and fluorouracil. Lancet 354(9173):130–131

Crawford J, Althaus B, Armitage J et al (2007) Myeloid growth factors. Clinical practice guidelines in oncology. J Natl Compr Canc Netw 5(2):188–202

Crivellari D, Bonetti M, Castiglione-Gertsch M et al (2000) Burdens and benefits of adjuvant cyclophosphamide, methotrexate, and fluorouracil and tamoxifen for elderly patients with breast cancer: the international breast cancer study group trial VII. J Clin Oncol 18:1412–1422

De Maio E, Gravina A, Pacilio C et al (2005) Compliance and toxicity of adjuvant CMF in elderly breast cancer patients: a single-center experience. BMC Cancer 5:30

Dees EC, O'Reilly S, Goodman SN et al (2000) A prospective pharmacologic evaluation of age-related toxicity of adjuvant chemotherapy in women with breast cancer. Cancer Invest 18:521–529

Diab SG, Elledge RM, Clark GM (2000) Tumor characteristics and clinical outcome of elderly women with breast cancer. J Natl Cancer Inst 92:550–556

Dominguez-Ventura A, Cassivi SD, Allen MS et al (2007) Lung cancer in octogenarians: factors affecting long-term survival following resection. Eur J Cardiothorac Surg 32:370–374

Elkin EB, Hurria A, Mitra N et al (2006) Adjuvant chemotherapy and survival in older women with hormone receptor-negative breast cancer: assessing outcome in a population-based, observational cohort. J Clin Oncol 24:2757–2764

Fargeot P, Bonneterre J, Roche H et al (2004) Disease-free survival advantage of weekly epirubicin plus tamoxifen versus tamoxifen alone as adjuvant treatment of operable, node-positive, elderly breast cancer patients: 6-year follow-up results of the French Adjuvant Study Group 08 trial. J Clin Oncol 22:4674–4682

Gianni L, Herman EH, Lipshultz SE et al (2008) Anthracycline cardiotoxicity: from bench to bedside. J Clin Oncol 26:3777–3784

Giordano SH, Duan Z, Kuo Y-F et al (2006a) Use and outcomes of adjuvant chemotherapy in older women with breast cancer. J Clin Oncol 24:2750–2756

Giordano SH, Duan Z, Hortobagyi G, Goodwin J (2006b) Congestive heart failure (CHF) in older women treated with anthracycline (A) chemotherapy (C). Journal of Clinical Oncology, 2006 ASCO annual meeting proceedings part I, vol. 24(18S) (June 20 supplement), p 521

Gridelli C, Maione P, Illiano A et al (2007) Cisplatin plus gemcitabine or vinorelbine for elderly patients with advanced non small-cell lung cancer: The MILES-2P studies. J Clin Oncol 25:4663–4669

Early Breast Cancer Trialists Collaborative Group (2005) Effects of chemotherapy and hormonal therapy for early breast cancer on recurrence and 15-year survival: an overview of the randomised trials. Lancet 365:1687–1717

Harbeck N, Jakesz R (2007) St. Gallen 2007: breast cancer treatment consensus report. Breast Care 2:130–134

Hurria A, Fleming MT, Baker SD et al (2006a) Pharmacokinetics and toxicity of weekly docetaxel in older patients. Clin Cancer Res 12:6100–6105

Hurria A, Rosen C, Hudis C et al (2006b) Cognitive function of older patients receiving adjuvant chemotherapy for breast cancer: a pilot prospective longitudinal study. J Am Geriatr Soc 54:925–931

Hurria A, Goldfarb S, Rosen C et al (2006c) Effect of adjuvant breast cancer chemotherapy on cognitive function from the older patient's perspective. Breast Cancer Res Treat 98:343–348

Hurria A, Wong FL, Villaluna D et al. (2008) Influence of age and health status on oncologists' and geratricians' adjuvant treatment recommendations for older adults with breast cancer. J Clin Oncol 26(20 Suppl); abstr 9643

Jones SE, Savin MA, Holmes FA et al (2006) Phase III trial comparing doxorubicin plus cyclophosphamide with docetaxel plus cyclophosphamide as adjuvant therapy for operable breast cancer. J Clin Oncol 24:5381–5387

Jones S, Holmes F, O'Shaughnessy J, et al. (2008) Extended follow-up and analysis by age of the US oncology adjuvant trial 9735: docetaxel/cyclophosphamide is associated with an overall survival benefit compared to doxorubicin/cyclophosphamide and is well-tolerated in women 65 or older. Breast Cancer Res Treat (abstr 12)

Muss HB, Woolf S, Berry D et al (2005) Adjuvant chemotherapy in older and younger women with lymph node-positive breast cancer. JAMA 293:1073–1081

Muss HB, Berry DA, Cirrincione C et al (2007) Toxicity of older and younger patients treated with adjuvant chemotherapy for node-positive breast cancer: the Cancer and Leukemia Group B experience. J Clin Oncol 25:3699–3704

Muss HB, Berry DA, Cirrincione CT et al (2009) Adjuvant chemotherapy in older women with early-stage breast cancer. N Engl J Med 360:2055–2065

Patt DA, Duan Z, Fang S et al (2007) Acute myeloid leukemia after adjuvant breast cancer therapy in older women: understanding risk. J Clin Oncol 25:3871–3876

Perez EA, Suman VJ, Davidson NE et al (2008) Cardiac safety analysis of doxorubicin and cyclophosphamide followed by paclitaxel with or without trastuzumab in the North Central Cancer Treatment Group N9831 adjuvant breast cancer trial. J Clin Oncol 26:1231–1238

Ries LAG, Melbert D, Krapcho M et al. (2008) SEER cancer statistics review, 1975–2005. National Cancer Institute, Bethesda, MD, http://SEER.CANCER.GOV/CSR/1975_2005/, based on November 2007 SEER data submission, posted to the SEER web site

Romond EH, Perez EA, Bryant J et al (2005) Trastuzumab plus adjuvant chemotherapy for operable HER2-positive breast cancer. N Engl J Med 353:1673–1684

Slamon D, Eiermann W, Robert N, et al. (2007) BCIRG 006: 2nd interim analysis phase III randomized trial comparing doxorubicin and cyclophosphamide followed by docetaxel (ACT) with doxorubicin and cyclophosphamide followed by docetaxel and trastuzumab (ACTH) with docetaxel, carboplatin and trastuzumab (TCH) in Her2neu positive early breast cancer patients. Breast Cancer Res Treat 2007 (abstr 52)

Smith TJ, Khatcheressian J, Lyman GH et al (2006) 2006 update of recommendations for the use of white blood cell growth factors: an evidence-based clinical practice guideline. J Clin Oncol 24:3187–3205

Tan-Chiu E, Yothers G, Romond E et al (2005) Assessment of cardiac dysfunction in a randomized trial comparing doxorubicin and cyclophosphamide followed by paclitaxel, with or without trastuzumab as adjuvant therapy in node-positive, human epidermal growth factor Receptor 2-overexpressing breast cancer: NSABP B-31. J Clin Oncol 23:7811–7819

Thomas S, Rich MW (2007) Epidemiology, pathophysiology, and prognosis of heart failure in the elderly. Heart Fail Clin 3:381–387

Wildiers H, Kunkler I, Biganzoli L et al (2007) Management of breast cancer in elderly individuals: recommendations of the International Society of Geriatric Oncology. Lancet Oncol 8:1101–1115

Chapter 17
Adjuvant Radiotherapy

Pierre G.M. Scalliet

17.1 Introduction

The goal of cancer care for elderly patients with breast cancer should include a plan for long-term control of the cancer (cure), maintenance of a maximum level of patient independence, freedom from symptoms, and maintenance of personal dignity and lifestyle (Wanebo et al. 1997). Radiotherapy (RT) after breast conserving surgery (BCS) or after mastectomy (post-mastectomy radiotherapy or PMRT) achieves improved local control and better survival than surgery alone, independent from other adjuvant interventions (Clarke et al. 2005). However, up to 30% of all breast cancer cases are reported to occur in patients over 70 years of age (Sader et al. 1999), a group that has often been excluded from the trials that have contributed to establishing the current standard of care. Although available age-specific clinical trials data demonstrate that treatment efficacy is not modified by age, this evidence is limited by the lack of inclusion of substantial numbers of older women, particularly those of advanced age and those with co-morbidities.

As life expectancy shortens with age, the question arises as to whether the treatment of breast cancer cannot be "de-escalated" to fit the remaining years to live rather than to stick to the "maximal" treatment model established for younger patients.

In particular, is it safe to omit the tedious RT treatment, as it only seems to add a few percent to the excellent level of local control already achieved with appropriate surgery. Quoting B. Fisher: "Breast cancer is a systemic disease involving a complex spectrum of host-tumor interactions; ... variations in effective local regional treatment are unlikely to affect survival substantially. Only systemic treatment is" (Fisher 1980).

P.G.M. Scalliet (✉)
Department Radiation Oncology, Cliniques Universitaires Saint Luc,
Avenue Hippocrate 10, Brussels, 1200, Belgium
e-mail: Pierre.scalliet@uclouvain.be

M.W. Reed and R.A. Audisio (eds.), *Management of Breast Cancer in Older Women*,   263
DOI 10.1007/978-1-84800-265-4_17, © Springer-Verlag London Limited 2011

17.2 Role of Radiotherapy in Breast Cancer

Several trials have been conducted in Europe and North America, establishing BCS followed by RT as the standard of care. RT has been considered for many years as an adjuvant "cosmetic" treatment to ensure maximal local control after BCS rather than an essential element contributing to long-term survival (Cuzick et al. 1987; Cuzick et al. 1994; Early Breast Cancer Trialists' Collaborative Group (EBCTCG) 1995; Early Breast Cancer Trialists' Collaborative Group (EBCTCG) 2000). It took decades to accumulate sufficient clinical data to assess various beneficial and deleterious effects of breast or chest RT.

The current view has been remodeled by a series of recent trials using RT techniques with a better control of the dose to the heart (Overgaard et al. 1997; Overgaard et al. 1999; Ragaz et al. 1997), allowing exploration of its curative impact without "contamination" by long-term lethal toxicity (Hojris et al. 1999). The EBCTCG, therefore, undertook the complex task of reviewing breast cancer clinical trials that began by 1995, uncovering the favorable effect of adjuvant RT after surgery to its full extent (Clarke et al. 2005). It is a rich report, exploring numerous aspects of local treatment (RT vs. no RT, more vs. less surgery, more surgery vs. RT). A short conclusion was that "differences in local treatment that affect local recurrence rates would, in the hypothetical absence of any other cause of death, avoid about one breast cancer death over 15 years for every four local recurrences avoided." In other words, the general finding was that a 20% absolute reduction in 5-year local recurrence risk led to a 5% reduction in 15-year breast cancer mortality.

Five-year isolated local recurrences were 6.7 vs. 22.9% in RT vs. no RT trials after BCS and node-negative disease, and 11 vs. 41.1% in node-positive women. Fifteen-year breast cancer mortality rates were 26.1 vs. 31.2% with and without RT in node-negative (Logrank $2p=0.006$), and 47.9 vs. 55.0% in node-positive cases (Logrank $2p=0.01$), respectively. The picture was similar after mastectomy in women with positive axillary nodes, both for 5- and 10-year isolated local recurrence and 15-year survival. Even in women with negative nodes, the risk of local recurrence, though small, was favorably influenced by adjuvant RT (6.3 vs. 2.3% at 5 years).

The issue of life-threatening side effects (mainly heart disease and secondary lung cancer) cannot be fully explored in recent trials, but there is a strong attempt to minimize both heart and lung dose with modern breast irradiation techniques.

These findings are very much in line with Hellman's view: "Breast cancer is a heterogeneous disease—a spectrum ranging from a disease that remains local throughout its course to a disease which is systemic when first detectable. Thus there could be situations where metastases would develop as a consequence of residual inadequately treated loco-regional disease" (Hellman 1994).

Hence, the significance of a local recurrence can be somewhat benign, a simple "accident" in the patient's history (if handled properly), or it can become the source of metastasis. The former case has no impact on the life expectancy of the patient, whereas the latter is eventually lethal. But in both case, the quality of life (QoL) of the patient is seriously disturbed.

17.3   Omitting RT After BCS

After BCS or mastectomy, the risk of local recurrence is a function of several tumor characteristics, including tumor size, grade, receptor status (including HER2), surgical margins, and the extent of nodal invasion.

In the last EBCTCG meta-analysis, the following factors were found to be significant predictors of local control: grade, size, ER status, and number of nodes (Table 17.1) (Clarke et al. 2005).

The local recurrence rates remained strikingly significant in the treatment arms without adjuvant RT even in women with a good prognostic disease. The lowest rate of recurrence was observed in women over 70, but a further analysis of the age effect was not possible as a result of the (inappropriate) policy of excluding older patients from randomized trials. Still, in this age group, the recurrence rate was a two-digit figure whenever RT was omitted.

Moreover, local recurrences after BCS was an early event, with a significant difference between irradiated and un-irradiated patients evident after just 1 year.

Attempts to replace RT by an adjuvant hormonal treatment did not offer a similar level of local control. In a Canadian randomized trial comparing tamoxifen (TAM) to RT after BCS in 769 T1-T2 node negative patients, the rate of local relapse was 7.7% at 5 years in the TAM group vs. only 0.6% in the RT group. At 8 years, the rate of relapse increased to 17.6 vs. 3.5% (Hughes et al. 2004).

A similar trial was conducted by the CALGB, RTOG, and ECOG in 636 women 70 years of age and older, but restricted to T1N0, ER+ tumors. In the TAM arm, the local recurrence rate at 5 years was 4 vs. 1% in the TAM+RT arm (Fyles et al. 2004).

Table 17.1 Effect of age and tumor characteristics on 5-year risk of local recurrence in trials of radiotherapy after breast conserving surgery in women with node-negative disease (Clarke et al. 2005)

Age (years)	RT (%)	Control (%)
<50	11	33
50–59	7	23
60–69	4	16
≥70	3	13
Tumor grade		
Well-differentiated	4	14
Moderately differentiated	9	26
Poorly differentiated	12	34
Tumor size (T category)		
1–20 mm (T1)	5	20
21–50 mm (T2)	14	35
ER status		
ER poor	12	30
ER positive	6	25

Another piece of the puzzle has been added in a recent update of the EORTC 22881–10882 data (the so-called boost vs. no boost trial) (Bartelink et al. 2007). 5,318 patients were randomized after BCS to RT alone (50 Gy) or followed by a boost dose (16 Gy) on the tumor site. T stage was 51.5% of T1 and 48% of T2; N stage was 90% of N0 (remaining N1–2 or Nx). About half of the population had positive estrogen receptors. With a median follow-up of 10 years the cumulative incidence of local recurrence was 10.2 (no boost) vs. 6.2% (boost) ($P<0.0001$). A significant absolute risk reduction was recorded in all age groups (<40, 41–50, 51–60, >60). The figure for the 60+ group was 7.3 vs. 3.8%. Although this does not directly demonstrate the usefulness of post-BCS RT, it indicates that radiation dose matters, and that recurrence rates, within the framework of a clinical trial with extensive quality control of surgery (margins) are far from insignificant, even after appropriate RT. This does surely not lend support to omit RT beyond the age of 60.

Preliminary results from the PRIME trial in UK were published in 2007, with quite a short follow-up period of 15 months. Within this short time frame, no local recurrences (LRs) were recorded. RT was therefore considered to be a non-cost-effective intervention after BCS in T1–2N0 elderly patient. Conversely, it was also shown that overall QoL was not substantially modified by the use of RT as compared to RT omission. It is important to note that women enrolled in the trial also benefit from adjuvant hormonal therapy that might delay the occurrence of LR. Also, statistical considerations around the trial indicate that a long-term reduction of LR by 5% would be sufficient to reverse the conclusion regarding cost-effectiveness (Prescott et al. 2007). At this stage, the PRIME trial has not matured sufficiently to deliver its full conclusions.

An Italian randomized trial enrolling 579 women with tumors ≤2.5 cm compared BCS with and without adjuvant RT. The rate of LR was strongly dependent on the use of RT, although the benefit seemed to decrease with age. The subgroup of women aged 65+ had no apparent benefit because of an already very low LR rate without RT. The trial however was not designed to investigate such questions (no stratification), and the population sampled was quite small (underpowered analysis) (Veronesi et al. 2001).

Smith et al. searched the SEER database, looking at the prevention of local relapse in patients (66 and older) with ductal carcinoma in situ (DCIS) treated with or without irradiation after conservative surgery. In this group of elderly women, RT significantly reduced the 5-year local relapse rate, both in high-risk and low-risk DCIS patients (Smith et al. 2006a).

The same group investigated the effect of RT after conservative surgery for invasive breast cancer (Smith et al. 2006b). 8,724 women aged 70 and older were identified in the SEER database, treated in the 1992–1999 period with a small invasive, lymph-node-negative, estrogen-receptor-positive (or unknown) tumor. All women benefited from BCS, followed or not by RT. Two endpoints were used: incidence of second ipsilateral cancer and/or a subsequent mastectomy. RT significantly reduced the composite outcome in all age groups, but more so in the 70–79 age group.

Truong et al. conducted another epidemiological survey in the cancer database of British Columbia Cancer Agency (Truong et al. 2006). 4,836 women aged

50 to 89 were treated with BCS for T1-T2, Nx-N1, M0 invasive breast cancer (period 1989–1998). Median follow-up was 7.5 year. Relapse rates, overall survival, and cancer survival were significantly correlated with the use or not of adjuvant RT, even in the women aged 75 years and older. For instance, 5-year breast-cancer-specific survival was 91 vs. 94%, without and with RT ($P=0.002$) in the entire cohort, and 88 vs. 94% in the 75-year and older cohort ($P=0.004$).

These last two communications point to a very relevant element, namely that elderly women are not aged 65, but rather 75 or more. The relevance of data comparing women aged <65 with >65 is limited regarding the question of making treatment decisions in elderly women.

17.4 Substituting BCS and RT by Radical Surgery

The conclusions of the many trials that established BCS + RT as an equivalent treatment to mastectomy can be reversed: in patients who want to avoid the long RT treatment that follows BCS, mastectomy offers an alternative with equal chance for cure.

In old or frail patients, or in women that, for whatever reason, do not want to spend 5 or 6 weeks in RT, mastectomy is a valid approach. Yet, one has to remember that women aged 70 and over are usually not included in prevention campaigns. As a consequence, they are often diagnosed at a more advanced stage (tumor can be palpated), with a higher rate of nodal involvement. In Flanders, for the period 2000–2001, the cancer registry has recorded an incidence of stage 0 (in situ) and stage 1 larger than 50% in women aged 50–69 vs. a little more than 30% in women over 70 (Van Eycken and De Wever 2006). And then, mastectomy or not, if the lymph nodes contain tumor cells, adjuvant RT is indicated to prevent the high risk of chest recurrence.

The complete picture is thus that (1) substituting BCS by mastectomy will not *automatically* prevent the need for adjuvant RT and (2) mastectomy in node-positive patients could have been avoided as RT is still indicated.

For instance, Lee et al., from the British Columbia Cancer Agency retrospectively reviewed clinical charts from 233 women aged 70+, and treated between 1989 and 1997 (Lee et al. 2005). All had locally advanced cancer (tumor >5 cm or ≥4 invaded nodes), and received hormonal therapy. 147 received post-mastectomy RT (PMRT) and 86 not. Despite a less favorable tumor profile, women after PMRT had a 16% recurrence rate vs. 26% without PMRT ($P=0.03$, median follow-up time 5.5 years).

Smith et al., recently reviewed SEER data in 11,594 women aged 70 years and older, treated with mastectomy for invasive breast cancer (Smith et al. 2006c). A total of 502 (7%) of 7,416 low-risk, 242 (11%) of 2,145 intermediate-risk, and 785 (38%) of 2,053 high-risk patients received PMRT. Median follow-up was 6.2 years. PMRT was associated with a significant improved survival in the high-risk group. Five-year adjusted survival was 50% after mastectomy without adjuvant therapy, 56% with PMRT, and 59% with both PMRT and chemotherapy, respectively. Randomized clinical trials are urgently needed to confirm this finding and define optimal treatment strategies for this patient group.

However, the subgroup most likely to benefit the most from PMRT is apparently not the one with the least favorable characteristics. In a recent analysis of the DBCG 82b&c trial, Kyndi et al. (2009) have shown that the largest benefit in terms of LR prevention and survival was in a favorable group (≤3 positive nodes, size <5 cm, positive hormonal receptors, Grade 1, and negative for HER2). In this group, an 11% reduction in LR probability was seen, with a similar reduction in 15-year breast cancer mortality. In the high-risk group (>3 nodes, size >5 cm, Grade 3, all receptors negative and HER2 positive), the reduction in LR probability was 36%, but it did not translate into a significant reduction in 15-year mortality, presumably because systemic disease already prevailed at the time of diagnosis. In an intermediate prognostic group, LR and survival were also improved by PMRT, to the same extent as in the low-risk group. Unfortunately, the relevance of these observations to the elderly population is unknown, as the inclusion criteria fixed 70 as upper age limit.

This is an important finding, as the common attitude of physicians is to prescribe PMRT only to patients with bad prognostic factors. For instance, in the SEER cohort, the risk factors for PMRT omission included advanced age, moderate to severe co-morbidity, *smaller tumor size, fewer positive lymph nodes,* and geographic region, with adjusted use rates ranging from 63.5% in San Francisco to 44.9% in Connecticut (Smith et al. 2008).

Conflicting data have been published by McCammon (McCammon et al. 2008), using the SEER database. It seems that PMRT is not improving cancer-specific survival in elderly women with T3N0 tumors. T3N0 should not be considered high-risk.

The EORTC now participates to the MRC SUPREMO of the Scottish Cancer Trials Breast Group (Selective Use of Postoperative Radiotherapy after MastectOmy) trial, a phase III randomized trial to assess the role of adjuvant chest wall irradiation in "intermediate risk" operable breast cancer following mastectomy. The goal is to include 3,700 patients after mastectomy. Since there is no age constraint in the inclusion criteria it is anticipated that analysis by age group will add some clarification to the question (www.eortc.be).

Last but not least, the common belief that older women do not seek conservative surgery is wrong. When *offered* the choice, the vast majority of women aged 70+ prefer conservative surgery (Sandison et al. 1996).

17.5 Shortening RT

An option frequently discussed is hypofractionation. It has the advantage of limiting the number of sessions (better cost-effectiveness, less burden to the patient), but the disadvantage of being more damaging to normal tissues with more long-term morbidity. In the specific case of breast cancer, hypofractionation, if properly adjusted for the tumor BED, would result in more breast edema and fibrosis, or so is predicted.

In the absence of a standard fractionation schedule—breast conserving trials actually used diverging fractionation schedules—the NCIC and Ontario Clinical Oncology Group designed a trial to compare two fractionation regimen (50 Gy in 25 fractions vs. 42.5 Gy in 16 fractions), in women treated with lumpectomy and with negative nodes (breast irradiation only). 1,234 women were randomized and, after a median follow-up of 69 months it was concluded that the two arms were equivalent in term of local control, disease-free, and overall survival. The percentage of patients with good or excellent cosmetic outcome after 3 years was 76.8 and 77%; this result remained unchanged at 5 years. About 17% of enrolled women were over 70; there was no apparent difference between them and the other age groups (Whelan et al. 2002).

Therefore, it seems that a 22-day schedule is equivalent to a 35-day one. In countries with long distances and/or in elderly women with difficulties to daily travel to the hospital, this could make a substantial difference. Indeed, it could help to convert mastectomies without RT into conservative treatments with RT, or so suggests Whelan (Whelan et al. 2002).

17.6   Co-Morbidities and Treatment of Recurrences

Although overall survival remains the Grail in oncology, the morbidity associated with local or loco-regional recurrences should not be overlooked.

First of all, a recurrence is a source of considerable psychological distress in cancer patients. Adjusting to the diagnosis of breast cancer is a painful process, and the rate of severe distress and depression is particularly high in this group of patients (Razavi 2005). In this context, it is not inconceivable that a recurrence will have a deeper negative impact on the patient's psychological status, and turn distress into depression in a substantial proportion of women.

Recurrences are early events, a few years only in most cases (Clarke et al. 2005), but they will happen at an older age, an age at which co-morbidities might have worsened and/or the cognitive functioning can be deteriorated. Therefore, recurrences might cause additional distress due to poor understanding on the side of the patient, and their treatment will be more complicated, if possible at all.

Indeed, a recurrence is likely to submit the patient to a second surgical intervention (mastectomy after BCS), and probably a change in the systemic treatment (substitution of tamoxifen by an aromatase inhibitor). The cumulative costs of the successive interventions for a recurrence are likely to be more expensive than a simple RT treatment.

Actual prices vary widely from country to country, but in Belgium, 1 year of aromatase inhibitor (anastrozole, letrozole, exemestane) costs about the same as a simple breast treatment of RT with two tangential beams (1.600 vs. 1.800€). The recommended duration of such a treatment, in the eventuality of a recurrence, is not clear yet. However, assuming a treatment of 5 years, the cost of a single aromatase inhibitor treatment would approximately balance the cost of five RT treatments. Therefore, the omission of RT in a population of women with a 20% risk of local recurrence would not save any cost to the social security system.

This is far from an economical analysis, barely a rough estimate, but it helps to fix orders of magnitude. More detailed investigation through the SEER database have estimated the cost of a local recurrence, a distal recurrence, or a contralateral breast cancer at 11.450, 19.596, and 19.183 U$, respectively (Stokes et al. 2008). Similar findings have been reported by others (Lamerato et al. 2008).

One needs to add a more specific consideration to elderly patients: the increasing frequency of co-morbidities with age renders the prescription of anticancer treatments more difficult, if not simply contraindicated (Van Weel and Schellevis 2006). Simple guidelines, validated in a younger population through appropriate clinical trials, never take account of potentially competing age-related diseases because, as said before, such patients are excluded from cancer research.

Co-morbidities have been prospectively recorded in the population-based Eindhoven Cancer Registry (Coebergh et al. 1999). The proportion of patients with one or more serious coexistent disease at the time of diagnosis of breast cancer was recently derived from this database (and updated); it ranged from 9% for patients younger than 50 years to 55% for patients aged 80 years and older (Table 17.2) (Louwman et al. 2005). The most frequent conditions were cardiovascular disease (7%), diabetes (7%), and previous cancer (6%).

As expected, 5-year survival was lower in patients with two or more co-morbid conditions than in those without: 72 vs. 84% in patients less than 50 years, 65 vs. 84% in the patients aged 50–69, and 35 vs. 68% in patients ≥70 years, respectively. Whether this loss of survival was related to the co-morbid conditions or to under-staging/under treatment of breast cancer, or to both was further explored by using relative survival to estimate disease-specific survival. This showed significantly lower 5-year survival rates for most of the recorded coexistent diseases, with rates up to 50% lower. An independent prognostic effect of age was also observed, presumably related to other factors (decreased performance status, lower organ reserves, diminished mental conditions, unfavorable social factors) (Louwman et al. 2005).

Table 17.2 Incidence of serious concomitant conditions by age of consecutive breast cancer patients diagnosed 1995–2001 in southeastern Netherlands (Fyles et al. 2004)

Number of concomitant conditions	Age at diagnosis (years)			
	<50	50–69	70–79	≥80
	Incidence of concomitant conditions (%)			
0	79	67	50	35
1	8	16	27	34
≥2	1	4	14	22
unknown	13	12	9	9

Lastly, the common belief that QoL is negatively affected by a long and strenuous RT treatment after breast surgery is contradicted by data from the PRIME trial, where the expected improvements in QoL scores when RT was omitted were not recorded (Prescott et al. 2006).

17.7 Making Individual Decisions

Obviously, breast cancer patients are at risk of dying from breast cancer as well as from competing causes. Assessing cancer stage, age, and coexistent diseases will help to allocate individual patients to particular subgroups with respective survival probabilities for each of these factors. Using, for example, Charlson's classification of co-morbidities and their severity (as used in (Louwman et al. 2005)), it is possible to estimate the life expectancy of patients, independently of their cancer stage (Charlson et al. 1987). Other predictors of 1-year mortality have been developed since, that can be used and combined with known recurrence rates for an estimate of the probability of breast cancer to recur within the expected lifespan of an individual patient (predictive scores are discussed elsewhere in this book).

However, predictions are probabilistic in nature, whereas the decision to treat or not is binary. An important element of clinical judgment will always remain necessary, together with a multidisciplinary discussion with other cancer specialists (including the geriatrician), the patient, and her family.

This is the ideal view. However, in the real world, the decision to offer postoperative RT continues to depend on other factors. For instance, the effect of distance to a treatment facility is detectable at 25 miles and substantial at 75 miles, with odds to benefit from adjuvant RT at 0.58 only compared to patient living within 25 miles. (Punglia et al. 2006). In another study in Florida, the distance to the closest radiation therapy facility was negatively associated with BCS and RT, with the odds ratio (OR) of receiving BCSR decreasing by approximately 3% for every 5-mile increase in the distance to radiation treatment facilities. Also, the age at diagnosis was a predictor of BCSR for local breast carcinoma, reducing the odds by 1% per year of increase in age. (Voti 2006).

Policy makers and oncologists should be made aware of these facts, both at the time of individual decision, and, in a broader perspective, regarding the policy for health infrastructure development.

17.8 Conclusions

1. Local recurrence is an early event after breast cancer surgery. The EBCTCG reports on a 5-year recurrence rate of 25.9% after BCS without RT. In the node-positive subgroup, the recurrence rate at 5 years is 41.1% (Clarke et al. 2005)
2. Local recurrence can be the source of further cancer dissemination (metastasis)

3. The treatment of locally recurrent or metastatic breast cancer incurs a high cost (psychological and financial)
4. This treatment might become difficult to prescribe in elderly patients because of competing co-morbidities, likely to be less or even absent at the time of primary surgery

Survival is unlikely to be affected by adjuvant RT after adequate breast cancer surgery in patients with a life expectancy shorter than 5 years. At 5 years, the survival curves after BCS with or without adjuvant RT already begin to diverge, particularly in node-positive patients. The number needed to treat for one life saved is 20 in the node-negative disease at 15 years; it is 14 in node-positive patients (Clarke et al. 2005). However, if one considers local recurrence instead of survival, differences between irradiated and non-irradiated patients are already visible after 1 year only.

These considerations should help the radiation oncologist to form an opinion to withhold RT or not after BCS in node-negative patients with an otherwise short life expectancy.

In all other patients with an increased risk of local recurrence (positive margins, bulky tumors, unfavorable histology, etc.), *it is unwise to omit RT,* unless there is a clear consent of the patient to accept mastectomy. Even then, RT might remain indicated, in case axillary lymph nodes are found to be positive at histology.

In the future, it is unlikely that new epidemiological studies will emerge that establish age as a single (and simple) prognostic criterion, offering guidance for the use of adjuvant RT. Rather than age, biological characteristics will probably emerge, detected by specific signatures of receptors, genes, or other relevant elements (Kyndi et al. 2008).

References

Bartelink H, Horiot JC, Poortmans P et al (2007) Impact of a higher radiation dose on local control and survival in breast conserving therapy of early breast cancer: 10 year results of the randomized boost versus no boost EORTC 22881–10882 trial. J Clin Oncol 25:3259–3265

Charlson ME, Pompei P, Ales KL, McKenzie CR (1987) A new method of classifying prognostic comorbidity in longitudinal studies: development and validation. J Chronic Dis 40:373–383

Clarke M, Collins R, Darby S et al (2005) Early Breast Cancer Trialists' Collaborative Group (EBCTCG). Effects of radiotherapy and of differences in the extent of surgery for early breast cancer on local recurrence and 15-year survival: an overview of the randomized trials. Lancet 366:2087–2106

Coebergh JW, Janssen-Heijnen ML, Post PN et al (1999) Serious co-morbidity along unselected cancer patients newly diagnosed in the southeastern part of The Netherlands in 1993–1996. J Clin Epidemiol 52:1131–1136

Cuzick J, Stewart H, Peto R et al (1987) Overview of randomized trials of postoperative adjuvant radiotherapy. Cancer Treat Rep 71:15–29

Cuzick J, Stewart H, Rutqvist L et al (1994) Cause-specific mortality in long-term survivors of breast cancer who participated in trials of radiotherapy. J Clin Oncol 12:447–453

Early Breast Cancer Trialists' Collaborative Group (EBCTCG) (1995) Effects of radiotherapy and surgery in early breast cancer: an overview of the randomized trials. N Eng J Med 333:1444–1455

Early Breast Cancer Trialists' Collaborative Group (EBCTCG) (2000) Favorable and unfavourable effects on long-term survival of radiotherapy for early breast cancer: an overview of the randomized trials. Lancet 355:1757–1770

Fisher B (1980) Laboratory and clinical research in breast cancer—a personal adventure: the David A Karnofsky memorial lecture. Cancer Res 40:3863–3874

Fyles AW, McCready DR, Lee A et al (2004) Tamoxifen with or without breast irradiation in women 50 years of age or older with early breast cancer. N Eng J Med 351:963–70

Hellman S (1994) Karnofsky Memorial Lecture. Natural history of small breast cancers. J Clin Oncol 12:2229–34

Hojris D, Overgaard M, Christensen JJ, Radiotherapy Committee of the Danish Breast Cancer Cooperative Group et al (1999) Morbidity and mortality of ischaemic heart disease in high-risk breast-cancer patients after adjuvant postmastectomy systemic treatment with or without radiotherapy: analysis of DBCG 82b and 82c randomised trials. Lancet 354:1425–1430

Hughes KS, Schnaper LA, Berry D et al (2004) Lupectomy plus tamoxifen with or without irradiation in women 70 years of age or older with early breast cancer. N Eng J Med 351:971–977

Kyndi M, Sorensen FB, Knudsen H et al (2008) Impact of BCL2 and p53 on postmastectomy radiotherapy response in high-risk breast cancer. A subgroup analysis of DBCG82 b&c. Acta Oncologica 47:608–617

Kyndi M, Overgaard M, Nielen HM et al (2009) High local recurrence risk is not associated with large survival reduction after postmastectomy radiotherapy in high-risk breast cancer: A subgroup analysis of DBCG 82 b&c. Radiother Oncol 90(1):74–79

Lamerato L, Havstad S, Gandhi S et al (2008) Economic burden associated with breast cancer recurrence. Cancer 106:1875–1882

Lee JC, Truong PT, Kader HA et al (2005) Postmastectomy radiotherapy reduces locoregional recurrence in elderly women with high-risk breast cancer. Clin Oncol 17:623–9

Louwman WJ, Janssen-Heijnen ML, Houterman S et al (2005) Less extensive treatment and inferior prognosis for breast cancer patients with comorbidity: a population-based study. Eur J Cancer 41:779–785

McCammon R, Finlayson C, Schwer A, Rabinovitch R (2008) Impact of postmastectomy radiotherapy in T3N0 invasive carcinoma of the breast: a Surveillance, Epidemiology, and End Results database analysis. Cancer 113:683–689

Overgaard M, Hansen PS, Overgaard J et al (1997) Postoperative radiotherapy in high-risk premenopausal women with breast cancer who receive adjuvant chemotherapy. N Eng J Med 337:949–955

Overgaard M, Jensen M-B, Overgaard J et al (1999) Postoperative radiotherapy in high-risk postmenopausal breast cancer patients given adjuvant tamoxifen: Danish Breast Cancer Cooperative Group DBCG 82c randomized trial. Lancet 353:1641–1648

Prescott HRJ, Kunkler IH, Williams LJ et al. (2006) PRIME I: assessing the impact of adjuvant breast radiotherapy on quality of life in low-risk older patients following breast conservation. In: Abstract 4080of the proceedings of 29th annual san antonio breast cancer symposium, December 2006

Prescott RJ, Kunkler IH, Williams LJ et al (2007) A randomised controlled trial of postoperative radiotherapy following breast-conserving surgery in a minimum-risk older population. The PRIME trial. Health Technol Assess 11:1–149

Punglia RS, Weeks JC, Neville BA, Earle CC (2006) Int J Radiat Oncol Biol Phys 66:56–63

Ragaz J, Jackson SM, Le N et al (1997) Adjuvant radiotherapy and chemotherapy in node-positive premenopausal women with breast cancer. N Eng J Med 337:956–962

Razavi D (2005) Étude des besoins et de l'organisation du soutien psychosocial des patients atteints d'un cancer et de leurs proches, Etude Fédérale, Ministère de la santé (www.fgov. health.be) avril

Sader C, Ingram D, Hastrich D (1999) Management of breast cancer in the elderly by complete local excision and tamoxifen alone. Aust N Z J Surg 69:790–793

Sandison AJ, Gold DM, Wright P, Jones PA (1996) Breast conservation or mastectomy: treatment choice of women aged 70 years and older. Br J Surg 83:994–996

Smith BD, Haffty BG, Buchholtz TA et al (2006a) Effectiveness of radiation therapy in older women with ductal carcinoma in situ. J Nat Cancer Inst 98:1302–10

Smith BD, Haffty BG, Hurria A et al (2006b) Postmastectomy radiation and survival in older women with breast cancer. J Clin Oncol 24:4901–7

Smith BD, Gross CP, Smith GL et al (2006c) Effectiveness of radiation therapy for older women with early breast cancer. J Nat Cancer Inst 98:681–90

Smith BD, Haffty BG, Smith GL et al (2008) Use of postmastectomy radiotherapy in older women. Int J Radiat Oncol Biol Phys 71:98–106

Stokes ME, Thompson D, Montoya EL et al (2008) Ten-year survival and cost following breast cancer recurrence: Estimates from SEER-Medicare data. Value Health 11:213–220

Truong PT, Bernstein V, Lesperance M et al (2006) Radiotherapy omission after breast-conserving surgery is associated with reduced breast cancer-specific survival in elderly women with breast cancer. Am J Surg 191:749–55

Van Eycken E, De Wever N. (2006) Cancer incidence and survival in Flanders, 2000–2001. Flemish Cancer Registry Network, VLK, Brussels

Van Weel C, Schellevis FG (2006) Comorbidity and guidelines: conflicting interests. Lancet 367:550–551

Veronesi U, Marubini E, Mariani L et al (2001) Radiotherapy after breast-conserving surgery in small breast carcinoma: Long-term results of a randomized trial. Ann Oncol 12:997–1003

Voti L (2006) Richardson LC. Reis IM et al. Treatment of local breast carcinoma in Florida: the role of the distance to radiation therapy facilities. Cancer 106:201–207

Wanebo HJ, Cole B, Chung M et al (1997) Is surgical management compromised in elderly patient with breast cancer? Ann Surg 225:579–589

Whelan T, McKenzie R, Julian J et al (2002) Randomized trial of breast cancer irradiation schedules after lumpectomy for women with lymph node-negative breast cancer. J Natl Canc Inst 94:1143–1150

Chapter 18
Prevention and Treatment of Skeletal Complications

Matthew C. Winter, Helen L. Neville-Webbe, and Robert E. Coleman

18.1 Early Breast Cancer

Management of early breast cancer has become increasingly successful, leading to current 10-year survival rates of around 80–85%. Approximately 75% of breast cancers are hormone-receptor-positive, and these patients are usually managed in the adjuvant setting with targeted hormonal agents, and if indicated, cytotoxic chemotherapy. These treatments are not without side effects, and of particular relevance to the older woman is their impact on skeletal health.

The rate of bone loss naturally increases with increasing age, with 1 in 3 women over the age of 50 years sustaining an osteoporotic fracture of the wrist, hip, or vertebrae (figures from the National Osteoporosis Society [NOS] 2002). The World Health Authority (WHO) defines osteoporosis by bone mineral density (BMD), with a T-score of ≤ -2.5 SD (that is, 2.5 standard deviations or more below that expected for young healthy women) as indicating osteoporosis; a T-score of ≥ -1.0 as normal BMD and a T-score between -1.0 and -2.5 as osteopenic (Kanis 1994). However, though osteoporotic fractures increase with decreasing T-score, an analysis of nearly 150,000 healthy postmenopausal women found that 82% of fractures occurred in non-osteoporotic women (T-score > -2.5) and 52% of fractures occurred in women with osteopenia (T-score -1.0 to -2.5) (Siris et al. 2004). Therefore, the WHO working group has identified risk factors for osteoporotic fracture, including increasing age, female sex, smoking, personal history of fracture over the age of 50 years, a parental history of hip fracture, a low body mass index (<20 mg/m^2), >3 units of alcohol per day, corticosteroid use, and other diseases such as rheumatoid arthritis (Kanis et al. 2007). These risk factors may be more prevalent in an older woman undergoing treatment for breast cancer. Furthermore, an osteoporotic hip fracture is associated with a 20% risk of dying within 12 months (Cummings and Melton 2002), and this risk may be increased with the potential

M.C. Winter (✉)
Academic Unit of Clinical Oncology, Weston Park Hospital,
The University of Sheffield, Sheffield, UK
e-mail: m.c.winter@sheffield.ac.uk

M.W. Reed and R.A. Audisio (eds.), *Management of Breast Cancer in Older Women*,
DOI 10.1007/978-1-84800-265-4_18, © Springer-Verlag London Limited 2011

toxicities associated with breast cancer treatment. Hence, it is imperative for clinicians treating elderly women with breast cancer to be aware of the risks to bone and to act appropriately to protect and treat the skeleton.

18.1.1   Current Adjuvant Treatment of Early Breast Cancer

Until recently, tamoxifen has been the cornerstone of hormonal therapy in postmenopausal women. However, aromatase inhibitors (AIs) have now largely superseded tamoxifen in this treatment setting. Post-menopausal women have a low level of circulating estrogen, resulting from the conversion of androgens to estrogen in peripheral tissues by the enzyme aromatase. Aromatase inhibition by the nonsteroidal reversible inhibitors (anastrozole and letrozole) or by the steroidal, irreversible inhibitor (exemestane) reduces circulating estrogen to nearly undetectable levels. Estrogen is important for bone health, as it inhibits osteoclastic resorption of bone and induces osteoclast apoptosis. Therefore, such low levels of estrogen induced by the AIs were expected to have a negative impact on skeletal health.

Large randomized trials have shown superiority of the AIs over tamoxifen in the adjuvant treatment of breast cancer in terms of disease-free survival, cancer recurrence, and a number of important toxicities such as thrombo-embolic and endometrial complications. However, their use is not without side effects. Most postmenopausal hormone-receptor-positive early breast cancer patients now receive an AI as part of their management; either upfront for 5 years, or following 2 years of treatment with tamoxifen. An AI is also the treatment of choice for elderly women receiving primary endocrine therapy instead of surgery. Only the excellent, or very good risk hormone-receptor-positive breast cancers, are now treated with tamoxifen alone.

18.1.2   Aromatase-Inhibitor-Induced Bone Loss

All AIs may induce bone loss. As part of the "Arimidex, Tamoxifen alone, or in Combination" (ATAC) trial, a bone sub-study evaluated 308 women who were investigated for the comparative effects of Arimidex on bone (Eastell et al. 2008). Lumbar spine and total hip BMD were assessed at baseline, and at 1, 2, and 5 years, by dual energy X-ray absorptiometry (DXA) scan. In anastrozole treated patients, there was a loss of BMD at 5 years of 6.08% at the lumbar spine, and 7.24% at the hip, compared to the tamoxifen-treated patients who had an increase of BMD of 2.77% (lumbar spine) and 0.74% (total hip). However, whilst anastrozole is associated with an accelerated loss of bone, those women with a normal BMD at baseline did not develop osteoporosis. The 100-month analysis of ATAC has recently been published (Forbes et al. 2008), which shows the increased annual rate of fractures in the anastrozole group compared to the tamoxifen group

(2.93% vs. 1.9%, respectively, incidence rate ratio 1.55 [1.31–1.83], $p<0.0001$), whilst on treatment. However, fracture rates between the groups were not different following completion of treatment.

Combined results of further anastrozole trials (the Australian Breast and Colorectal Study Group [ABCSG]-8 and Arimidex-Nolvadex [Arno]-95), also show a significant increase in fracture for patients going on to receive anastrozole following 2 years of tamoxifen, compared to the group who continued on tamoxifen ($p=0.015$) (Jakesz et al. 2005).

The National Cancer Institute of Canada Clinical Trials Group MA-17 study investigated the benefit of letrozole vs. placebo, after a 5-year standard treatment with tamoxifen. Those in the letrozole group had a significantly greater incidence of (newly) diagnosed osteoporosis than in the placebo group (8.1% vs. 6%, respectively, $p=0.003$), and a nonsignificant increase in fractures compared to the placebo group (5.3% vs. 4.6%, $p=0.25$) (Goss et al. 2005). The MA-17 trial also had a bone sub-protocol evaluating BMD in 226 women. The letrozole-treated patients had a significant decrease in BMD, both at the hip ($p=0.044$), and lumbar spine ($p=0.008$) (Perez et al. 2006).

In a recent further analysis of elderly women in the BIG 1–98 trial, potential efficacy of letrozole and adverse events were assessed according to age (Crivellari et al. 2008). The age categories were: "younger" postmenopausal patients (<65 year, $n=3,127$), "older" patients (65–74 year, $n=1,500$), and "elderly" patients (>75 years, $n=295$). As with the overall trial results, letrozole significantly improved disease-free survival, and, importantly for considering the use of AIs in the elderly, this was not adversely affected by age. In the elderly (>75 year) group, whilst those receiving letrozole had a significantly greater number of grade 3–5 adverse events, compared to tamoxifen, fracture rates within the letrozole group did not differ by age. This differs from analysis of the ATAC study, whereby 3 age groups (<60 years, 60–70 years, and >70 years) were assessed for risk of fracture due to an aromatase inhibitor. Eastell et al. showed that the incidence of fracture increased over time and with increasing age, with the over-70-years age group being the most at risk (Eastell et al. 2008). This is the more likely scenario: a combination of the natural ageing process and an aggravating factor (aromatase inhibition) is more likely to increase risk of bone loss.

Exemestane was compared with tamoxifen in the Intergroup Exemestane Study (IES), which randomized postmenopausal women with breast cancer to adjuvant tamoxifen for 5 years or tamoxifen for 2–3 years, followed by exemestane for 2–3 years (Coombes et al. 2007). Exemestane is a steroidal AI, having weak androgenic activity and as such, was anticipated to have less adverse effects on bone than the nonsteroidal AIs letrozole and anastrozole. However, with 58 months follow-up, there has been an increase in fracture risk with exemestane, with an incidence of 7% in the sequential group, compared to 4.9% in the tamoxifen group ($p=0.003$). In fact, in the Letrozole, Exemestane, and Anastrozole Pharmacodynamics (LEAP) study in postmenopausal women, there was no difference between any of the AIs (letrozole, anastrozole, and exemestane) on bone metabolism, as measured by biochemical markers of bone resorption (McCloskey et al. 2007).

Therefore, it is accepted that it is a class effect of AIs to induce bone loss and fractures, in addition to other risk factors including age. Furthermore, a proportion of these women will also receive chemotherapy which may well have a direct effect on bone. Greep et al. measured BMD scores, by DXA scan, of 130 postmenopausal women, 36 of whom received adjuvant chemotherapy, whilst 94 did not. Mean adjusted bone density scores at the hip and spine were significantly lower in patients who had received chemotherapy compared to those who had not (Greep et al. 2003). Finally, another risk to consider is that imposed by chest wall radiotherapy. In a retrospective study of over 1,600 patients, chest wall radiotherapy induced an increased, albeit small, risk of rib fracture (1.8% incidence) 12 months post-radiation (Pierce et al. 1992). This study assessed patients between 1968 and 1985, when AIs were not in use, and is not known whether their use will further increase this risk.

18.1.2.1   Management of Aromatase-Inhibitor-Induced Bone Loss

All women prescribed an AI should undergo assessment of bone density. DXA scanning of the hip and lumbar spine is the preferred imaging technique, as it is sensitive, accurate, and generally available.. Other techniques, such as quantitative computed tomography, quantitative ultrasound, high-resolution magnetic resonance imaging, and ultrasound transmission velocity densitometry, are not currently used routinely, but may have scope for the future. The 2003 American Society of Clinical Oncology (ASCO) update on the role of bisphosphonates (BPs) and bone health issues in women with breast cancer [16] includes a management algorithm for treatment-induced bone loss. These guidelines use only BMD, as measured by DXA scan, to recommend treatments. They recommend that all women prescribed an AI should receive calcium and vitamin D supplements. Women with a T score of >-2.5 are monitored yearly by DXA; women with a T score of ≤ -2.5 are recommended to receive a BPs. However, as seen by the study by Siris et al. (2004), risks to skeletal health and risk of fracture in older women being treated for early breast cancer is not solely related to BMD. Therefore, all women about to start treatment with an AI should be clinically assessed for risk factors outlined above. These issues are addressed by recently published UK guidelines and are further discussed below, along with recommendations of treatment with BPs for AI-induced bone loss.

18.1.3   Current UK Guidelines and Recommendations for the Management of Breast Cancer Treatment-Induced Bone Loss

The National Institute for Health and Clinical Excellence (NICE) has recommendations for the management of secondary prevention of osteoporotic fractures in postmenopausal women. These women are preferably treated with one of the following BPs: alendronate, etidronate or risedronate (NICE 2005). NICE guidelines are not available for the primary prevention of osteoporosis, and the draft guidance does not currently address the impact of AI use and breast cancer. Thus, specific guidance was required to aid clinicians involved in the management of early breast cancer. A UK expert panel (Reid et al. 2008) concluded that the 2003 ASCO guidelines do not sufficiently reflect other contributing risk factors, more recently accrued data, nor the increased risk with age alone and developed an evidence-based guidance document. The panel performed a systematic literature search, assessing randomized controlled trials, meta-analyses, and observational studies, from 1960 to 2005. The resulting guidance and management algorithms has been reviewed and endorsed by the National Cancer Research Institute Breast Cancer Group and the National Osteoporosis Society (NOS).

The guidelines recommend that women over 75 years of age receiving an AI should receive a BP for bone protection, if they have at least 1 or more risk factors (other than being female), as discussed above, for osteoporotic fracture regardless of BMD score (Fig. 18.1). These women are at greater risk for having secondary osteoporosis, and should be investigated for this, by measuring full blood count, erythrocyte sedimentation rate, bone and liver function (calcium, phosphate, alkaline phosphatase, albumin, AST/gamma GT), serum urea and creatinine, endomysial antibodies, and serum thyroid stimulating hormone. This will screen for conditions such as hyperparathyroidism, hyperthyroidism, chronic renal failure, and chronic liver failure, which may be overlooked or not clinically apparent in the elderly. If the patient is deficient in calcium, calcium and vitamin D supplementation should be prescribed. This is particularly important as elderly, housebound women are prone to vitamin D deficiency.

Management of postmenopausal women younger than 75 years depends on BMD which should be measured by DXA within 3 months of starting AI therapy. Three groups are defined: high-risk (T-score < -2), medium-risk (T score between -1 and -2), and low-risk (T score > -1). Low-risk patients can be reassured and do not need any specific additional monitoring during a 5-year treatment period. At the other end of the spectrum, the high-risk group should receive bone protection with a BP, calcium and vitamin D supplements, and given lifestyle advice regarding diet, smoking, and exercise. Patients of medium risk require regular monitoring of BMD every 2 years in addition to lifestyle advice, plus calcium and vitamin D supplementation if necessary. If BMD drops below $T = < -2$ or the annual rate of bone loss exceeds 4% then bone protection with a BP is recommended.

As yet there are no specific monitoring requirements for those postmenopausal women receiving tamoxifen, chemotherapy alone, or no adjuvant endocrine treatment.

18.1.4 Bisphosphonates for the Treatment of Aromatase-Inhibitor-Induced Bone Loss

Three parallel designed trials to assess the efficacy of zoledronic acid in the prevention of aromatase inhibitor (letrozole) induced bone loss, have shown that

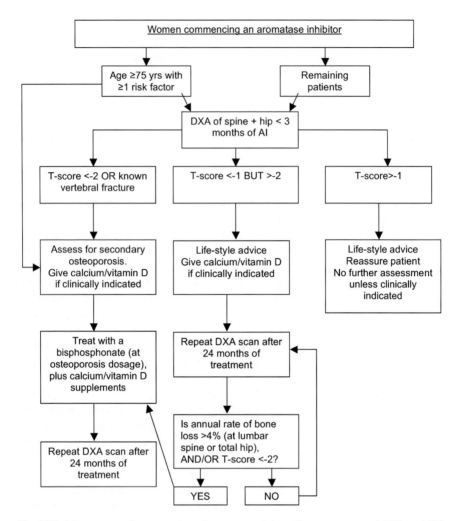

Fig. 18.1 Management of postmenopausal women receiving adjuvant aromatase inhibitors (AIs), including the over 75-year age group. Adapted from Reid et al. (2008) with permission from Elsevier

zoledronic acid inhibits letrozole-induced bone loss in postmenopausal women. The Zometa-Femara Adjuvant Synergy Trials included 602 women in the Z-FAST trial in the USA and Canada (Brufsky et al. 2007), 1,066 women in the ZO-FAST trial in Europe (Bundred et al. 2008), and 527 women in the E-ZO-FAST trial (Schenk et al. 2007) in various other countries, including the Far East and South America. All trials randomized postmenopausal women with either normal BMD or osteopenia (T-score > −2) and who were planned to receive adjuvant letrozole to immediate or delayed zoledronic acid (4 mg intravenously every 6 months). The delayed group received zoledronic acid when BMD score at the lumber spine or hip decreased to less than −2, or they incurred a nontraumatic (osteoporotic) fracture.

In all three trials mean BMD increased in those receiving immediate zoledronic acid and fell in those in the delayed group. At 12 months the differences in lumbar spine BMD between the groups were 4.4% (95% CI, 3.7–5%, $p < 0.0001$) in Z-FAST, 5.7% (95% CI 5.2–6.1%, $p = 0.0001$) in ZO-FAST, and 5.4% in E-ZO-FAST. Similarly, at the hip BMD was 3.3% higher (95% CI 2.8–3.8%, $p < 0.0001$) in Z-FAST, 3.6% (95% CI 3.3–4%, $p = 0.0001$) in ZO-FAST, and 3.3% in E-ZO-FAST. No specific information is provided on the effects in older women but there is no reason to anticipate that the response to zoledronic acid would be significantly influenced by age. Subsequent reports have confirmed that these BMD advantages to immediate zoledronic acid are maintained. However, to date there are no data on the impact of the two different strategies on fracture incidence.

The oral BP, risedronate, is NICE-approved for the treatment of postmenopausal osteoporosis, and has recently been investigated in 234 postmenopausal women with early breast cancer receiving the aromatase inhibitor anastrozole, as part of the SABRE study (Study of Anastrozole with the Bisphosphonate RisedronatE) (Eastell et al. 2007). This study randomized postmenopausal women ($n = 234$), receiving anastrozole to either oral risedronate (35 mg weekly) or placebo, having initially been stratified by fracture risk, based on initial hip and lumbar spine T-score. Women with a T-score of > −1.0 (low risk of fracture) or < −2.0 (high risk of fracture), were enrolled in an open-label design and received anastrozole alone or anastrozole plus risedronate, respectively. Patients who were osteopenic, and so at moderate risk of fracture, were enrolled in a double-blind fashion and randomized to anastrozole and risedronate or anastrozole and placebo. The primary endpoint was BMD at 12 months. Risedronate increased BMD both in the osteopenic group (by 1.7%) and in those patients classed as osteoporosis at baseline. Those receiving placebo in the osteopenic group had a decrease in BMD of 0.41%.

The ARIBON study ("Prevention of anastrozole induced bone loss with monthly oral ibandronate during adjuvant aromatase inhibitor therapy for breast cancer") (Lester et al. 2007) is a randomized, double-blind, placebo-controlled trial, evaluating the efficacy of oral ibandronate on BMD in postmenopausal women taking anastrozole, for early breast cancer. Patients were stratified according to baseline BMD at the lumbar spine and total hip. All patients received anastrozole and calcium and vitamin D supplements daily. Further management depended on baseline BMD. Women with a normal BMD (T-score> −1 at spine and hip) ($n = 68$) were observed and underwent follow-up DXA scan at 2 years. Women with osteoporosis (T-score< −2.5, at either the hip or spine) received open-label ibandronate (150 mg, every 28 days, orally), ($n = 13$). Women labeled as osteopenic (T-score > −2.5 and < −1.0, either at hip or spine), were randomized to receive oral ibandronate (150 mg every 28 days, $n = 25$) or (identically appearing) placebo tablets, every 28 days ($n = 25$). The primary endpoint evaluated change in BMD at 1 and 2 years. The median age of the ibandronate group was 67.8 years and that of the placebo group, 67.5 years. For osteopenic patients treated with anastrozole and ibandronate, the increases in BMD at the lumbar spine and total hip were 2.76 and 0.49%, respectively, at 2 years. For the anastrozole and placebo group, the changes in BMD at 2 years were −3.4 and −4.02%) at the spine and hip respectively. All differences between the treated and placebo groups were statistically significant ($p < 0.01$). Furthermore, 7 osteopenic patients developed a normal BMD with ibandronate, whilst none of those in the placebo group did.

Clodronate has not been investigated in the treatment of AI-induced bone loss but has been shown to increase BMD in postmenopausal women receiving anti-estrogens (tamoxifen or toremifene), compared to women receiving anti-estrogens alone (Saarto et al. 1997). Alendronate has been approved for treatment of postmeno-pausal osteoporosis and has also been investigated in postmenopausal women being treated for early breast cancer. However, the studies were small or did not reach statistical significance so definite conclusions cannot currently be drawn.

18.1.4.1 Current Recommendation for Choice of Bisphosphonate

If a BP is indicated, the UK expert group (Reid et al. 2008) recommends that the choice of BP should be directed by local funding and protocols. Based on best available evidence for managing osteoporosis, the panel considered the following as appropriate choices: weekly oral alendronate 70 mg or risedronate 35 mg, monthly oral ibandronate 150 mg, 3-monthly intravenous ibandronate 3 mg, or 6-monthly intravenous zoledronic acid 4 mg. From osteoporosis data BPs generally confer a relative risk reduction (RRR) of 45% for vertebral fractures and approxi-mately 16% RRR for nonvertebral fractures. Adherence to oral osteoporotic treatments remains suboptimal, which not surprisingly has a direct relationship with increasing fracture risk (Rabenda et al. 2008). In Belgian postmenopausal women, greater adherence to BP medication was associated with being older and type of initial dosing, with weekly BP treatment being preferable to daily (Beest et al. 2008). Improved patient understanding of the potential gain in benefit, in terms of fracture risk reduction, is likely to improve compliance in older patients despite the risk of side effects (de Bekker-Grob et al. 2008). This may explain why medication prescribed by a specialist is associated with greater compliance following a fully informed discussion.

18.1.5 Other Lessons to be Learnt from the Management of Age-Related Osteoporosis

Elderly women are at risk of osteoporosis from age alone, regardless of whether they have other risk factors, such as those imposed by breast cancer treatments, coexisting conditions, or medication causing bone loss. For this reason various screening tools have been set up for assessment of osteoporotic fracture risk, which can be applied to elderly women seen in the breast cancer clinic, regardless of whether DXA scan is available. The EPISEM database (Hans et al. 2008) assessed approximately 13,000 (Caucasian) women aged over 70 years. They were followed prospectively for clinical risk factors that could be used to determine hip fracture risk and which, when combined with quantitative ultrasound (QUS) measurement of the stiffness index (SI) (Z-score) of the heel, could estimate a 10-year probability of osteoporotic hip fracture. Clinical risk factors in elderly women that predicted future hip fracture included low BMI, previous history of fracture, an impaired chair test, diabetes, current cigarette smoking, and history of recent fall. Combining a clinical risk factor score with the SI score enhanced the predictive value of either score alone, and was not dependent on DXA scanning.

Another screening tool for osteoporotic fracture risk assessment (for men and women) is the FRAX™, developed by the WHO Collaborating Center for Metabolic Bone Diseases (Kanis et al. 2008). Like the EPISEM database, this tool gives a 10-year probability of fracture risk. FRAX™, however, takes into account country of origin of patient and cultural identity (USA only). The tool uses clinical risk factors identified from previous meta-analyses (age, sex, BMI, previous history of fracture, a parental history of fracture, rheumatoid arthritis, use of glucocorticoids, current smoking, alcohol >3 units/day, and other secondary causes of osteoporosis), either alone or combined with BMD T score, if DXA scan is available, to give a 10-year fracture risk. The tool does not advise on treatments, which should be based on clinical judgment, but is a very useful adjunct in the clinic when faced with an elderly women who is about to start an AI, especially if DXA is either not available or may take some time. Assessment can be done on-line at www.shef.ac.uk/FRAX/.

18.2 Advanced Breast Cancer

Breast cancer commonly metastasizes to the skeleton, representing the most commonly affected organ and the first site of metastases in approximately half of patients developing recurrent disease. Furthermore, 65–75% of women with metastatic breast cancer have skeletal involvement (Coleman 2001). In stark contrast to first relapse at a visceral site, the median survival of patients with first relapse in the skeleton is associated with a more prolonged clinical course measurable in years, and therefore the presence of bone metastases is associated with considerable morbidity and significant demands on healthcare systems.

18.2.1 Causes of Bone Metastases

Bone is a fertile soil for metastatic tumor growth. Bone metastases from breast cancer are most common in the axial skeleton and limb girdles, thought to be as a result of the drainage of blood via the vertebral-venous plexus. Additionally, of considerable importance are the biological and molecular characteristics of tumor cells that promote their colonization in the bone microenvironment. Furthermore, more recently, the multidirectional interactions of tumor cells with bone cells in the bone microenvironment have been the focus of intense research. The presence of tumor cells inside the bone microenvironment destroys the normally balanced coupling of osteoclastic bone resorption and osteoclastic bone formation. The release of tumor cell-derived factors, such as PTHrP, and a variety of growth factors and cytokines stimulate osteoclastic activity, leading to accelerated bone resorption and the formation of lytic and destructive bone lesions. This mainly occurs through the osteoblastic activation of receptor activator of nuclear factor κβ [kappa beta] ligand (RANKL) and subsequent binding to its cognitive receptor, RANK, which is present on osteoclasts. Increased levels of bone-derived growth factors from the bone matrix, such as TGF-β [beta], are released as a result of accelerated bone resorption and in turn stimulate tumor growth. This creates the formation of a self-sustaining vicious cycle of cancer-induced bone disease. Inhibition of bone resorption and blockade of these molecular pathways within the vicious cycle have become therapeutic targets and strategies in both the treatment of bone metastases and, more recently, in their prevention.

18.2.2   Diagnosis

Bone metastases commonly cause severe pain, but can also be painless in many patients. In older patients, the diagnosis of bone metastases can be problematic, due to the potential coexistence of more common bone disorders such as degenerative disease, traumatic fractures, and osteoporosis. In elderly women with a previous history of breast cancer presenting with back pain, it may be very difficult to ascertain the etiology as both malignant osteolytic destruction and osteoporotic collapse would be differential diagnoses. The implications for the patient are clear and, consequently, a patient should only be labeled with a diagnosis of metastatic skeletal disease in the presence of confirmatory investigations. To ascertain the correct diagnosis, it is imperative that the clinical presentation and relevant medical history are interpreted alongside appropriate imaging and investigations. In addition, the measurement of metabolic bone markers in serum, such as bone alkaline phosphatase (bALP), propeptides of procollagen type 1 (all markers of bone formation), and markers of bone resorption and the breakdown of type I collagen, such as serum C-telopeptide (CTX) and N-telopeptide (NTX) in urine, are of value in predicting skeletal morbidity and clinical outcome (Coleman 2006).

18.2.3   Skeletal Morbidity

Breast cancer patients with bone metastases are at significant risk of skeletal morbidity associated with debilitating consequences that complicate the clinical course and contribute to reduced survival. Complications include pain that may require narcotic analgesia, reduced mobility, hypercalcemia, pathological fracture, spinal cord or nerve root compression, bone marrow infiltration, hypercalcemia of malignancy (HCM), and the need for orthopedic intervention or palliative radiotherapy. The resulting skeletal morbidity can significantly reduce the patient's quality of life, social and functional independence and, additionally, impact on their careers and healthcare resources. In the placebo arms of two randomized phase III studies of women with breast carcinoma and osteolytic bone metastases (with approximately one-third of randomized patients >65 years old) over the course of 2-year follow-up, almost 70% of patients had 1 or more skeletal complication. The commonest skeletal related event was pathological fracture, in approximately 50% of patients. In essence, patients experienced an average of four skeletal events, including two pathological fractures, per year (Lipton et al. 2000) with more events with progressive disease and as therapeutic options reduce (Coleman 2006).

18.2.4 Approach to the Treatment of Bone Metastases in Older Breast Cancer Patients

Bone metastases from breast cancer represent incurable disease, but as the median survival of patients with metastatic disease confined to the skeleton is measurable in years, both symptomatic treatment and prevention of longer-term risks of bone-related events form essential parts of clinical care (Table 18.1). The primary goals of treatment of bone metastases are to palliate symptoms and reduce the risk of bone events, thereby maintaining quality of life. Patients require input from a multidisciplinary team setting including involvement of medical and radiation oncologists, general and family physicians, radiologists, orthopedic surgeons, palliative care physicians, and specialist nurses.

There are special considerations in older patients that should also be taken into account. Ageing is associated with a progressive physiological decline in the functional reserve of organ systems, e.g., age-related decline in glomerular filtration rate. In addition, there is an increased prevalence of coexisting comorbidities

Table 18.1 Options and goals of therapy in the management of bone metastases from breast cancer

Options of therapy	Goal of therapy
Traditional therapies	
Analgesia	Palliation of bone pain
Radiotherapy/radionuclides	Palliation of bone pain
Orthopedic Surgery	Stabilization/repair of bone
Endocrine therapy	Anti-tumor effect
Chemotherapy	Anti-tumor effect
Tumor targeted therapies	Anti-tumor effect
Complementary therapy	
Bone-specific treatments	Inhibit bone cell function

that are associated with the challenging problem of polypharmacy, including the potential concomitant administration of medications, such as non-steroidal anti-inflammatory drugs (NSAIDs) for pain, and anti-hypertensive, lipid-lowering, and anti-diabetic drugs.

18.2.5   Treatment of Bone Pain

Many patients with metastatic skeletal disease experience severe bone pain, which remains a clinically challenging problem to treat rapidly and effectively. The pathophysiology of cancer-induced bone pain (CIBP) is not well understood although animal models have revealed potential mechanisms that may be used as strategies for targeted therapies. CIBP may be due to a combination of a neuropathic type nerve injury, due to direct tumor compression or ischemia, and sensitization of peripheral nociceptors or primary afferent neurons as a result of the release of a variety of growth factors and cytokines, such as prostaglandins, endothelins, and TGF-β [beta] (reviewed in Colvin and Fallon 2008). In general, the treatment of CIBP initially requires analgesia, following the principles of the WHO analgesic ladder, starting with non-opioid analgesia, including paracetamol and NSAIDs, followed by weak and strong opioids, and the addition of adjuvant analgesics at any stage including glutamate inhibitors and NMDA antagonists.

Beyond analgesics, treatment for metastatic skeletal disease includes external beam radiotherapy, radioisotopes, local surgery, and systemic therapies including endocrine treatment, chemotherapy, and BPs. The choice of therapy often depends on whether the disease is focal or widespread and on the presence or absence of visceral metastases. The clinical course may be characterized by periods of disease response or stability, interspersed by progressive disease, at which point changes in therapy are warranted in an attempt to gain disease control. However, ultimately resistance to treatment is inevitable.

18.2.5.1   Radiation Therapy

External beam radiotherapy is an effective treatment for metastatic bone pain, with up to 80% of patients having some pain relief and approximately one-third experiencing complete pain relief (Wu et al. 2003). The optimal radiotherapy regimen has been debated over several years. Numerous published studies have reported equal efficacy of pain relief between single and multiple fractions in the management of painful bone metastases. A meta-analysis showed no significant difference in pain-relief palliation of uncomplicated bone metastases among different fractionation schedules of localized radiotherapy from 8 Gy in a single fraction to 40 Gy in 15 fractions, with overall response rates of 73% in both the single and multifractionation arms (Wu et al. 2003). However, there appears to be a higher retreatment rate and pathological fracture rate with the use of single, large fractions. Despite this, many patients may prefer the convenience of a single fraction radiotherapy regimen and this should be a significant consideration, especially in elderly patients who may have coexisting co-morbidities. In patients who have disease extending to one region of the body, wide-field radiotherapy may be suitable although this is invariably associated with significant toxicities.

Complete pain relief is not achieved in approximately two-thirds of patients with bone metastases following external beam radiotherapy (Sze et al. 2004). The use of radioisotopes such as strontium-89 and samarium-153 in the palliative setting in patients with widespread painful bone metastases have been shown to reduce bone pain (Finlay et al. 2005). Radioisotopes are administered systemically and preferentially bind to bone matrix in areas of active bone turnover. Most of the published data relates to studies in hormone-resistant prostate cancer, and as yet, only small studies of breast cancer patients have been reported but indicate improvement in pain and reduction of analgesic use with acceptable hematological toxicities (thrombocytopenia and neutropenia). Repeated dosing is possible, and further research in breast cancer patients is certainly warranted.

18.2.5.2 Surgery

Metastatic destruction of bone causes a reduction in load-bearing capability and the accumulation of microfractures leads to pathological fractures, most commonly occurring in ribs and vertebrae. However, the most devastating disability of metastatic skeletal disease results from fractures of a long bone or epidural extension of tumor into the spine. These represent the main complications that require surgical intervention, when the main aims of surgery are to relieve pain, provide structural stability, restore mobility, and in the case of vertebral metastases, reduce neurological deficit or risk of nerve compression. Increased attention is focused on the prediction of long-bone metastatic sites at risk of fracture, and in these patients, referral to an orthopedic surgeon should be considered to evaluate the need for prophylactic surgery. Prophylactic internal fixation should be generally followed by radiotherapy. Spinal instability causes debilitating pain that is mechanical in origin and can be refractory to radiotherapy or systemic therapy. Referral to a spinal surgeon is justified for consideration of spinal stabilization in an appropriately selected patient group.

Spinal cord or cauda equina compression is a medical emergency and requires immediate attention and treatment, including high-dose steroids and urgent referral for radiotherapy or surgical decompression and spinal stabilization. Early diagnosis is paramount to successful rehabilitation.

18.2.6 Systemic Therapy

Systemic therapy for the treatment of bone metastases from breast cancer can potentially have direct or indirect anti-tumor effects. Endocrine therapy, cytotoxic chemotherapy, biologically targeted agents, and radionuclides, aim to directly reduce skeletal tumor burden and the release of tumor cell-derived growth factors and cytokines. Alternatively, bone-targeted treatment, e.g., BPs, may be aimed at inhibiting the effects of these tumor cell-derived factors on host bone cells, such as osteoclasts and osteoblast/stromal cells.

Endocrine treatment is the preferred initial treatment option in the treatment of patients with hormone-receptor-positive breast cancer and metastases isolated to bone. There are few data specific to elderly patients, but a single trial has reported that letrozole, as first-line treatment, is as effective in older postmenopausal women (≥70 years) as in younger postmenopausal women (<70 years) in analyses of time to progression and objective response rate, and was more effective than tamoxifen in both older and younger patients (Mouridsen and Chaudri-Ross 2004).

Chemotherapy is indicated in patients with hormone-insensitive tumors, in those with rapidly progressing life-threatening disease (in whom it is not possible to wait approximately six weeks for potential response) and in those patients who progress after endocrine therapy. Women over the age of 70 treated with chemotherapy for metastatic disease gain similar benefits to younger patients, and therefore should not be excluded from chemotherapy treatment on the basis of age alone (Wildiers et al. 2007). The use of trastuzumab (herceptin) should be considered in patients with HER2/neu positive disease. Treatment decisions should be based on the severity of co-morbidities and the wishes of the patient.

The chief aim of palliative chemotherapy is palliation of symptoms, with the main goals being pain relief and resumption of functional activity. In general, responses to treatment are only partial, with a median duration of response of up to a year. Strict on-treatment review of these patients is required to ensure avoidance of overtreatment and to monitor impact on quality of life, toxicity, and the need for dose modification and supportive care. Chemotherapy may be potentially hazardous in those with disease-induced poor bone marrow reserve and the use of hematopoietic growth factors may be required. Recommendations of the International Society of Geriatric Oncology suggest that preference should be given to monotherapy using chemotherapy drugs with safer profiles such as weekly taxane regimens, anthracyclines formulations with less cardiotoxicity, and capecitabine, gemcitabine, and vinorelbine (Wildiers et al. 2007).

18.2.6.1 Bisphosphonates

Bisphosphonates (BPs), as potent inhibitors of osteoclast-mediated bone resorption, have become firmly established in the treatment of breast cancer patients with bone metastases, and represent the current standard of care (Pavlakis et al. 2005). The indications for their use in the metastatic skeletal setting are for the treatment of HCM, treatment of metastatic bone pain and for the prevention of the complications of malignant skeletal disease. Guidelines suggest that starting BPs should be considered in patients with breast cancer as soon as bone metastases are confirmed by radiographs, even in absence of symptoms (Hillner et al. 2003; Aapro et al. 2008).

Both intravenous and oral BPs have shown significant clinical benefit in breast cancer patients with bone metastases and are approved in this treatment setting (Table 18.2), but to date, studies of oral BPs have not reported consistent and statistically significant improvements across multiple end-points. Oral clodronate and ibandronate are approved in the management of patients with breast cancer and bone metastases, and an oral regimen should be considered for patients who are not able to attend regular hospital care (Aapro et al. 2008). The use of oral BPs is complicated by complex dosing requirements needed to minimize gastrointestinal toxicities and to ensure adequate absorption. Oral BPs are poorly absorbed from the gut and absorption is negatively affected by food intake. Furthermore, oral formulations need to be taken on an empty stomach in the upright position, and patients should continue to fast and remain upright for at least 30 min post dosing. Recent recommendations of an international expert panel on the use of BPs in solid tumors suggest that the intravenous route is preferable as compliance can be more effectively monitored (Aapro et al. 2008).

Clinical trials that have investigated the benefits of BPs in the setting of bone metastases from breast cancer have used a variety of clinical end-points. End-points such as assessments of quality of life and pain can be affected by subjective bias and therefore trials have assessed measurement of skeletal-related events (SRE) as a composite end-point. These are defined as events including pathological fracture, spinal cord compression, irradiation of or surgery on bone, and HCM (Coleman 2005). Effective treatment that prevent or delay these events would clearly be of clinical importance, impacting positively on quality of life and clinical outcome. Numerous clinical trials of BPs have demonstrated the beneficial effects on skeletal morbidity in patients with breast cancer and skeletal metastases, including reducing the risk and rate of development of a skeletal event and increasing the time to first SRE and rate of subsequent events (Table 18.3) (Bellahcene et al. 1996; Body et al. 2003; Body et al. 2004; Hortobagyi et al. 1998; Kohno et al. 2005; Kristensen et al. Jul 1999; Paterson et al. 1993; Theriault et al. 1999; Tubiana-Hulin et al. 2001). A Cochrane meta-analysis of 8 trials, including 2,276 women with breast cancer and clinically evident bone metastases, demonstrated a 21% reduction in the risk of developing a skeletal event for patients on BP therapy (at recommended dosing) compared with placebo (RR 0.79; 95% CI 0.74–0.86, $p < 0.0001$) (Fig. 18.2) (Pavlakis et al. 2005), but as can be seen in Fig. 18.2 the greatest risk reduction of SREs was observed with zoledronic acid. Further potential clinical benefits include improvement in quality of life and effective reduction in bone pain, although BPs should be used as an addition to analgesia, rather than as first-line therapy for the treatment of bone pain (Coleman May 2005).

In the only direct comparison in an appropriately powered comparison of two BPs, zoledronic acid has been shown to reduce skeletal complications more effectively than pamidronate in patients with bone metastases from breast cancer. The proportion of patients with at least 1 SRE was similar for both drugs, but multiple event analysis showed that zoledronic acid significantly reduced the risk of SREs by an additional 20% over and above that achieved with pamidronate ($p = 0.025$) (Rosen et al. 2004).

Table 18.2 Current bisphosphonates (BPs) licensed for treatment of bone metastases in breast cancer

BP choice	Formulation	Dose and schedule	Considerations in the elderly patient
Clodronate[a]	Oral	1,600 mg daily (single or 2 divided doses)	Reduce dose to 800 mg daily in severe renal impairment (<30 mls/min)
			Contraindicated if cr. cl <10mls/min
		Range: 800 mg–3,200 mg	High incidence of gastrointestinal adverse events/difficulty swallowing may limit compliance
			Avoidance of food for 1 h before and after medication
Pamidronate	Intravenous infusion over 2 h	90 mg every 3–4 weeks	Monitor renal function prior to each dose
			Not recommended if cr. cl <30 ml/min
			Withhold until renal function returns to within 10% of baseline value
			Caution when used concurrently with other potential nephrotoxic drugs
Zoledronic acid	Intravenous infusion over 15 min	4 mg every 3–4 weeks	Monitor renal function prior to each dose
			Not recommended if cr. cl <30 mls/min
			Withhold treatment in patients with renal deterioration
			Caution when used concurrently with other potential nephrotoxic drugs
Ibandronate[a]	Oral or intravenous infusion over 1 h	Oral: 50 mg daily Intravenous: 6 mg every 3–4 weeks	Renal monitoring at physician's discretion
			Reduce dose if cr. cl <30 mls/min: 2 mg IV every 3–4 weeks or 50 mg PO weekly
			No dosing restrictions with other potential nephrotoxic drugs
			Oral formulation to be given upright after overnight fast, before food

[a]approved in Europe but not USA, cr. cl=creatinine clearance
Compiled from recommendations of the International Society of Geriatric Oncology of the use of BPs in elderly patients Kohno et al. 2005

Table 18.3 Randomized placebo-controlled trials demonstrating the effects of BPs (at currently recommended doses) on skeletal morbidity

BP and formulation	No. of patients	Results
Clodronate 1600 mg/day PO Paterson et al. (1993)	173	Significantly reduced combined event rate of all morbid skeletal events: SMR 305 vs. 219 events/100 women years ($p<0.001$)
Clodronate 1600 mg/day PO Kristensen et al. (1999)[a]	100	Significantly delayed time to 1st SRE ($p=0.015$) Reduced fracture incidence ($p=0.02$)
Clodronate 1600 mg/day PO Tubiana-Hulin et al. (2001)	144	Significantly delayed time to 1st SRE (244 days vs. 180 days, $p=0.05$) Reduction in pain intensity and use of analgesia
Pamidronate 90 mg, 3–4 weekly IV Hortobagyi et al. (1998)	382	Significantly reduced percentage of patients experiencing SRE (65% vs. 46%, $p<0.001$) Significantly delayed time to 1st SRE (13.1 months vs. 7.0 months, $p=0.0005$)
Pamidronate 90 mg, 4 weekly IV Theriault et al. (1999)	374	Significantly reduced percentage of patients experiencing SRE (67% vs. 56%, $p=0.027$) Significantly delayed time to 1st SRE (10.4 months vs. 6.9 months, $p=0.049$)
Ibandronate 2 or 6 mg, 3–4 weekly IV Body et al. (2003)	466	6 mg dose vs. placebo: significantly reduced SMPR[b] by 20% (1.48 vs. 1.19 periods with events per patient year, $p=0.004$) 2 mg dose: no significant clinical benefit Significantly delayed time to 1st SRE (50.6 weeks vs. 33.1 weeks, $p=0.018$) Reduction in pain intensity and use of analgesia
Ibandronate 50 mg/day PO Body et al. (2004)	564	Significantly reduced SMPR[b] (1.18 vs. 0.95, $p=0.004$)
Zoledronic acid 4 mg, 4 weekly IV Kohno et al. (2005)	228	Significantly reduced percentage of patients experiencing SRE[b] (50% vs. 30%, $p=0.003$) Significantly delayed time to 1st SRE ($p=0.007$) Reduction of risk of SREs by 41%[b] in multiple event analysis ($RR=0.59$, $p=0.019$) Significantly improved pain scores compared to placebo

SMR, skeletal morbidity rate,
[a] not placebo-controlled, SMPR, skeletal morbidity period rate (the number of 12 week periods with new bone events, allowing for time on study,
[b] excludes HCM)

Optimum Use of Bisphosphonates in Metastatic Bone Disease

There remains uncertainty regarding the most appropriate duration and schedule of treatment, and factors that need to be taken into consideration, particularly in the older patient, include life expectancy, disease extent and the risk of developing

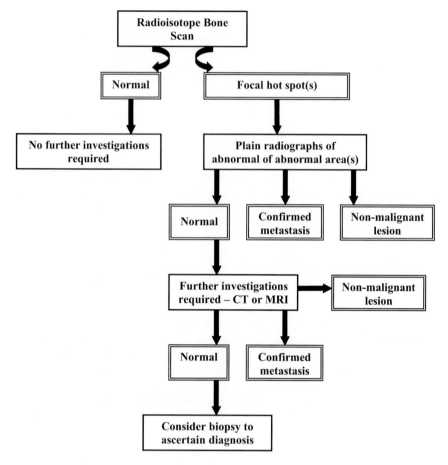

Fig. 18.2 Prevention of skeletal complications in metastatic breast cancer and existing bone metastases in placebo-controlled trials vs. bisphosphonate (at recommended dosing). Adapted from Pavlakis et al. (2005) Copyright Cochrane Collaboration, reproduced with permission

a SRE, the logistics and accessibility of treatment for the patient, and treatment cost. BPs should certainly not be stopped following the development of a first skeletal-related event whilst on treatment; this should not be considered a failure of treatment, as BPs show a significant reduction in second and subsequent complications. The role of bone-marker-directed therapy, using markers such as the collagen breakdown product N-terminal cross-linked type 1 collagen telopeptide (NTX), is currently under investigation in a large prospective randomized phase III trial (BISMARK).

Prescribing Bisphosphonates in the Elderly Patient

There are limited data on the use of BPs specifically in elderly breast cancer with bone metastases. However, a recently published population-based analysis of the use of intravenous BPs in older women treated for breast cancer reported that women

≥75 years old were less likely to receive treatment than patients <70 years old (Giordano et al. 2008). However, following a consideration of life expectancy and potential benefit, their use is recommended with no specific limitations. Clearly, it is important that the treating physician chooses the most appropriate BP with the most acceptable toxicity profile (Body et al. 2007), weighed up against the patient's co-morbidities, functional status, and concomitant medications. Unfortunately, comparative safety and efficacy data of BPs are lacking. However, the choice and implications of administration may be of considerable importance in the elderly patient, and specific considerations in the elderly are presented in Table 18.2.

Elderly patients may be at higher risk of developing renal impairment due to reduced hydration, and the use of concomitant nephrotoxic drugs such as NSAIDs and anti-hypertensives. The use of concomitant nephrotoxic agents with BPs should be limited if possible. An International Society of Geriatric Oncology task force (Body et al. 2007) recommends that in patients being treated with pamidronate or zoledronic acid, creatinine clearance should be monitored in every patient, even when serum creatinine is within the normal range, with evaluation and optimization of hydration status and review of concomitant medications.

In addition, the elderly have an increased incidence of dental problems, and therefore are potentially at higher risk of osteonecrosis of the jaw. This is an emerging complication characterized by the appearance of exposed bone in the maxillofacial region with failure of healing after 8 weeks. It is increasingly suspected to be a potential complication of BP therapy (Khosla et al. 2007), and seems to be particularly related to potency, intravenous formulation, and duration of treatment, co-incident with the occurrence of a dental intervention, e.g., extraction. The risk appears to be approximately 1% per year on monthly intravenous therapy. It is therefore recommended before starting BP therapy, that patients are reviewed by a dentist and any pre-existing dental problems treated (Body et al. 2007).

18.2.7 Other Potential Targets in the Treatment of Metastatic Bone Disease

We now have a greater understanding of the complex cellular and molecular signaling pathways that occur between bone cells, and between bone cells and tumor cells in the establishment of the vicious cycle of malignant bone destruction. Consequently, drugs inhibiting these targets in the treatment of bone metastases are in development. Osteoclast-mediated bone resorption is regulated by receptor activator of nuclear factor κβ [kappa bta] ligand (RANKL), which is essential for osteoclast formation, function, and survival. Currently the most promising new agent is denosumab, a fully humanized monoclonal antibody that specifically inhibits RANKL, leading to inhibition of osteoclast function and bone resorption. A 4-weekly dose of 120 mg s.c. has been defined in a recent phase II trial in breast cancer patients with bone metastases, and taken through to phase III studies (Lipton et al. 2007). Other potential targets include the inhibition of cathepsin K, a proteinase secreted by osteoclasts and is essential for osteolysis, and PTHrP, an abundant and important osteoclast-activating factor.

18.3 Summary

Older patients represent a significant proportion of the breast cancer population and are unfortunately substantially underrepresented in clinical trials. Patients with bone metastases from breast cancer are at significant risk of skeletal morbidity, associated with debilitating consequences complicating the clinical course and contributing to reduced survival. There are important considerations specific to this population, and the optimal management of bone metastases requires an experienced multidisciplinary input to ensure appropriate and timely diagnosis and the coordination of both local and systemic therapeutic strategies.

References

Aapro M, Abrahamsson PA, Body JJ et al (2008) Guidance on the use of bisphosphonates in solid tumors: recommendations of an international expert panel. Ann Oncol 19(3):420–432
Beest FJ, Erkens JA, Herings RM (2008) Determinants of noncompliance with bisphosphonates in women with postmenopausal osteoporosis. Curr Med Res Opin 24(5):1337–1344
Bellahcene A, Menard S, Bufalino R, Moreau L, Castronovo V (1996) Expression of bone sialoprotein in primary human breast cancer is associated with poor survival. Int J Cancer 69(4):350–353
Body JJ, Diel IJ, Lichinitzer M et al (2004) Oral ibandronate reduces the risk of skeletal complications in breast cancer patients with metastatic bone disease: results from two randomized, placebo-controlled phase III studies. Br J Cancer 90(6):1133–1137
Body JJ, Coleman R, Clezardin P, Ripamonti C, Rizzoli R, Aapro M (2007) International society of geriatric oncology (SIOG) clinical practice recommendations for the use of bisphosphonates in elderly patients. Eur J Cancer 43(5):852–858
Body JJ, Diel IJ, Lichinitser MR et al (2003) Intravenous ibandronate reduces the incidence of skeletal complications in patients with breast cancer and bone metastases. Ann Oncol 14(9):1399–1405
Brufsky A, Harker WG, Beck JT et al (2007) Zoledronic acid inhibits adjuvant letrozole-induced bone loss in postmenopausal women with early breast cancer. J Clin Oncol 25(7):829–836
Bundred NJ, Campbell ID, Davidson N et al (2008) Effective inhibition of aromatase inhibitor-associated bone loss by zoledronic acid in postmenopausal women with early breast cancer receiving adjuvant letrozole: ZO-FAST Study results. Cancer 112(5):1001–1010
Coleman RE (2001) Metastatic bone disease: clinical features, pathophysiology and treatment strategies. Cancer Treat Rev 27(3):165–176
Coleman RE (2005) Bisphosphonates in breast cancer. Ann Oncol 16(5):687–695
Coleman RE (2006) Clinical features of metastatic bone disease and risk of skeletal morbidity. Clin Cancer Res 12(20 Pt 2):6243s–6249s
Colvin L, Fallon M (2008) Challenges in cancer pain management-bone pain. Eur J Cancer 44(8):1083–1090
Coombes RC, Kilburn LS, Snowdon CF et al (2007) Survival and safety of exemestane versus tamoxifen after 2–3 years' tamoxifen treatment (Intergroup Exemestane Study): a randomized controlled trial. Lancet 369(9561):559–570
Crivellari D, Sun Z, Coates AS et al (2008) Letrozole compared with tamoxifen for elderly patients with endocrine-responsive early breast cancer: the BIG 1–98 trial. J Clin Oncol 26(12):1972–1979
Cummings SR, Melton LJ (2002) Epidemiology and outcomes of osteoporotic fractures. Lancet 359(9319):1761–1767

de Bekker-Grob EW, Essink-Bot ML, Meerding WJ, Pols HA, Koes BW, Steyerberg EW (2008) Patients' preferences for osteoporosis drug treatment: a discrete choice experiment. Osteoporos Int 19(7):1029–1037

Eastell R, Van Poznak CH, Hannon RA (2007) The SABRE (study of Anastrozole with the Bisphosphonate Risedronate) study: 12 month analysis. J Bone Miner Res 22(suppl. 1):S113 (abstract number 300)

Eastell R, Adams JE, Coleman RE et al (2008) Effect of anastrozole on bone mineral density: 5-year results from the anastrozole, tamoxifen, alone or in combination trial 18233230. J Clin Oncol 26(7):1051–1057

Finlay IG, Mason MD, Shelley M (2005) Radioisotopes for the palliation of metastatic bone cancer: a systematic review. Lancet Oncol 6(6):392–400

Forbes JF, Cuzick J, Buzdar A, Howell A, Tobias JS, Baum M (2008) Effect of anastrozole and tamoxifen as adjuvant treatment for early-stage breast cancer: 100-month analysis of the ATAC trial. Lancet Oncol 9(1):45–53

Giordano SH, Fang S, Duan Z, Kuo YF, Hortobagyi GN, Goodwin JS (2008) Use of intravenous bisphosphonates in older women with breast cancer. Oncologist 13(5):494–502

Goss PE, Ingle JN, Martino S et al (2005) Randomized trial of letrozole following tamoxifen as extended adjuvant therapy in receptor-positive breast cancer: updated findings from NCIC CTG MA.17. J Natl Cancer Inst 97(17):1262–1271

Greep NC, Giuliano AE, Hansen NM, Taketani T, Wang HJ, Singer FR (2003) The effects of adjuvant chemotherapy on bone density in postmenopausal women with early breast cancer. Am J Med 114(8):653–659

Hans D, Durosier C, Kanis JA, Johansson H, Schott-Pethelaz AM, Krieg MA (2008) Assessment of the 10-year Probability of Osteoporotic Hip Fracture Combining Clinical Risk Factors and Heel Bone Ultrasound: The EPISEM Prospective Cohort of 12958 Elderly Women. J Bone Miner Res 23(7):1045–1051

Hillner BE, Ingle JN, Chlebowski RT et al (2003) American Society of Clinical Oncology 2003 update on the role of bisphosphonates and bone health issues in women with breast cancer. J Clin Oncol 21(21):4042–4057

Hortobagyi GN, Theriault RL, Lipton A et al (1998) Long-term prevention of skeletal complications of metastatic breast cancer with pamidronate. Protocol 19 Aredia breast cancer study group. J Clin Oncol 16(6):2038–2044

Jakesz R, Jonat W, Gnant M et al (2005) Switching of postmenopausal women with endocrine-responsive early breast cancer to anastrozole after 2 years' adjuvant tamoxifen: combined results of ABCSG trial 8 and ARNO 95 trial. Lancet 366(9484):455–462

Kanis JA (1994) Assessment of fracture risk and its application to screening for postmenopausal osteoporosis: synopsis of a WHO report. WHO Study Group. Osteoporos Int 4(6):368–381

Kanis JA, Johnell O, Oden A, Johansson H, McCloskey E (2008) FRAX and the assessment of fracture probability in men and women from the UK. Osteoporos Int 19(4):385–397

Kanis JA, Oden A, Johnell O et al (2007) The use of clinical risk factors enhances the performance of BMD in the prediction of hip and osteoporotic fractures in men and women. Osteoporos Int 18(8):1033–1046

Khosla S, Burr D, Cauley J et al (2007) Bisphosphonate-associated osteonecrosis of the jaw: report of a task force of the American Society for Bone and Mineral Research. J Bone Miner Res 22(10):1479–1491

Kohno N, Aogi K, Minami H et al (2005) Zoledronic acid significantly reduces skeletal complications compared with placebo in Japanese women with bone metastases from breast cancer: a randomized, placebo-controlled trial. J Clin Oncol 23(15):3314–3321

Kristensen B, Ejlertsen B, Groenvold M, Hein S, Loft H, Mouridsen HT (1999) Oral clodronate in breast cancer patients with bone metastases: a randomized study. J Intern Med 246(1): 67–74

Lester JE, Dodwell D, Purohit OP, et al (2007) Effect of monthly oral ibandronate on anastrozole-induced bone loss during adjuvant treatment for breast cancer: one year results from the ARIBON study. J Clin Oncol 25(suppl. 18S): abstract 553

Lipton A, Theriault RL, Hortobagyi GN et al (2000) Pamidronate prevents skeletal complications and is effective palliative treatment in women with breast carcinoma and osteolytic bone metastases: long term follow-up of two randomized, placebo-controlled trials. Cancer 88(5): 1082–1090

Lipton A, Steger GG, Figueroa J et al (2007) Randomized active-controlled phase II study of denosumab efficacy and safety in patients with breast cancer-related bone metastases. J Clin Oncol 25(28):4431–4437

McCloskey EV, Hannon RA, Lakner G et al (2007) Effects of third generation aromatase inhibitors on bone health and other safety parameters: results of an open, randomized, multi-centre study of letrozole, exemestane and anastrozole in healthy postmenopausal women. Eur J Cancer 43(17):2523–2531

Mouridsen H, Chaudri-Ross HA (2004) Efficacy of first-line letrozole versus tamoxifen as a function of age in postmenopausal women with advanced breast cancer. Oncologist 9(5):497–506

NICE (2005) Bisphosphonates (alendronate, etidronate, risedronate), selective estrogen receptor modulators (raloxifene) and parathyroid hormone (teriparatide) for the secondary prevention of osteoporotic fragility fractures in postmenopausal women: National Institute for Health and Clinical Excellence technology appraisal guidance 161

Paterson AH, Powles TJ, Kanis JA, McCloskey E, Hanson J, Ashley S (1993) Double-blind controlled trial of oral clodronate in patients with bone metastases from breast cancer. J Clin Oncol 11(1):59–65

Pavlakis N, Schmidt R, Stockler M (2005) Bisphosphonates for breast cancer. Cochrane Database Syst Rev (3):CD003474

Perez EA, Josse RG, Pritchard KI et al (2006) Effect of letrozole versus placebo on bone mineral density in women with primary breast cancer completing 5 or more years of adjuvant tamoxifen: a companion study to NCIC CTG MA.17. J Clin Oncol 24(22):3629–3635

Pierce SM, Recht A, Lingos TI et al (1992) Long-term radiation complications following conservative surgery (CS) and radiation therapy (RT) in patients with early stage breast cancer. Int J Radiat Oncol Biol Phys 23(5):915–923

Rabenda V, Mertens R, Fabri V et al (2008) Adherence to bisphosphonates therapy and hip fracture risk in osteoporotic women. Osteoporos Int 196:811–818

Reid D, Doughty J, Eastell R et al (2008) Guidance for the Management of Breast Cancer Treatment Induced Bone Loss. A consensus position statement from a UK Expert Group. Cancer Treat Rev 34(Suppl 1):S3–S18

Rosen LS, Gordon D, Tchekmedyian NS et al (2004) Long-term efficacy and safety of zoledronic acid in the treatment of skeletal metastases in patients with nonsmall cell lung carcinoma and other solid tumors: a randomized, Phase III, double-blind, placebo-controlled trial. Cancer 100(12):2613–2621

Saarto T, Blomqvist C, Valimaki M, Makela P, Sarna S, Elomaa I (1997) Clodronate improves bone mineral density in post-menopausal breast cancer patients treated with adjuvant antioe-strogens. Br J Cancer 75(4):602–605

Schenk N, Llombart A, Frassoladti A (2007) The E-ZO-FAST trial: zoledronic acid (ZA) effectively inhibits aromatase inhibitor associated bone loss (AIBL) in postmenopausal women (PMW) with early breast cancer (EBC) receiving adjuvant letrozole (Let). Eur J Cancer 5:186

Siris ES, Chen YT, Abbott TA et al (2004) Bone mineral density thresholds for pharmacological intervention to prevent fractures. Arch Intern Med 164(10):1108–1112

Sze WM, Shelley M, Held I, Mason M (2004) Palliation of metastatic bone pain: single fraction versus multifraction radiotherapy – a systematic review of the randomized trials. Cochrane Database Syst Rev (2):CD004721

Theriault RL, Lipton A, Hortobagyi GN et al (1999) Pamidronate reduces skeletal morbidity in women with advanced breast cancer and lytic bone lesions: a randomized, placebo-controlled trial. Protocol 18 Aredia Breast Cancer Study Group. J Clin Oncol 17(3):846–854

Tubiana-Hulin M, Beuzeboc P, Mauriac L et al (2001) Double-blinded controlled study comparing clodronate versus placebo in patients with breast cancer bone metastases. Bull Cancer 88(7):701–707

Wildiers H, Kunkler I, Biganzoli L et al (2007) Management of breast cancer in elderly individuals: recommendations of the International Society of Geriatric Oncology. Lancet Oncol 8(12): 1101–1115
Wu JS, Wong R, Johnston M, Bezjak A, Whelan T (2003) Meta-analysis of dose-fractionation radiotherapy trials for the palliation of painful bone metastases. Int J Radiat Oncol Biol Phys 55(3):594–605

Chapter 19
Medical Management of Advanced Disease

Hans P.M.W. Wildiers

19.1 Introduction

Breast cancer is the most common cancer site in women in the world with 1.15 million new cases, of which 3,61,000 are in Europe and 2,30,000 in North America (Parkin et al. 2005). In 2002, 4,11,000 women died of breast cancer worldwide. For women aged 65 years and older, breast cancer incidence rates are 432.7 per 1,00,000 females in North America and 295.0 per 1,00,000 in Europe; corresponding breast cancer mortality figures are 121.2 and 135.0 per 1,00,000 females, respectively. About a third of the global breast cancer cases occur in patients above age 65, and in more developed countries this is more than 40%. Breast cancer can recur many years after the initial diagnosis and treatment, so within the "metastatic breast cancer" population, the percentage of elderly women will be even higher.

The terminology of "advanced disease" is understood in this chapter as being an incurable/metastatic disease. In contrast, locally advanced breast cancer has a reasonable chance of cure if it is appropriately treated, but it will not be discussed here. Although metastatic breast cancer can be treated and is often sensitive to therapy, it is generally not curable. Many treatment options are available for patients with metastatic breast cancer. Since metastatic breast cancer is considered a systemic disease, the role of local therapy such as surgery, radiotherapy, or radiofrequency ablation is limited in controlling the global disease, although in selected patients and for symptom control, there can certainly be an indication for local therapy in metastatic breast cancer. Systemic therapy such as hormone therapy and chemotherapy, and more recently also targeted therapy is in general the treatment of choice since the global disease, including micrometastases can be treated and controlled. The main aims in treating elderly patients, as in younger patients with metastatic breast cancer, are to maintain quality of life, minimize symptoms from disease, and prolong survival

H.P.M.W. Wildiers (✉)
Department of General Medical Oncology, Uz Leuven—Gasthuisberg,
Herestraat 49, B-3000, Leuven, Belgium
e-mail: hans.wildiers@uzleuven.be

M.W. Reed and R.A. Audisio (eds.), *Management of Breast Cancer in Older Women,*
DOI 10.1007/978-1-84800-265-4_19, © Springer-Verlag London Limited 2011

without causing excessive toxicity. This chapter describes possible treatment options in elderly breast cancer patients with advanced/metastatic disease.

19.2   Local Therapy

Local therapy can be used with two goals in metastatic disease: to improve outcome by locally treating metastases or the primary tumor and to improve symptom control.

Local treatment of metastases can be an option in selected patients. Several case reports and small patients' series show that progression-free survival can be very long, up to many years, when solitary metastases (Caralt et al. 2008; Thelen et al. 2008) are resected or irradiated. There are no randomized studies, and selection bias was certainly present in these studies. In selected patients, local therapy of limited metastases might lead to a long period of disease control. The chance that this local therapy will cure patients with metastatic breast cancer is very small however, and this information should be clearly explained to patients before starting (sometimes debilitating) local therapy.

Also the role of primary breast tumor resection in patients with metastatic breast cancer has been an issue of controversy. In renal cancer, resection of the primary tumor can cause shrinkage of distant metastases, and is considered standard practice in many institutions. In breast cancer, distant metastases shrinkage after resection of the primary tumor has not been reported, and this intervention is generally considered as futile surgery without impact on outcome. Two recent retrospective analyses in patients with metastatic breast cancer (Khan et al. 2002; Rapiti et al. 2006) suggest that resection of the primary tumor has a better outcome compared to patients who did not have breast cancer surgery. Selection bias and the retrospective nature of the data do not allow to generalize this attitude, and prospective studies are warranted before adopting this in general clinical practice.

A second goal of local therapy is symptom control. Local therapy can be very effective in local symptom control; antalgic radiotherapy has a high chance of relieving pain when painful bone metastases are present, orthopedic surgery for pathological fractures or bone metastases at risk of fracture can be crucial in maintaining a good quality of life, hygienic mastectomy can relieve important wound problems from local breast tumors with cutaneous invasion. Local therapy for symptom relief in metastatic breast cancer should be considered in elderly patients in the same way as for younger patients.

19.3   Hormone Therapy

Breast tumors are hormone-receptor-positive in about 80% of patients, and in elderly even higher percentages (up to 90%) have been reported. When antihormonal treatment is administered, patients with ER/PR-positive tumors have a 50–60%

chance of clinical benefit (Muss et al. 1994; Mouridsen et al. 2003a), compared to 5–10% in those with ER/PR-negative tumors (Taylor et al. 1986) (although this percentage might be lower at present due to improved immunohistochemical staining techniques). The most important classes of antihormonal therapies used and studied in metastatic breast cancer are: selective estrogen receptor modulators (mainly tamoxifen), steroidal anti-estrogens (mainly fulvestrant), and estrogen-deprivation therapies (mainly aromatase inhibitors).

The selective estrogen receptor modulator (SERM) tamoxifen has been the standard of care for the past decades for hormone-responsive advanced breast cancer due to its favorable safety profile and good efficacy. For postmenopausal women, more recent studies have shown that estrogen depletion might represent a slightly more effective strategy than tamoxifen; Aromatase inhibitors are associated with an increased median time to progression (TTP) of about 2–3 months compared to tamoxifen, while there were no differences in overall survival (Mouridsen et al. 2003b; Milla-Santos et al. 2003). The presence of ER and PR expression are the most important predictive factors for response and benefit. Other factors that predict responsiveness to endocrine therapy in the metastatic setting include a long relapse-free interval, isolated bone involvement, and a prior response to endocrine therapy. Many patients with hormone-responsive advanced breast cancer undergo sequential endocrine treatments for second-line, third-line, and even fourth-line therapy, reserving chemotherapy until all endocrine options have been exhausted. There is no hard evidence that the sequence of the different treatment modalities makes a difference in outcome. As mentioned, aromatase inhibitors are slightly more effective in terms of progression-free survival compared to tamoxifen, but it might well be that aromatase inhibitors after first-line tamoxifen are more effective than tamoxifen after first-line aromatase inhibitors, thus neutralizing the initial benefit of upfront aromatase inhibitors which are more costly than tamoxifen.

Therefore, also in elderly breast cancer patients with metastatic disease, hormone therapy should be the treatment of choice for women with ER-positive and/or PR-positive tumors without life-threatening disease. Most studies have not been performed or analyzed specifically for the elderly. One study by Mouridsen et al. (Mouridsen and Chaudri-Ross 2004) looked in a preplanned sub-analysis at age-related differences between tamoxifen and letrozole as first-line therapy in younger (<70 years) and older (≥70 years) postmenopausal women with advanced breast cancer. Nine hundred and seven patients with advanced breast cancer were randomly assigned to receive 2.5 mg letrozole ($n=453$) or 20 mg tamoxifen ($n=454$) once daily in a double-blind, multicenter, international trial. Among the prospectively planned analyses were analyses of (TTP) and overall response rate (ORR) by age (<70 and ≥70 years). The ORR in the older subgroup was significantly higher in patients treated with letrozole (38%) than in patients treated with tamoxifen (18%). In the younger subgroup of postmenopausal patients, the ORRs were not significantly different (letrozole, 26%; tamoxifen, 22%). TTP was significantly longer for letrozole than for tamoxifen in both age groups (younger: letrozole median TTP, 8.8 months; tamoxifen, 6.0 months; older: letrozole median TTP, 12.2 months; tamoxifen, 5.8 months). This study demonstrates that aromatase inhibitors such as letrozole are at least as effective in older, postmenopausal women as in younger postmenopausal women with advanced breast cancer.

It is also of interest that aging has been shown to be related to alterations in the metabolism of tamoxifen resulting in higher levels of tamoxifen and its metabolites in elderly women. Whether this leads to altered efficacy or side effects is unknown (Sheth et al. 2003). In metastatic disease this might be less relevant, but in the adjuvant setting this may be more significant.

When looking at tolerability, tamoxifen is associated with a higher risk of endometrial cancer and thromboembolic events such as deep venous thrombosis, pulmonary embolism, and cerebrovascular accidents. Patients with advanced disease are at increased risk of thrombosis, and tamoxifen might further increase this risk. However, the absolute risk and certainly the risk of mortality from endometrial cancer and thromboembolic episodes is very small and certainly much smaller than the mortality reduction induced by tamoxifen in these patients with metastatic disease.

Side effects related to aromatase inhibitors are muscle and osteoarticular pain, osteoporosis, and bone fractures. In case of aromatase-inhibitor-induced osteoporosis, or in case of (osteolytic) bone metastases, bisphosphonates to prevent bone loss and skeletal related events are recommended. There is some controversy on the increased risk of cardiovascular events caused by aromatase inhibitors when compared to tamoxifen. However, this difference might be more related to the cardioprotective and lipid-lowering effects of tamoxifen than to the aromatase inhibitors by themselves.

In conclusion, aromatase inhibitors are generally slightly superior compared to tamoxifen in terms of disease-free survival but not overall survival. Tamoxifen can be a valuable alternative over aromatase inhibitors if adverse events or cost are a concern. In case of subsequent progression after first-line hormonal therapy, patients who initially responded or who have prolonged stable disease can have significant benefit from a subsequent line of non-cross-resistant hormone therapy. Treatment options include tamoxifen, an aromatase inhibitor, a pure anti-estrogen such as fulvestrant, a non-cross-resistant aromatase inhibitor (steroidal aromatase inhibitor when a non-steroidal aromatase inhibitor has been used or vice versa), or progestins. There is no evidence that hormone therapy should be differently used in elderly breast cancer patients with metastatic disease compared to younger postmenopausal patients.

19.4   Chemotherapy

Since hormonal therapy is less toxic than chemotherapy, and since a significant proportion of (elderly) patients can have longer-term benefit from hormonal therapy in metastatic setting, this is generally the treatment of choice when metastases are diagnosed. However, a smaller proportion of breast tumors (10–20%) are hormone-receptor-negative. Moreover, all patients with hormone-receptor-positive tumors will eventually develop resistance to hormonal therapy. In these cases, chemotherapy is in general the most appropriate therapy.

Patient selection is an important issue for elderly patients. Physicians are sometimes reluctant to use chemotherapy in elderly patients with metastatic (breast) cancer because of concerns of inducing toxicity without having much benefit. However, one study found that women older than 70 years who are treated with chemotherapy for metastatic disease derive similar benefits to their younger counterparts (Christman et al. 1992). This case-comparison study of patients with metastatic breast cancer treated in five clinical trials of the Piedmont Oncology Association compared outcome in relation to age. Seventy patients 70 years or older were compared with 60 patients aged 50 through 69 years and 40 patients less than 50 years. Women 70 years or older who were enrolled in these trials were similar to their younger counterparts in response rates, time to disease progression, survival, and toxic effects. The authors concluded that women in this age group should not be excluded, based on age alone, from clinical trials involving chemotherapy for advanced breast cancer. For fit patients, it is generally quite obvious that chemotherapy is likely to be beneficial in contrast to real frail patients where the disadvantages of chemotherapy will probably be greater than the advantages. The most difficult category is the category in between, also called "vulnerable" patients. A full comprehensive geriatric assessment (discussed elsewhere in this book) is certainly required in this patient category in order to have a better view on the global health situation which may ultimately allow to make a more appropriate decision on the indication of chemotherapy.

Choosing the most appropriate chemotherapy regimen for a specific older patient is also a major challenge. It is not really possible to provide strict guidelines on which specific regimen or which order of regimens should be used in sequential situations (first line, second line, third line, etc.). This is quite similar to the situation in metastatic breast cancer in the general (not elderly) population; there have never been specific or concrete international consensus/guidelines on how metastatic breast cancer patients should be treated. For elderly more than in younger patients preference should be given in general to chemotherapeutic agents with safer profiles. The choice of a specific regimen depends on different factors: Is there a need for urgent response (might be a reason to take the most active regimens first)? Is it a slow growing disease in a vulnerable patient where toxicity should be avoided in any case (soft oral regimens or even wait-and-see attitude)? Is co-morbidity present that excludes specific regimens (e.g., no anthracyclines in case of cardiac failure; no taxanes in case of existing significant neuropathy)? Which drugs are available/reimbursed in the country? Which regimens is the oncologist familiar with? Table 19.1 shows a selection of the largest phase II studies and one phase III study that have been performed in elderly patients with metastatic breast cancer. First of all, most studies had a small sample size and radiological response was not centrally reviewed (which generally decreases response rate). Moreover, it is difficult to generalize the results of these trials to the whole elderly population, since selection bias was probably highly prevalent, indicated by the fact that the large majority of the population in all these studies had a WHO performance

Table 19.1 Selection of the largest clinical trials in elderly women with metastatic breast cancer (based on Hamberg et al. 2007)

Reference	Agent	Dosage	Number of pts, age (years)	Response rate (%)	Most important gr III-V toxicities
(Biganzoli et al. 2007)	Pegylated liposomal doxorubicin	50 mg/m2 q4w	28, ≥70	39[a]	Stomatitis14%, HFS 11%
(Barzacchi et al. 1994)	Mitoxantrone	10–14 mg/m2 q3w	27, <67	26	Neutropenia 29%, asthenia 7%, nausea 7%
(Mammoliti et al. 1996)	MFL[c]	[c]q4w	24, ≥70	50	Leucopenia 4%
(Perez et al. 2002)	Paclitaxel	80 mg/m2 qw	73, ≥65	20	Asthenia 5%; Neutropenia 15%
(Hainsworth et al. 2001)	Docetaxel	36 mg/m2 qw, 6w/8	41, ≥65	36	Fatigue 20%; diarrhea 10%, edema 7%; Leucopenia 4%
(Vogel et al. 1999)	Vinorelbine	30 mg/m2 d1–8 q3w	56, ≥60	40	Neutropenia 80%, N/V 10%, asthenia 7%, 1 toxic death
(Bajetta et al. 2005)	Capecitabine	1,000 mg/m2 po d1–14q3w	43, ≥65	47	Fatigue 12%, dyspnea 5%, N/V 5%, neutropenia 2%
(Gelman & Taylor 1984)	CMF[b]	[b]q4w	92, ≥65	42	N/V 58%, mucositis 18%, diarrhea 10%, infection 10%, 3 toxic deaths
(Feher et al. 2005) Phase III	Gemcitabine vs. Epirubicin	1,200 mg/m2 qw 3/4w; 35 mg/m2 qw 3/4w	198, ≥60; 199, ≥60	16; 40	Neutropenia 25%, thrombopenia 9%, N/V 7%, 3 toxic deaths; Neutropenia 18%, N/V 7%, 0 toxic deaths

[a] also included 34 pts with 60–70 mg/m2 q6w, where much higher toxicity was observed

[b] CMF=cyclophosphamide, methotrexate and fluorouracil; dose of CM based on creatinine clearance, dose of F 600 mg/m2; C d1–14 po, MF d1–8

[c] MFL=mitoxantrone, fluorouracil and levo-leucovorin; dose M 10 mg/m2 d1; F 500 mg/m2 d15–16, L 250 mg/m2 d15–16

status of 0 or 1, which is not representative for a general older population. Also, age cut-off was 65 or even 60 in most of these studies, and a large part of the so-called elderly patients were below the age of 70, which is more or less an accepted threshold for the elderly with cancer. Another issue is that the pharmacology of these drugs might change in the elderly. Indeed, age can affect most pharmacokinetic parameters, including absorption, volume of distribution, hepatic drug metabolism, and excretion (Wildiers et al. 2003). Atrophic gastritis, decreased gastric motility and secretions, or decreased intraluminal surface area, can cause diminished *absorption* of oral agents, possibly resulting in reduced effectiveness, although whether decreased absorption actually occurs with age is still controversial. Polypharmacy with multiple concomitant medications can alter absorption by binding drugs in the gastrointestinal tract, changing adsorption or pH, and by competition for carrier sites. The following paragraphs will discuss the clinical and pharmacological data on the most frequently used cytostatic drugs in breast cancer in the elderly and is reviewed more in detail elsewhere (Wildiers et al. 2003).

19.4.1   Anthracyclines

Anthracyclines have been one of the basic treatments of breast cancer for many years. Anthracyclines are mainly metabolized and eliminated in the liver. Decreased early clearance and increased plasma peak levels have been observed in the elderly, without a clear difference in total doxorubicin clearance. The lack of age-related differences in the total clearance of doxorubicin was confirmed in another study of 44 women aged 35–79 years. Doxorubicin is about 70% bound to plasma proteins, so a case for dose adjustment can be made in elderly patients with hypoalbuminemia.

More myocardial toxicity and myelosuppression is observed in the elderly. The increased incidence of anthracycline-related cardiomyopathy over the age of 70 is most likely due to a combination of factors, including a higher prevalence of preexisting conditions restricting the functional reserve of the myocardium.

In clinical practice, doxorubicin is often avoided in the elderly. Nevertheless, a reasonable amount of data is available on the use of doxorubicin in elderly patients. In adjuvant setting, doxorubicin-based chemotherapy was well-tolerated in a study of 65 elderly patients (>65 years) of good performance status with breast cancer and a normal cardiac ejection fraction, and overall survival was similar to those of 325 younger patients (50–64 years) (Ibrahim et al. 1999). However, the dose of doxorubicin was limited to 40 mg/m^2 per cycle, and no information was provided concerning dose reduction. In a previous large retrospective study from the same authors of 244 elderly patients (>65 years) with metastatic breast cancer, doxorubicin was usually given at 50 mg/m^2. There were no significant differences in toxicity and efficacy in older patients (>65 years) and younger patients (50–64 years) (Ibrahim et al. 1996). However, caution is warranted because the delivered dose was less in the older group, while the leucocyte and platelet nadir counts were similar, suggesting

Table 19.2 Strategies to reduce toxicity of anthracyclines in vulnerable elderly cancer patients

Use protracted infusion rate since this might decrease cardiac toxicity

Prophylactic use of CSF (colony stimulating growth factors) if classical 3-weekly regimens are used (e.g., AC, FEC75) with the aim of reducing the risk of febrile neutropenia

Use desrasoxane as cardioprotecting agent; concerns exist however that also antitumor efficacy might decrease as well.

Use weekly low dose regimens (e.g., epirubicine 35 mg/m2 qw) instead of 3-weekly regimens

Use "softer" anthracyclines, such as mitoxantrone, which have much less toxicity but also lower antitumor effect compared to classical anthracyclines

Use liposomal anthracyclines, which have less alopecia, neutropenia, and most importantly less cardiac toxicity compared to classical anthracyclines

increased hematological toxicity in this group. Moreover, all patients were in phase II studies, which may have excluded elderly patients with comorbid conditions.

Certainly in more vulnerable of frail patients, the use of classical anthracyclines is debatable, and a significant proportion of this population may have more harm than benefit from this treatment. Several strategies are available to use anthracyclines in this population while minimizing the risk of toxicity. A summary is shown in Table 19.2.

- When doxorubicin is administered by continuous infusion or in small daily doses, the incidence of drug-related cardiotoxicity is reduced significantly.
- Hematological support with leucocyte growth factors (G-CSF or GM-CSF) is effective in reducing hematological toxicity and increasing dose intensity. Whether it also increases outcome/survival is not known at present in metastatic breast cancer. There is more evidence for the use of CSF in secondary prophylaxis than in primary prophylaxis for elderly patient with metastatic breast cancer receiving classical anthracyclines.
- Desrazoxane can also reduce cardiac toxicity, but this needs to be confirmed and investigated specifically in the elderly population, and there are concerns that the efficacy of anthracyclines might decrease as well when desrazoxane is administered.
- Weekly epirubicine is the best studied drug in elderly patients with metastatic breast cancer. In the only phase III study performed in this population (Feher et al. 2005), epirubicin was superior compared to gemcitabine in first-line treatment. "Elderly" was defined however as age greater or equal to 60 years (median 68 years) so this is not really representative of the general elderly population. In this randomized, phase III study, patients with clinically measurable disease received either gemcitabine 1,200 mg/m^2 ($n=198$) or epirubicin 35 mg/m^2 ($n=199$) on days 1, 8, and 15 of a 28-day cycle. Epirubicin demonstrated statistically significant superiority in TTP (6.1 and 3.4 months, $P=0.0001$), overall survival (19.1 and 11.8 months, $P=0.0004$), and independently assessed response rate (40.3 and 16.4% in 186 and 183 evaluable patients, $P<0.001$). For gemcitabine ($n=190$) and epirubicin ($n=192$), respectively, common WHO grade 3/4 toxicities were neutropenia (25.3 and 17.9%) and leukopenia

(14.3 and 19.3%). Of the 28 on-study deaths (17 gemcitabine, 11 epirubicin), three were considered possibly or probably related to treatment (gemcitabine). The authors concluded that epirubicin was superior to gemcitabine in the treatment of metastatic breast cancer in women age ≥60, confirming that anthracyclines remain important drugs for first-line treatment of MBC. Whether epirubicine is a more effective drug than its cheaper analogue doxorubicin remains a matter of debate.

- Mitoxantrone is considered as an anthracycline with somewhat reduced efficacy, but also much lower toxicity compared to doxorubicine. In general, there is no alopecia or nausea and vomiting, and also neutropenia is much less common. It is also an attractive treatment option for elderly patients although some concerns exist on the potency of this drug compared to classical anthracyclines and taxanes.
- Liposomal formulations of doxorubicin have been shown to decrease significantly the risk of cardiotoxicity, while providing comparable antitumor activity. The EORTC trial (see Table 19.1) with liposomal doxorubicin shows a reasonable efficacy with limited toxicity, apparently less than observed with classical anthracyclines, but formal comparison in the elderly population is lacking. Liposomal anthracyclines are an attractive treatment option in elderly patients with metastatic breast cancer.

In conclusion, anthracyclines are still an important treatment modality in elderly patients with metastatic breast cancer. There are no strict guidelines for the dose adjustment of doxorubicin on the basis of age, but great care is recommended in the elderly, given the observed increased toxicity, and doses higher than 50 mg/m^2 should probably be avoided in the majority of the 70+ population. It has been suggested that in patients over the age of 70, regardless of coexisting heart disease, a cumulative doxorubicin dose of 450 mg/m^2 should not be exceeded, whereas in younger patients, a 550 mg/m^2 threshold is used. Several strategies to reduce toxicity are available, such as prolonged infusion rate, prophylactic use of CSF, weekly regimens, or liposomal anthracyclines.

19.4.2 Taxanes

Taxanes are considered to be the most effective drugs in breast cancer, and as the weekly regimens seem at least as effective as the 3-weekly regimens but with less toxicity, these weekly regimens are very attractive for elderly breast cancer patients. Several different doses have been used for the weekly taxane regimens in phase II trials. Although large comparative studies are lacking, pharmacological studies are suggestive for a decreased clearance of unbound paclitaxel in elderly patients compared to nonelderly patients (Smorenburg et al. 2003) while clearance of docetaxel seems rather unaffected by age (ten Tije et al. 2005). It seems safe to use the lower range of proposed doses of the weekly regimens until further data provide stronger evidence for optimal dosing in elderly patients. A dose of paclitaxel 80 mg/m2/week (see Table 19.1) and docetaxel 36 mg/m2/week seems tolerable for elderly patients without excessive toxicity and with high response rates. The dose limiting toxicity for 3-weekly taxanes, severe neutropenia, is generally very limited in weekly regimens, also in the elderly or frail patients. However, neuropathy (paclitaxel) or fatigue and fluid retention (docetaxel) can be troublesome, and eventually require dose modifications. In general, however, weekly taxanes are a reasonable option for older patients with metastatic breast cancer (Wildiers and Paridaens 2004).

19.4.3   Vinorelbine

Vinorelbine is a semisynthetic vinca alkaloid and causes less neurotoxicity than the older compounds in this group. The Vd, terminal half-life, and elimination rate of vinorelbine in 25 elderly patients (>65 years) with metastatic breast cancer were similar to those reported in younger patients, implying that dose reduction in elderly patients is unnecessary. Conflicting data have been reported by Gauvin et al. In 12 elderly patients (>65 years) with advanced breast cancer, a high correlation was found between age and total clearance, while the area under the curve (AUC) correlated with the decrease in Hb level and neutrophil count. Full dose vinorelbine (30 mg/m² day 1 and day 8) has been shown to have a favorable tolerance profile in general (Sorio et al. 1997), but in elderly patients, the amount of grade III-IV neutropenia was high (80%). It might be more prudent to use a lower dose, e.g., 25 mg/m2 d1–8, but formal dose finding studies in elderly patients are lacking (Wildiers et al. 2003).

19.4.4   Capecitabine

Capecitabine is an oral prodrug of 5-FU and has been developed to increase the therapeutic index and improve convenience and flexibility of dosing. It has clear activity in breast cancer and is associated with palmar-plantar erythrodysesthesia, as seen with a continuous 5-fluorouracil infusion. Initial pharmacokinetic and efficacy data were obtained in the non-fasting state, but food has since been shown to significantly decrease the AUC and peak levels of capecitabine. It is important to give the drug with food to avoid unexpected pharmacokinetic effects. One study found that the effect of age and creatinine clearance (CrCl) on the pharmacokinetics of capecitabine was negligible, but patients with severe renal impairment were not included (Wildiers et al. 2003). A study specifically investigating the effect of renal function clearly demonstrated increased toxicity with renal impairment, and as a result dose adjustment guidelines were proposed: avoid in severe renal impairment (CrCl <30 ml/min); 75% of the regular dose in moderate renal impairment (CrCl 30–50 ml/min); and if the CrCl >50 ml/min then no dose adjustment is needed (Poole et al. 2002). Significant drug interactions have been reported, e.g., with warfarin, so great care is warranted in the elderly population who often take lots of other drugs concomitantly.

19.4.5 Metronomic Chemotherapy

Although not specifically investigated for the elderly population, metronomic cyclophosphamide (C) and methotrexate (M) (Colleoni et al. 2006) in patients with metastatic breast cancer might be a very attractive treatment option, especially in vulnerable/frail patients where any significant toxicity may result in severe morbidity or even mortality. In a phase II study from the IBCSG, patients with advanced breast cancer received oral C (50 mg daily) and M (2.5 mg twice daily on days 1 and 4). In 90 evaluable patients, 3 complete remissions and 15 partial remissions were observed, resulting in an overall response of 20.9% (95% confidence interval [CI] 12.9–31%). Toxicity was generally very mild.

In metastatic breast cancer, there is no proof that high-dose chemotherapy or combination of strong chemotherapeutic agents provides real benefit above using sequential monotherapy regimens. For instance, the combination of anthracyclines and taxanes in younger patients only prolongs TTP slightly compared to sequential anthracyclines and taxanes, without prolonging overall survival, and at the cost of much higher toxicity. So also in elderly patients, it is acceptable to use softer regimens rather than aggressive regimens. The goal of chemotherapy in metastatic breast cancer is to control disease as long as possible without causing excessive toxicity/harm. Since elderly patients are more susceptible to toxicity, great care is warranted when a specific regimen is chosen for a specific patient, keeping in mind the delicate balance between gains in efficacy (tumor control) and losses by inducing morbidity and even treatment-related mortality. The choice of chemotherapy regimens and agents is dependent on individual patient characteristics and also on drug availability/reimbursement by the health system. Since chemotherapy in this situation is only palliative, the quality of life is paramount, and significant toxicity is generally not acceptable. Elderly patients should also be followed more closely than younger patients for toxicity since the incidence of toxicity is higher, and since they have less reserve capacities to deal with toxicities. For instance, when elderly have vomiting or severe diarrhea, they dehydrate much faster and can develop renal failure and related complications, which will bring them to a downward vicious circle. In principle, dose reductions in the elderly are not systematically recommended, but should be considered based on pharmacological parameters and altered according to observed toxicity (Wildiers et al. 2003; Lichtman et al. 2007a; Lichtman et al. 2007b). Strict follow-up is essential in this population in particular to avoid overtreatment and debilitating side effects. Particular attention should be paid to supportive care, as older patients are more likely to develop neutropenia than younger patients (Dees et al. 2000), and generally have less functional reserve than their younger counterparts. Bisphosphonates can also provide symptomatic relieve in patients with bone metastases. This topic is discussed elsewhere in this book. The safety of long-term administration of bisphosphonates in elderly cancer patients has been established.

19.5   Targeted Therapies

Targeted therapies have been a breakthrough in the treatment of (metastatic) breast cancer. Trastuzumab, a monoclonal antibody against the HER-2/neu receptor, increases the response rate of chemotherapy significantly, and combination of taxanes and trastuzumab can achieve response rates about 60–70% in HER-2/neu positive disease. Also combinations with vinorelbine and capeticabine have been shown to be very effective. Trastuzumab is generally very well-tolerated. The main side effect is cardiac failure. The highest incidence of cardiac failure with trastuzumab has been observed in combination with anthracyclines, and for this reason these two drugs are generally not used together. In contrast to conventional anthracyclines, it seems safe to combine trastuzumab with liposomal anthracyclines. Age is a documented risk factor for congestive heart failure in patients receiving trastuzumab, but depends probably more on pre-existing comorbidities than on age by itself (Giuliani 2004).

Lapatinib, an oral HER-1 and HER-2 tyrosine kinase inhibitor, also has activity in case of trastuzumab resistance, both in monotherapy and in combination with capecitabine (Geyer et al. 2006). No specific efficacy or toxicity data for elderly patients are available. However, lapatinib can cause diarrhea, which occasionally can be severe. Elderly patients are more vulnerable to dehydration, and fluid should be replaced as soon as possible, if appropriate by intravenous infusion.

Also antiangiogenic therapy has been studied in metastatic breast cancer. Most data are available for bevacizumab, a monoclonal antibody against vascular endothelial growth factor (VEGF). In a study of patients of all ages, the addition of bevacizumab to paclitaxel as first-line therapy for metastatic breast cancer demonstrated an improvement in response rate and disease-free survival (Miller 2005). There are few data specific to the risks and benefits of bevacizumab in older patients with breast cancer; however, a pooled analysis of patients with all types of cancer from 5 randomized trials demonstrated that patients >age 65 are at increased risk of arterial thromboembolic events, particularly when bevacizumab is given in combination with chemotherapy (Skillings et al. 2005). Concerns exist for elderly patients who are treated with anti-angiogenic therapy, since the modest benefit in disease control might be counterbalanced by increased toxicity, as was demonstrated in lung cancer (Ramalingam et al. 2008).

19.6   Conclusion

The goals of treating metastatic breast cancer in older patients are not different from those in younger patients. For the majority of patients with hormone-receptor-positive breast cancer, hormonal therapy should be the first choice. The use of chemotherapy should be considered in patients with hormone-receptor-negative, hormone-refractory or life-threatening disease. Choice of chemotherapy regimens and agents is dependent on individual patient characteristics, preferences, and drug availability.

References

Bajetta E, Procopio G, Celio L, Gattinoni L, la Torre S, Mariani L, Catena L, Ricotta R, Longarini R, Zilembo N, Buzzoni R (2005) Safety and efficacy of two different doses of capecitabine in the treatment of advanced breast cancer in older women. Journal of Clinical Oncology 23:2155–2161

Barzacchi MC, Nobile MT, Sanguineti O, Sertoli MR, Chiara S, Repetto L, Forno G, Lavarello A, Rosso R (1994) Treatment of Metastatic Colorectal-Carcinoma with Lymphoblastoid Interferon and 5-Fluorouracil—Data of A Phase-Ii Study. Anticancer Research 14:2147–2149

Biganzoli L, Coleman R, Minisini A, Hamilton A, Aapro M, Therasse P, Mottino G, Bogaerts J, Piccart M (2007) A joined analysis of two European Organization for the Research and Treatment of Cancer (EORTC) studies to evaluate the role of pegylated liposomal doxorubicin (Caelyx (TM)) in the treatment of elderly patients with metastatic breast cancer. Critical Reviews in Oncology Hematology 61:84–89

Caralt M, Bilbao I, Cortes J, Escartin A, Lazaro JL, Dopazo C, Olsina JJ, Balsells J, Charco R (2008) Hepatic resection for liver metastases as part of the "oncosurgical" treatment of metastatic breast cancer. Ann Surg.Oncol 15:2804–2810

Christman K, Muss HB, Case LD, Stanley V (1992) Chemotherapy of Metastatic Breast-Cancer in the Elderly—the Piedmont-Oncology-Association Experience. Jama-Journal of the American Medical Association 268:57–62

Colleoni M, Orlando L, Sanna G, Rocca A, Maisonneuve P, Peruzzotti G, Ghisini R, Sandri MT, Zorzino L, Nole F, Viale G, Goldhirsch A (2006) Metronomic low-dose oral cyclophosphamide and methotrexate plus or minus thalidomide in metastatic breast cancer: antitumor activity and biological effects. Ann Oncol 17:232–238

Dees EC, O'Reilly S, Goodman SN, Sartorius S, Levine MA, Jones RJ, Grochow LB, Donehower RC, Fetting JH (2000) A prospective pharmacologic evaluation of age-related toxicity of adjuvant chemotherapy in women with breast cancer. Cancer Invest 18:521–529

Feher O, Vodvarka P, Jassem J, Morack G, Advani SH, Khoo KS, Doval DC, Ermisch S, Roychowdhury D, Miller MA, von Minckwitz G (2005) First-line gemcitabine versus epirubicin in postmenopausal women aged 60 or older with metastatic breast cancer: a multicenter, randomized, phase III study. Annals of Oncology 16:899–908

Gelman RS, Taylor SG (1984) Cyclophosphamide, methotrexate, and 5-fluorouracil chemotherapy in women more than 65 years old with advanced breast cancer: the elimination of age trends in toxicity by using doses based on creatinine clearance. J Clin Oncol 2:1404–1413

Geyer CE, Forster J, Lindquist D, Chan S, Romieu CG, Pienkowski T, Jagiello-Gruszfeld A, Crown J, Chan A, Kaufman B, Skarlos D, Campone M, Davidson N, Berger M, Oliva C, Rubin SD, Stein S, Cameron D: Lapatinib plus capecitabine for HER2-positive advanced breast cancer. N.Engl.J Med 2006, 355:2733–2743.

Hainsworth JD, Burris HA III, Yardley DA, Bradof JE, Grimaldi M, Kalman LA, Sullivan T, Baker M, Erland JB, Greco FA (2001) Weekly docetaxel in the treatment of elderly patients with advanced breast cancer: a Minnie Pearl Cancer Research Network phase II trial. J Clin Oncol 19:3500–3505

Hamberg P, Verweij J, Seynaeve C (2007) Cytotoxic therapy for the elderly with metastatic breast cancer: A review on safety, pharmacokinetics and efficacy. European Journal of Cancer 43:1514–1528

Ibrahim NK, Frye DK, Buzdar AU, Walters RS, Hortobagyi GN: Doxorubicin-based chemotherapy in elderly patients with metastatic breast cancer. Tolerance and outcome. Arch Intern.Med 1996, 156:882–888.

Ibrahim NK, Hortobagyi GN, Ewer M, Ali MK, Asmar L, Theriault RL, Fraschini G, Frye DK, Buzdar AU: Doxorubicin-induced congestive heart failure in elderly patients with metastatic breast cancer, with long-term follow-up: the M.D. Anderson experience. Cancer Chemother. Pharmacol. 1999, 43:471–478.

Khan SA, Stewart AK, Morrow M (2002) Does aggressive local therapy improve survival in metastatic breast cancer? Surgery 132:620–626

Lichtman SM, Wildiers H, Launay-Vacher V, Steer C, Chatelut E, Aapro M (2007a) International Society of Geriatric Oncology (SIOG) recommendations for the adjustment of dosing in elderly cancer patients with renal insufficiency. European Journal of Cancer 43:14–34

Lichtman SM, Wildiers H, Chatelut E, Steer C, Budman D, Morrison VA, Tranchand B, Shapira I, Aapro M: International Society of Geriatric Oncology Chemotherapy Taskforce: evaluation of chemotherapy in older patients—an analysis of the medical literature. J.Clin.Oncol. 2007, 25:1832–1843.

Mammoliti S, Merlini L, Caroti C, Gallo L (1996) Phase II study of mitoxantrone, 5-fluorouracil, and levo-leucovorin (MLF) in elderly advanced breast cancer patients. Breast Cancer Research and Treatment 37:93–96

Milla-Santos A, Milla L, Portella J, Rallo L, Pons M, Rodes E, Casanovas J, Puig-Gali M (2003) Anastrozole versus tamoxifen as first-line therapy in postmenopausal patients with hormone-dependent advanced breast cancer—A prospective, randomized, phase III study. American Journal of Clinical Oncology-Cancer Clinical Trials 26:317–322

Miller KD (2005) WMGJDMCMPESTDNE: A randomized phase III trial of paclitaxel versus paclitaxel plus bevacizumab as first-line therapy for locally recurrent or metastatic breast cancer: a trial coordinated by the Eastern Cooperative Oncology Group (E2100) In: Abstractof the san antonio breast cancer symposium

Mouridsen H, Chaudri-Ross HA (2004) Efficacy of first-line letrozole versus tamoxifen as a function of age in postmenopausal women with advanced breast cancer. Oncologist 9:497–506

Mouridsen H, Gershanovich M, Sun Y, Perez-Carrion R, Boni C, Monnier A, Apffelstaedt J, Smith R, Sleeboom HP, Jaenicke F, Pluzanska A, Dank M, Becquart D, Bapsy PP, Salminen E, Snyder R, Chaudri-Ross H, Lang R, Wyld P, Bhatnagar A (2003a) Phase III study of letrozole versus tamoxifen as first-line therapy of advanced breast cancer in postmenopausal women: analysis of survival and update of efficacy from the International Letrozole Breast Cancer Group. J Clin Oncol 21:2101–2109

Mouridsen H, Gershanovich M, Sun Y, Perez-Carrion R, Boni C, Monnier A, Apffelstaedt J, Smith R, Sleeboom HP, Jaenicke F, Pluzanska A, Dank M, Becquart D, Bapsy PP, Salminen E, Snyder R, Chaudri-Ross H, Lang R, Wyld P, Bhatnagar A: Phase III study of letrozole versus tamoxifen as first-line therapy of advanced breast cancer in postmenopausal women: analysis of survival and update of efficacy from the International Letrozole Breast Cancer Group. J.Clin.Oncol. 2003, 21:2101–2109.

Muss HB, Case LD, Atkins JN, Bearden JD III, Cooper MR, Cruz JM, Jackson DV Jr, O'Rourke MA, Pavy MD, Powell BL (1994) Tamoxifen versus high-dose oral medroxyprogesterone acetate as initial endocrine therapy for patients with metastatic breast cancer: a Piedmont Oncology Association study. J Clin Oncol 12:1630–1638

Parkin DM, Bray F, Ferlay J, Pisani P (2005) Global cancer statistics, 2002. CA Cancer J Clin 55:74–108

Perez EA, Vogel CL, Irwin DH, Kirshner JJ, Patel R (2002) Weekly paclitaxel in women age 65 and above with metastatic breast cancer. Breast Cancer Research and Treatment 73:85–88

Poole C, Gardiner J, Twelves C, Johnston P, Harper P, Cassidy J, Monkhouse J, Banken L, Weidekamm E, Reigner B (2002) Effect of renal impairment on the pharmacokinetics and tolerability of capecitabine (Xeloda) in cancer patients. Cancer Chemotherapy and Pharmacology 49:225–234

Giuliani R (2004) AMMMPJYLMRJDJPKADLMJPLB: Is age a risk factor of congestive heart failure (CHF) in patients receiving trastuzumab (H)? Results from two Belgian compassionate use programs in metastatic breast cancer (MBC) patients (pts) [abstract]. Proc Am Soc Clin Oncol 22: 838

Ramalingam SS, Dahlberg SE, Langer CJ, Gray R, Belani CP, Brahmer JR, Sandler AB, Schiller JH, Johnson DH (2008) Outcomes for elderly, advanced-stage non small-cell lung cancer patients treated with bevacizumab in combination with carboplatin and paclitaxel: analysis of Eastern Cooperative Oncology Group Trial 4599. J Clin Oncol 26:60–65

Rapiti E, Verkooijen HM, Vlastos G, Fioretta G, Neyroud-Caspar I, Sappino AP, Chappuis PO, Bouchardy C (2006) Complete excision of primary breast tumor improves survival of patients with metastatic breast cancer at diagnosis. Journal of Clinical Oncology 24:2743–2749

Sheth HR, Lord G, Tkaczuk K, Danton M, Lewis LM, Langenberg P, Lim CK, Flaws JA: Aging may be associated with concentrations of tamoxifen and its metabolites in breast cancer patients. J.Womens Health (Larchmt.) 2003, 12:799–808.

Skillings JR, Johnson DH, Miller K, Kabbinavar F, Bergsland E, Holmgren E, Holden SN, Hurwitz H, Scappaticci F: Arterial thromboembolic events (ATEs) in a pooled analysis of 5 randomized, controlled trials (RCTs) of bevacizurnab (BV) with chemotherapy. Journal of Clinical Oncology 2005, 23:196S.

Smorenburg CH, ten Tije AJ, Verweij J, Bontenbal M, Mross K, van Zomeren DM, Seynaeve C, Sparreboom A: Altered clearance of unbound paclitaxel in elderly patients with metastatic breast cancer. Eur.J Cancer 2003, 39:196–202.

Sorio R, Robieux I, Galligioni E, Freschi A, Colussi AM, Crivellari D, Saracchini S, Monfardini S (1997) Pharmacokinetics and tolerance of vinorelbine in elderly patients with metastatic breast cancer. European Journal of Cancer 33:301–303

Taylor SG, Gelman RS, Falkson G, Cummings FJ (1986) Combination chemotherapy compared to tamoxifen as initial therapy for stage IV breast cancer in elderly women. Ann Intern Med 104:455–461

ten Tije AJ, Verweij J, Carducci MA, Graveland W, Rogers T, Pronk T, Verbruggen MP, Dawkins F, Baker SD (2005) Prospective evaluation of the pharmacokinetics and toxicity profile of docetaxel in the elderly. Journal of Clinical Oncology 23:1070–1077

Thelen A, Benckert C, Jonas S, Lopez-Hanninen E, Sehouli J, Neumann U, Rudolph B, Neuhaus P (2008) Liver resection for metastases from breast cancer. J Surg Oncol 97:25–29

Vogel C, O'Rourke M, Winer E, Hochster H, Chang A, Adamkiewicz B, White R, McGuirt C (1999) Vinorelbine as first-line chemotherapy for advanced breast cancer in women 60 years of age or older. Annals of Oncology 10:397–402

Wildiers H, Paridaens R (2004) Taxanes in elderly breast cancer patients. Cancer Treat Rev 30:333–342

Wildiers H, Highley MS, de Bruijn EA, van Oosterom AT (2003) Pharmacology of anticancer drugs in the elderly population. Clinical Pharmacokinetics 42:1213–1242

Chapter 20
The Use of Chemotherapy in Elderly Cancer Patients: Dose Adjusting, Drug Interactions, and Polypharmacy

Lazzaro Repetto and Claudia Di Bartolomeo

20.1 Introduction

In geriatric oncology, the progressive decline of the functional reserve of multiple organ systems and restriction in personal and social resources represent the most important variables in treatment choice. As aging process is highly individualized, the key to safe and effective management of cancer in the older patient is individualization of treatment. The application of this model requires proper evaluation of the global health status of the older patient. The most reliable and best validated assessment is referred to as comprehensive geriatric assessment (CGA) (Repetto et al. 2002; Extermann et al. 2005).

Older patients are generally more susceptible to treatment-related toxicity due to reduced organ functional reserves, changes in the body composition, comorbidities, polypharmacy, nutritional status, and dehydration. All these conditions may affect the pharmacokinetic (PK) and the pharmacodynamic (PD) properties of administered drugs and require the exclusion of certain drugs or dose adjustment. For drugs with a high therapeutic index, dose adjusting may be clinically unimportant, but for cytotoxic drugs, pharmacological changes occurring with age may be responsible for severe toxicity.

Due to the wide variation of the pharmacological parameters treatment-related toxicity is fairly predictable and continuous dose adjustment may be required.

The fear of chemotherapy-related side effects by physicians is frequently responsible for not offering adequate chemotherapy regimens to elderly cancer patients. Choosing the correct chemotherapy regimen and dose can be extremely difficult because of physiological changes, associated comorbidities, and polypharmacy. Treatment decisions need to be based on a patient's individual performance, functional status, and life expectancy. Currently, we lack accepted algorithms to guide management decisions in elderly cancer patients.

L. Repetto (✉) and C. Di Bartolomeo
Department of Oncology, INRCA-IRCCS, Rome, Italy
e-mail: l.repetto@inrca.it

M.W. Reed and R.A. Audisio (eds.), *Management of Breast Cancer in Older Women,*
DOI 10.1007/978-1-84800-265-4_20, © Springer-Verlag London Limited 2011

Most of the pharmacological data published in literature are obtained from young patients; thus, special care is recommended when cytotoxic chemotherapy is employed in elderly patients.

Although elderly patients are largely underrepresented in clinical trials, an increasing amount of information is available to support drug and dose choice in individual patients and to guide decision making (Wildiers 2007).

Waiting for evidence-based guidelines, few recommendations are discussed in this chapter, to reduce toxicity and to tailor the dose of chemotherapy.

20.2 The Use of Cytotoxic Chemotherapy in the Elderly Patient

Few studies, mostly retrospective, reported the feasibility and effectiveness of treating healthy elderly with the same regimen employed in younger cancer patients (Sargent et al. 2001; Langer et al. 2002). It must be underlined that these patients are at increased risk of treatment-related toxicity and require intensive supportive care, including prophylactic supportive treatment (Repetto 2003). The application of the CGA model allows more feasible recognition of such patients and proper cancer care prescription. These patients should be evaluated for standard treatment with special emphasis on supportive care.

Conversely, we lack evidence to support treatment choice in the vulnerable and frail elderly. These patients are "geriatric" and the most challenging for clinical oncologists, they should not be excluded from cancer care but rather receive individualized CGA-based treatment. Due to the growing number of this population, oncologists should be trained to face this emergency and to apply lessons from geriatrics and clinical pharmacology in the management of elderly cancer patients.

The epidemiological observations support that 75% of the patients aged 70 years are otherwise healthy and fit, as 35% at 80, and 10% at 90.

20.2.1 Physiological and Pharmacological Changes

Older patients are generally more susceptible to treatment-related toxicity for a number of reasons including reduced organ functional reserves, changes in the body composition with increase in body fat and decrease in lean body mass and total body water, comorbidities, polypharmacy and drug interactions, nutritional status, and dehydration. All these conditions may affect the PK of cytotoxic drugs, increase toxicity, and require the exclusion of certain drugs or dose adjustment (Repetto et al. 2002; Moscinski 1998; Lipschitz 1995; Iber et al. 1994; Allen 1992; Swain et al. 1997; Benjamin et al. 1995; Gill et al. 1995; Kaplan and Wiernik 1982; Zagonel et al. 1998; Fleck et al. 1990; Rubin et al. 1992; Schagen et al. 1999; Bonetti et al. 1994; Julis-Elysee and White 1990).

The normal tissues, whose susceptibility to chemotherapy increases with age, include the mucoses, the hemopoietic system, the heart, and the peripheral and central nervous systems (Balducci and Extermann 2001; Balducci and Corcoran 2000a; Schijvers et al. 1999; Repetto et al. 2003; Egorin 1993a; Jacobson et al. 2001).

The progressive decline of functional reserve is very individualized; thus, organ functions, especially liver and renal functions, should be always evaluated in the planning of chemotherapy treatment for older patients.

Most of the pharmacological data published in the literature are obtained from young patients; thus, special care must be recommended when extrapolating data from clinical trials to the general elderly population. Table 20.1 reports the most frequent toxic effect observed in elderly patients receiving chemotherapy. Factors that influence the pharmacokinetis of cytotoxic chemotherapy and recommendation for drugs selection in elderly cancer patients have been already addressed (John et al. 2003; Skirvin and Lichtman 2002; Wildiers et al. 2003).

The age of the patient may influence the choice of drugs and doses with frequent occurrence of undue dose reduction. Although age influences effectiveness and safety of cytotoxic chemotherapy, treatment choice should be based on pharmacologic considerations only.

The age-related decrease of the total body water affects the volume of distribution of water-soluble agents with a substantial increase in the risk of acute side effects (Balducci and Extermann 2001; Balducci and Corcoran 2000a).

Adequate counseling on proper fluid intake and/or intravenous fluid support reduces such risk.

The volume of distribution of water-soluble drugs is a function of the body composition, the albumin levels, and the hemoglobin concentration. Because many of the cytotoxic drugs are bound to red blood cells, a drop in red blood cell mass is associated with increased concentration of free drug in circulation (Schijvers et al. 1999). At least five studies showed that hemoglobin level is an independent risk factor for myelotoxicity for a number of agents, including anthracyclines, epipodo-phyllotoxins, and camptothecins (Balducci and Extermann 2001). Anemia is of special concern to elderly individuals because its prevalence increases with age and the decline in total body proteins and total body water hampers compensatory

Table 20.1 Chemotherapy-related toxicities whose incidence is increased in the older patient

Type of toxicity	Age-related changes
Hematologic	Due to reduced bone marrow stem cells and response to hematological growth factors
Gastroenteric	Increased risk of mucositis, dehydration, and inadequate nutritional support
Cardiovascular	Three-fold risk of anthracycline-related cardiomyopathy
Central Nervous System	Due to reduced neuronal cells or preexistent vascular and/or degenerative injuries
Peripheral Nervous System	Increased toxicity to Vinca alkaloids and platinum compounds. Comorbidity
Lung	Increased risk of interstitial pneumonitis and fibrosis

mechanisms to buffer the increase concentration of free drugs (Repetto et al. 2003). Treatment with hematological growth factors to target hemoglobin value to 12 g/L is recommended in older cancer patients.

The reduction in the glomerular filtration rate (GFR) occurs almost invariably with age and is correlated with creatinine clearance. Calculation of creatinine clearance allows proper dose adjustment of several drugs to reduce toxicity. Tables 20.2 and 20.3 show a number of cytotoxic agents eliminated by the kidney and the dose adjustments based on the GFR reduction, according to the formula of Kintzel and Dorr (Balducci and Corcoran 2000a).

Due to the wide variation of the area under the plasma concentration-time curve (AUC) of the same drugs in different patients of the same size, and of the ability of aging cells to catabolize drugs, the pharmacological consequences of administering chemotherapy in the older patients are fairly predictable.

Table 20.2 Glomerular filtration rate (GFR) declines with aging; as a consequence renal clearance of certain drugs is reduced

Reduced drug release:	
complete kidney excretion	Carboplatin, Methotrexate, Bleomycine
partial kidney excretion	Cyclophosphamide, Epipodophyllotoxine, Taxanes, Fludarabine
Reduced excretion of active metabolites	Idarubicinol, Daunorubicinol
Reduced excretion of toxic metabolites	Arauridine

Table 20.3 Suggested dose reduction of cytotoxic drugs excreted by the kidney according to creatinine clearance. Obviously such reductions do not apply to drugs excreted and/or inactivated by the liver, even in the case of impaired renal function

Cytotoxic drugs	Dose % of drug being excreted by the kidney as active/toxic metabolites	Suggested dose reduction according to Cr Cl (mL/min)		
		≤60	≤45	≤30
Bleomicine	62	0.70	0.60	–
Carboplatin	66	Calvert Formula[a]		
Carmustine	43	0.80	0.75	–
Lomustine	50	0.75	0.70	–
Semustine	47	0.75	0.70	–
Cisplatin	30	0.75	0.50	–
Cytarabine	76	0.60	0.50	–
Dacarbazine	41	0.80	0.75	0.70
Fludarabine	44	0.80	0.75	0.65
Hydrossiurea	36	0.85	0.80	0.75
Hyphosphamide	40	0.80	0.75	0.70
Melphalan	34	0.65	0.50	–
Methotrexate	77	Gelman e Taylor Formula[b]		
Etoposide	32	0.85	0.80	0.75

[a] Calvert Formula: Carboplatin (mg): AUC (mg/mL x min) x {GFR (mL/min) +25}
[b] Gelman e Taylor Formula: Dosaggio Methotrexate: Dose x $Cl\ Cr\ 70$

Thus after initial dose calculation based on GFR, further dose adjustment may be required according to treatment tolerance and observed toxicity (Kinzel and Dorr 1995; Levey et al. 1999; Tranchant 2002; Graham et al. 2000; Matsui et al. 2001; Mould et al. 2002; Nagai et al. 1998; Nakamura et al. 2000; Nguyen 2002; Kintzel and Dorr 1995; Koren et al. 1992).

Although the age-related changes in hepatic drug metabolism are controversial, there is substantial agreement on the reduction of liver size and liver blood flow with aging. Both these circumstances may affect the clearance of the drugs eliminated by the liver. The cytochrome P450 (CYP) microsomal system, which is responsible for phase I reaction, is substantially affected by age (Egorin 1993a). The levels of enzyme activity is genetically determined, several drugs both oncologic and nononcologic are metabolized via the CYP enzymes, thus the potential for drug interaction due to competition and/or interference with the enzyme systems is high, particularly in the older patient frequently treated with several drugs (Jacobson et al. 2001).

Tables 20.4 and 20.5 show a number of cytotoxic agents eliminated by the liver and the suggested dose adjustments according to the authors.

The occurrence of having at least one chronic disease or condition increases substantially with age: the number of comorbidities increases from 2.9 for patients age 55–64 years, to 4.2 in patients age 75 years and older (Yancik 1997). Compared with younger counterparts, elderly cancer patients generally have more comorbid conditions such as hypertension, arthritis, heart disease, and diabetes mellitus for which they are prescribed multiple medications (Gurwitz 2004).

Table 20.4 Cytotoxic drugs excreted or inactivated by the liver

Cytotoxic Drug	Drug % excreted by the kidney
Daunorubicine	<18
Doxorubicine, Epirubicin	<10
Idarubicin, Mitoxantron	<10
Amsacrine	>10
Paclitaxel, Docetaxel	<10
Vincristine, Vinblastine	10–11
Vindesine, Vinorelbine	13–14
Cytotoxic Drug	Drug % excreted by the kidney as active and/or toxic metabolites
Clorambucil	<1
Cyclophosphamide	16
Low dose Cytarabine	11
5-Fluorouracil	<10
Gemcitabine	<10
6-Mercaptopurine	21
Mitomycine C	5
Procarbazide	not detectable
Teniposide	<10
6-Tioguanine	not detectable

Table 20.5 Suggested evaluation criteria and dose adjustment for cytotoxic drugs excreted and/ or inactivated by the liver

	Trombotest	AST	Albuminemia	Bilirubin	Suggested dose reduction
Liver function	(%)	(U/L)	(g/L)	(mg/dL)	(%)
Good	>40	<51	>34	<1.2	100
Average	25–39	51–200	28–34	1.2–3.0	50–75
Impaired	<25	>200	>28	>3.0	25–50

It has been estimated that about 80% of patients older than 65 years are on medications, and about 40% regularly take five or more drugs (Jorgensen et al. 2001), while up to 90% consume over-the-counter (OTC) medications (Hanlon and Fillenbaum 2001).

Use of multiple medications predisposes elderly patients to adverse drug reactions (ADRs) (Repetto and Audisio 2006).

Drug interactions are thought to be a leading cause of ADRs, which also may be the results of changes in drug pharmacology in the senior adult.

20.3   Clinical Pharmacology

Elderly patients are at risk for ADRs because of the physiologic changes occurring with aging, which affect both PK and PD of drug, making older patients more sensitive (Beers 1999). These changes include decreased absorption, declining renal function, reduced liver mass, and metabolic clearance of medications.

The progressive decline of the functional reserve of multiple organ systems may influence PKs and PDs of antineoplastic drugs and reduce the tolerance of normal tissues for treatment complications (Balducci and Extermann 2000; Duthie 1998; Balducci and Corcoran 2000b).

20.3.1   Pharmacokinetics

PKs is the interaction between the drug and the body in terms of its absorption, distribution, metabolism, and excretion. All of these parameters may undergo age-related variations.

20.3.1.1   Absorption

Absorption is the process by which a medication enters the body and moves through the bloodstream and lymphatic system to its site of action. Age-related changes that affect absorption include decreased gastrointestinal motility, decreased splanchnic blood flow, decreased secretion of digestive enzymes, and mucosal atrophy (Baker and Grochow 1997; Moraca-Sawicki 1998). The net result of these changes is a reduction in the drug absorption rate rather than reduced overall absorption of drugs. The increased gastric pH exhibited by elderly patients may affect the absorption of medications that require an acidic pH. Medications such as ketoconazole and aspirin may have decreased bioavailability in elderly. The diffuse atrophy of the digestive mucosa described in persons of advanced age (>80 years) may significantly impair the oral absorption of drugs.

Drug absorption is now becoming a major concern due to the number of new oral agents introduced in the market such as Vinorelbine, Capecitabine, Idarubicin, Ftorafur, and Epipodophyllotoxins (Skirvin and Lichtman 2002).

20.3.1.2 Distribution

Distribution occurs after a medication reaches the systemic circulation. The volume of distribution (Vd) of drugs is a function of body composition and the concentration of circulating plasma proteins such as serum albumin and red blood cells (Vestal 1997). With age, there is a progressive decline in total body water and a progressive accumulation of total body fat, which results in a decreased Vd for water-soluble agents and an increased Vd for fat soluble compounds. For example, benzodiazepines and barbiturates, that are stored extensively in the fat-tissues, show a prolonged action by a slow release from the adipose tissue, resulting in increased duration of action and increased half-life of the medications, leaving patients with prolonged residual drowsiness in the morning.

Gentamicin is a water-soluble medication that is distributed mostly to lean body tissue and the aqueous parts. With less lean body tissue and total body water in the elderly, more gentamicin stays in bloodstream, resulting in increased medication concentration and potential toxicity (Larsen and Hoot Martin 1999).

Also, a progressive decline in the concentration of plasma proteins may further reduce the Vd of water-soluble drugs, especially of those that are heavily protein-bound, such as taxanes, anthracyclines, and vinca alkaloids. Plasma albumin may decrease by 15–20% or more, especially with chronic illness, malnutrition, and frailty. Anemia is the only component of Vd that can be manipulated, by beneficial correction with erythropoietin (Schrijvers and Highley 1999).

20.3.1.3 Metabolism

The liver is the main site of drug metabolism. The hepatic metabolism of drugs is a function of the hepatic blood flow, the rate of drug extraction by the hepatocytes, and the hepatocyte mass, in addition to the intracellular concentration and activity of drug-metabolizing enzymes (Durnas et al. 1990).

Liver size decreases with age and liver blood flow is reduced at a rate of 0.3–1.5% per year after age 25 (Egorin 1993b). This may lead to lower clearances of drugs that are dependent on blood flow for elimination.

Two types of drug-metabolizing reactions occur within the liver.

Type I reactions are oxido-reductive reactions, that may generate both active and inactive metabolites of drugs. Phase I metabolism occurs primarily via intracellular activity of P450 cytochrome enzymes, that decline with age. The CYP microsomal system enzymes, consisting of a number of isoenzymes, are heme-based enzymes located in the liver, small bowel, kidneys, lungs, and brain. Genetic variability accounts for differing levels of enzyme activity, which may lead to clinically important PD differences among individuals. The potential for drug interactions is high, particularly with the CYP3A4 enzyme, which is inhibited by a variety of common medications and is involved in the metabolism of a variety of anticancer agents. Cyclophosphamide, paclitaxel, and tamoxifen are all substrates of CYP3A4.

Type II reactions are conjugative reactions that give origin to water-soluble compounds excreted through the bile or urine. Phase II reactions appear to be unaffected by age.

So the risk of hepatic drug interactions may increase in older individuals as polypharmacy becomes common with age.

20.3.1.4 Excretion

Renal excretion is affected by the gradual decline in function with age. There is a decrease in the GFR by approximately 1 mL/min for every year over the age of 40 (Brenner et al. 1982). The majority of elderly individuals have a GFR of only 60–70% of normal (Larsen and Martin 1994).

The reduction in GFR is not reflected by an increase in serum creatinine because of the simultaneous loss of muscle mass.

Age-related reduction in blood flow and decreased GFR alter medication excretion and cause accumulation of medications and their toxic metabolites, particularly with water-soluble medications. Additionally, the active metabolites of the medication produced in the liver may depend on the kidneys for excretion and therefore will accumulate due to reduced renal function. Drugs with a narrow therapeutic range and high toxic potential are most affected by age-related changes to the renal system.

20.3.2   Pharmacodynamics

The PDs of a medication is the effect the medication has on the individual and how the medication interacts with receptors at the site of action.

PD changes may influence both toxicity and activity of cytotoxic agents (Balducci and Corcoran 2000b). Some researchers evidence that elderly patients may have increased sensitivity to some medications due to changes in receptor numbers or affinity, receptor alterations, or decreased homeostatic mechanisms (Swift 1990).

In particular, elderly patients seem to have a greater central nervous system response to the benzodiazepines as a result of changes in the blood-brain barrier.

Some evidence suggests that older individuals have greater response to narcotics, anticoagulants, heparin, and thrombolytic agents. On the other hand, beta blockers exhibit decreased sensitivity in elderly. Other medication categories may demonstrate simultaneously both increased and decreased sensitivity.

20.4 Dose Adjustments

The diversity of the elderly patient population in respect to age-related multisystem physiological changes has an effect on several aspects of pharmacology that need to be considered when tailoring chemotherapy regimens to minimize toxicity.

The excretion of most chemotherapeutic agents is via the biliary or renal routes. Patients with poor renal or hepatic function are often excluded from clinical trials, which results in many elderly patients being excluded. Declining renal function is an important contributor to drug toxicity in the elderly. It is not, however, a reason to withhold therapy, but these patients should have their treatment adapted. Appropriate dose adjustments have to be made according to the creatinine clearance, calculated with formulae such as Cockcroft-Gault. Patients with renal impairments need no dose adjustments of drugs excreted by the liver, and vice versa.

A progressive decline in GFR is one of the most consistent findings of normal aging. Comorbid conditions, such as hypertension and diabetes, may accelerate the development of renal insufficiency, and so may the chronic intake of certain drugs, such as acetaminophen and nonsteroidal anti-inflammatory drugs (NSAIDs).

The importance of GRF impairment in the management of older persons with cancer has been highlighted in several studies. In a retrospective analysis some authors demonstrated that the toxicity of a combination of methotrexate, cyclophosphamide, and 5-fluorouracil (CMF) was minimized, without reduction of the antineoplastic activity, when the doses of methotrexate and cyclophosphamide were adjusted to the GFR in women aged 65 and over.

Several drugs, such as etoposide, have a mixed hepatic and renal excretion. In these circumstances, a reduction of GFR of up to 25 mL/min does not seem to prevent adequate drug excretion, as long as biliary obstruction is not present.

In general, biliary excretion seems to be unaffected by age. Drugs such as anthracyclines, taxanes, and vinca alkaloids have hepatic excretion.

Patients with hepatic impairment have to be evaluated through biochemical parameters. According to these values dose adjustment of drugs is calculated.

20.5 Drug Interactions

Drug interactions are responsible for 15–20% of adverse drug reactions (Doucet et al. 1999), and according to some researchers, the incidence increases exponentially with the number of medications a patient takes (Nolan and O'Malley 1988); it has been shown to be the most consistent risk factor for ADRs (Montamat and Cusack 1992). Research suggests that the potential for an ADR to occur is 6% when patients take two medications, it increases to 50% when five or more medications are taken concomitantly and 100% when ≥8 medications are prescribed (Jones 1997).

Drug interactions are an emerging concern in oncology (Mc Leod 1998; Beijnen 2004), as the complex treatment of cancer coupled with increased comorbidity make older patients especially vulnerable to the risks associated with polypharmacy. Twenty to thirty percent of all adverse reactions are caused by interactions between drugs, and these reactions are clinically relevant in up to 80% of elderly patients (Beijnen 2004; Kohler et al. 2000).

Cytotoxic anticancer drugs are some of the strongest acting drugs. They have a complex pharmacological profile, a narrow therapeutic window, a steep dose-toxicity curve, and many PK and PD differences both within and between patients. In oncology such drugs are often used in combinations, especially in elderly patients (Kuhlmann and Mueck 2001). The use of such combinations and the number of drugs involved increases the potential for drug–drug interactions.

Drug interactions can be categorized as pharmaceutical, PK, or PD.

20.5.1 Pharmaceutical Interactions

Pharmaceutical interactions occur when two compounds interact because they are incompatible either physically or chemically. An example is the modulating effect of a vehicle on the PK and PD properties of a drug (Corcoran 1997). Encapsulation of doxorubicin into pegylated liposomes results in a lower incidence of cardiotoxicity (Ten Tije et al. 2003), and this process has a substantial effect on the PK profile of the drug. The AUC of the total drug concentration in plasma is about 300 times greater, clearance is 250 times lower, and the distribution volume is 60 times lower after this drug is encapsulated in these liposomes compared with free doxorubicin. As a consequence, the dose-limiting toxic-effects profile of encapsulated doxorubicin changes from bone marrow suppression and cardiac toxic effects with free doxorubicin, to palmar-plantar erythrodysesthesia with pegylated liposomal doxorubicin (Safra 2003).

When the cytotoxic active ingredient paclitaxel is dissolved in a mixture of polyoxyethylated castor oil and ethanol, the solvent greatly affects the PK behavior of drug (Gabison et al. 2003). The non-ionic polyoxyethylated castor oil forms micelles in the bloodstream, entrapping paclitaxel and thereby preventing distribution of the drug into tissues (Sparreboom et al. 1996), so that the AUC of paclitaxel is higher, with lower clearance and distribution volume. This effect should be taken in account when paclitaxel is combined with other drugs. Cardiotoxicity that is induced by anthracyclines is enhanced by concomitant use of paclitaxel, possibly because doxorubicin is modified pharmacokinetically by the polyoxyethylated castor oil in the paclitaxel solvent (Vaishampayan et al. 1999). The presence of the castor oil seems to lead to a significant increase of the AUC of doxorubicin and its active metabolite doxorubicinol, and could explain the higher incidence of cardiotoxicity when paclitaxel is combined with anthracyclines (Millward et al. 1998; Gennari et al. 1999).

20.5.2 Pharmacokinetic Interactions

PK drug interactions have been identified with several anticancer agents at the level of absorption, distribution, metabolism, and elimination.

For several reasons oral chemotherapy is preferred over other methods of administration. However, drug's bioavailability is limited and variable through this method of administration (Danesi et al. 2002). Drug transporters and CYP isozymes (CYP3A4 and CYP3A5) in the intestinal epithelium seem to be major obstacles for efficient drug uptake.

Entrapment of a drug in a vehicle such as liposome can substantially reduce the distribution volume. Anticancer drugs can also bind to several blood components (Kruijtzer et al. 2002), including albumin, lipoproteins, immunoglobulins, and erythrocytes. The unbound drug is regarded the biologically active fraction because it can extravasate to reach target tissues. Theoretically, drug displacement from blood components or tissue-binding sites increases the apparent distribution volume.

Cytotoxic drugs that are highly protein-bound such as paclitaxel and etoposide, have the potential to interact with other protein-bound drugs like warfarin.

The hepatic CYP system is the major site of drug metabolism, and most drug–drug interactions take place at this site. For drugs that are administered orally, gut wall CYP3A is also of major importance in drug–drug and drug–xenobiotic interactions. Many anticancer drugs are cleared by the CYP3A4 system. Therefore, a potential for drug–drug interaction with both cytotoxic and non-cytotoxic drugs that share the same CYP machinery exists. Anticancer drugs that are metabolized by CYP3A4 include the oxazaphosphorines (cyclophosphamide, ifosfamide) and the taxanes (paclitaxel, docetaxel). Treatments that include these agents are thus at risk when combined with other CYP3A4 substrates or inhibitors such as benzodiazepines, antifungals, antihistamines, and anticonvulsants (Stewart and Zamboni 1998).

In addition to the type of companion drug, the sequence of their administration can also affect the PK interaction. In a phase I study (Mather et al. 2000) researchers found that myelosuppression was more pronounced when paclitaxel was given after cisplatin compared with the alternate sequence. This finding was explained by a 25% lower paclitaxel clearance when cisplatin preceded paclitaxel than when given after this taxane, possibly because of its effect on paclitaxel metabolizing CYP enzymes.

Drug–drug interactions generally involve renal impairment, either by the drug itself or the concomitant (nephrotoxic) agent. Probenecid, salicylates, trimethoprim, and sulphamethoxazol can increase plasma concentrations of methotrexate to toxic levels (Rowinsky et al. 1991). NSAIDs have caused toxic effects when given with methotrexate or cisplatin (Bannwarth et al. 1996).

20.5.3 Pharmacodynamic Interactions

PK drug–drug interactions do not always have relevant clinical consequences. However, when two drugs show no PK interactions, they might still interact with each other pharmacodynamically (toxic effects or antitumor activity) in an additive, synergistic, or antagonistic manner. Anticancer drugs are given mostly in combination regimens.

Combination chemotherapy is often preferred to circumvent resistance, to reduce nonoverlapping toxic effects, and to benefit from any synergistic antitumor action.

One positive PD drug interaction has been found between 5-FU and folinic acid (Balis 1986).

5-FU induces its anticancer activity in part by inhibiting thymidylate synthase (TS) through formation of a ternary complex between 5-FU-TS and reduced folates. Many tumor cells have been found to have relatively low levels of reduced folates, thereby influencing the efficiency of TS inhibition by 5-FU. Administration of folinic acid prior to 5-FU therapy is commonly used as a mechanism to optimize the use of this anticancer therapy (Machover 1997).

20.6 Conclusions

The importance of proper assessment and management of elderly cancer patients to be evaluated for cytotoxic treatment is increasingly recognized.

Oncologists and practicing physicians must be aware that age-related conditions such as comorbidity, disability, and polypharmacy, are by no means absolute criteria to ban cancer treatment and the large proportion of older cancer patients can obtain some benefit from the application of geriatric-oncology model.

Choosing the correct regimen and dose for the older patient remains a challenge as there are no accepted algorithms to guide clinical decisions in these patients. Older cancer patients who have an adequate functional status, mild comorbidity, and a reasonable life expectancy should receive the same therapies as younger patients. For those older patients with a poor functional status, severe comorbidities, single- agent reduced dose chemotherapy options, and nonchemotherapeutic approaches should be considered, together with palliative and supportive care options. The publication of dedicated guidelines such as the National Comprehensive Cancer Network—Senior Adult Oncology guidelines would greatly aid the physicians treating older patients.

On the clinical setting we recommend:

- To perform geriatric assessment of patient aged >70 years.
- To modify the anticancer drug doses according to pharmacological factors (GFR, liver function) and observed toxicity.
- To use intensive supportive treatment to effectively prevent functional deterioration and disability.

References

Allen A (1992) The cardiotoxicity of chemotherapeutic drugs. Sem Oncol 19:529–542

Baker SD, Grochow LB (1997) Pharmacology of cancer chemotherapy in the older person. Clin Geriatr Med 13:169–183

Balducci L, Corcoran MB (2000a) Antineoplastic Chemotherapy of the older cancer patient. Hematol Oncol Clin N America 14:193–212

Balducci L, Corcoran MB (2000b) Antineoplastic chemotherapy of the older cancer patient. Hematol Oncol Clin North Am 14:193–212

Balducci L, Extermann M (2000) Cancer and aging.An evolving panorama. Hematol Oncol Clin North Am 14:1–16

Balducci L, Extermann M (2001) A practical approach to the older patient with cancer. Current problems in Cancer 25:1–76

Balis F (1986) Pharmacokinetic drug interactions of commonly used anticancer drugs. Clin Pharmacokinet 11:223–235

Bannwarth B, Pehourcq F, Schaverbeke T, Dehais J (1996) Clinical pharmacokinetics of low-dose pulse methotrexate in rheumatoid arthritis. Clin Pharmacokinet 30:194–210

Beers M H (1999) Aging as a risk factor for medication-related problems. www.ascp.com/public/pubs/tcp/1999/dec/aging.shtml. Accessed 16 May 2005

Beijnen JH (2004) Drug interactions in oncology. The Lancet Oncology 5(8):489–496

Benjamin RS, Feldman EJ, Lichtman SM et al (1995) Mitoxantrone in the older patients. Sem Oncol 22:11–28

Bonetti A, Franceschi T, Apostoli G et al (1994) Cisplatin pharmacokinetics in elderly patients. The Drug Montor 16:477–482

Brenner BM, Meyer TW, Hostetter Th (1982) Dietary protein intake and the progressive nature of kidney disease: the role of hemodynamically medicated glomerular injury in the pathogenesis of progressive glomerular sclerosis in aging, renal ablation, and intrinsic renal disease. N Engl J Med 307:652–659

Corcoran ME (1997) Polypharmacy in the older patient with cancer. Cancer Control 4:419–428

Danesi R, Innocenti F, Fogli S et al (2002) Pharmacokinetics and pharmacodynamics of combination chemotherapy with paclitaxel and epirubicin in breast cancer patients. Br J Clin Pharmacol 53:508–518

Doucet J, Capet C, Jègo A et al (1999) Les effects indesiderables des medicaments chez le sujet age: epidemiologie et prevention. La Presse Medicale 28(32):1789–1793

Durnas C, Loi CM, Cusack BJ (1990) Hepatic drug metabolism and aging. Clin Pharmacokinet 19:359–389

Duthie E (1998) Physiology of aging: relevance to symptom perceptions and treatment tolerance. In: Balducci L, Lyman GH, Ershler WB (eds) Comprehensive Geriatric Oncology. Harwood Academic Publishers, London, pp 247–262

Egorin MJ (1993a) Cancer Pharmacology in the elderly. Semin. Oncol. 20:43–9

Egorin MJ (1993b) Cancer pharmacology in the elderly. Semin Oncol 20:43–49

Extermann M, Aapro M, Bernabei R, Cohen HJ, Droz JP, Lichtman S, Mor V, Monfardini S, Repetto L, Sorbye L, Topinkova E (2005) Use of comprehensive geriatric assessment in older cancer patients: Recommendations from the task force on CGA of the International Society of Geriatric Oncology (SIOG). Crit Rev Oncol Hematol 55(3):241–252

Fleck JF, Einhorn LH, Lauer RC et al (1990) Is prophylactic cranial irradiation indicated in small cell lung cancer? J Clin Oncol 8:209–214

Gabison A, Shmeeda H, Barenholz Y (2003) Pharmacokinetics of pegylated liposomal doxorubicin: review of animal and human studies. Clin Pharmacokinetic 42:419–436

Gennari A, Salvadori B, Donati S et al (1999) Cardiotoxicity of epirubicin/paclitaxel-containing regimens: role of cardiac risk factors. J Clin Oncol 17:3596–3602

Gill PS, Espina BM, Muggia F et al (1995) Phase I/II clinical and pharmacokinetic evaluation of liposomal daunorubicin. J Clin Oncol 13:996–1003

Graham MA, Lockwood GF, Greenslade D et al (2000) Clinical pharmacokinetics of oxaliplatin: a critical review. Clin Cancer Res 6:1205–1218

Gurwitz JH (2004) Polypharmacy: A new paradigm for quality drug therapy in the elderly? ArchIntern Med 164:1957–1959

Hanlon JT, Fillenbaum GG (2001) RubyC, et al: Epidemiology of over-the-counter drug use in community dwelling elderly: United States perspective. Drugs Aging 18:123–131

Iber FL, Murphy PA, Connors ES (1994) Age-related changes in the gastrointestinal system. Drugs and aging 5:34–48

Jacobson SD; Cha S; Sargent DJ et al (2001) Tolerability, dose intensity and benefit of 5FU based chemotherapy for advanced colorectal cancer (CRC) in the elderly. A North Central Cancer Treatment Group Study. Proc Am Soc Clin Oncol 20: 384a, abstract 1534

John V, Mashru S, Lichtman SM (2003) Pharmacological factors influencing anticancer drug selection in the elderly. Drugs Aging 20(10):737–759

Jones B (1997) Decreasing polypharmacy in clients most at risk. AACN clin 8: 628

Jorgensen T, Johansson S, Kennerfalk A et al (2001) Prescription drug use, diagnoses, and healthcare utilization among the elderly. Ann Pharmacother 35:1004–1009

Julis-Elysee K, White DA (1990) Bleomycin-induced pulmonary toxicity. Clin Chest Med 11(1):1–20

Kaplan RS, Wiernik PH (1982) Neurotoxicity of antineoplastic drug. Sem Oncol 9:102–130

Kintzel PE, Dorr RT (1995) Anticancer drug renal toxicity and elimination: dosing guidelines for altered renal function. Cancer Treat. Rev. 21:33–64

Kinzel PE, Dorr RT (1995) Anticancer drug renal toxicity and elimination: dosing guidelines for altered renal function. Cancer Treat Rev 21:33–64

Kohler GI, Bode-Boger SM, Busse R et al (2000) Drug-drug interactions in medical patients: effects on in-hospital treatment and relation to multiple drug use. Int J Clin Pharmacol Ther 38:504–513

Koren G, Beatty K, Seto A, Einarson TR, Lishner M (1992) The effects of impaired liver function on the elimination of antineoplastic agents. Ann. Pharmacother. 26:363–371

Kruijtzer CMF, Beijnen JH, Schellens JHM (2002) Improvement of oral drug treatment by temporary inhibition of drug transporters and/or Cytochrome P450 in the gastrointestinal tract and liver: an overview. Oncologist 7:516–530

Kuhlmann J, Mueck W (2001) Clinical pharmacological strategies to assess drug interaction potential during drug development. Drug Saf 24:715–725

Langer CJ, Manola J, Bernardo P et al (2002) Cisplatin-based therapy for elderly patients with advanced non small cell lung cancer: implication of Easter Cooperative Group 5592, a randomized trial. J Natl Cancer Inst 94(3):173–181

Larsen PD, Hoot Martin JL (1999) Polypharmacy and elderly patients. AORN Journal 69(3):619–628

Larsen P, Martin J (1994) Renal system changes in the elderly. Aorn Journal 60:299

Levey AS, Bosch JP, Lewis JB et al (1999) A more accurate method to estimate glomerular filtration rate from serum creatinine: a new prediction equation. Ann Intern Med 130:461–470

Lipschitz DA (1995) Age-related decline in hemopoietic reserve capacity. Sem Oncol 22(1):3–6

Machover D (1997) A comprehensive review of 5-fluorouracil and leucovorin in patients with metastatic colorectal carcinoma. Cancer 80:1179–1187

Mather CG, Levy RH et al (2000) Metabolic drug interactions. In: Levy RH, Thummel KE, Trager WF (eds) Anticonvulsants. Lippincott, Williams and Wilkins, Philadelphia, pp 217–243

Matsui K, Masuda N, Yana T et al (2001) Carboplatin calculated with Chatelut's foprmul plus etoposide for elderly patients with small-cell liung cancer. Inter Med 40:603–606

Mc Leod HL (1998) Clinically relevant drug-drug interactions in oncology. Br J Clin Pharmacol 45:539–544

Millward MJ, Webster LK, Rischin D et al (1998) Phase I trial of cremophor EL with bolus doxorubicin. Clin Cancer Res 4:2321–2329

Moraca-Sawicki A (1998) Drug therapy and the older adult, in Pharmacotherapeutics: A Nursing Process Approach, Kuhn M (ed) (Philadelphia: FA Davis) pp 87

Montamat SC, Cusack B (1992) Overcoming problems with polypharmacy and drug misuse in the elderly. Clin Geriatr Med 8(1):143–158

Moscinski LC (1998) Hemopoiesis and aging. In: Balducci L, Lyman GH, Ershler WB: Comprehensive geriatric oncology. Hardwood Academic Publishers, London, pp 399–312

Mould DR, Holford NH, Schellens J et al (2002) Population pharmacokinetics and adverse event analysis of topotecan in patients with solid tumors. Clin Pharmacol Ther 71:334–348

Nagai N, Ogata H, Wada Y et al (1998) Population pharmacokinetics and pharmacodynamics of cisplatin in patients with cancer. Analysis with the NONMEM program. J Clin Pharmacol 38:1025–1034

Nakamura Y, Sekine I, Furuse K, Saijo N (2000) Restrospective comparison of toxicity and efficacy in phase II trials of 3-h infusion of paclitaxel for patients 70 years of age or older and patients under 70 years of age. Cancer Chemother Pharmacol 46:114–118

Nguyen L (2002) TranchandN, Puozzo C, Variol P: Population pharmacokinetics model and limited sampling strategy for intravenous vinorelbine derived from phase I clinical trials. Br J Clin Pharmacol 53:459–468

Nolan L, O'Malley K (1988) Prescribing for the elderly, part 1: Sensitivity of the elderly to adverse drug reactions. JAGS 36(2):142–149

Repetto L (2003) Accettura C. The importance of prophylactic management of chemotherapy-induced neutropenia Anti-Cancer Drugs 14(9):725–730

Repetto L, Audisio RA (2006) Elderly patients have become the leading drug consumers: it's high time to properly evaluate new drugs within the real targeted population. JCO 24(35): 62–63

Repetto L, Fratino L, Audisio RA et al (2002) Comprehensive geriatric assessment adds information to ECOG performance status in elderly patients: an italian group for geriatric oncology study. J Clin Oncol 20:494–502

Repetto L, Carreca I, Maraninchi D, Aapro M, Calabresi P, Balducci L (2003) Use of growth factors in the elderly patient with cancer: a report from the 2nd International Society for Geriatric Oncology (SIOG) 2001 meeting. Critical Rev Oncol Hematol 45(2):123–128

Rowinsky EK, Gilbert MR, McGuire WP et al (1991) Sequences of taxol and cisplatin: a phase I and pharmacologic study. J Clin Oncol 9:1692–1703

Rubin EH, Andersen JW, Berg DT et al (1992) Risk factors far high dose cytarabine neurotoxicity: an analysis of Cancer and Leukemia Group Trial in palients with acute myeloid Ieukemia. J Clin Oncol 10:948–953

Safra T (2003) Cardiac safety of liposomal anthracyclines. Oncologist 8(2):17–24

Sargent DJ, Goldberg RM, Jacobson SD et al (2001) A pooled analysis of adjuvant chemotherapy for resected colon cancer in elderly patients. N Engl J Med 345:1091–1097

Schagen SB, van Dam FSAM, Muller MJ et al (1999) Cognitive deficits after postoperative adjuvant chemotherapy for breast carcinoma. Cancer 85:640–650

Schijvers D, Highley M, DuBruyn E et al (1999) Role of red blood cell in pharmakinetics of chemotherapeutic agents. Anticancer Drugs 10:147–53

Schrijvers D, Highley M (1999) De Bruyn e et al: Role of red blood cells in pharmacokinetics of chemotherapic agents. Anticancer Drugs 10:147–153

Skirvin JA, Lichtman SM (2002) Pharmacokinetic considerations of oral chemotherapy in elderly cancer patients. Drugs Aging 19(1):25–42

Sparreboom A, Van Tellingen O, Nooijen WJ, Beijnen JH (1996) Non linear pharmacokinetics of paclitaxel in mice results from the pharmaceutical vehicle cremophor EL. Cancer Res 56:2112–2115

Stewart CF, Zamboni WC (1998) Plasma protein binding of chemotherapeutic agents. In: Grochow LB, Ames MM (eds) A Clinician's guida to chemotherapy pharmacokinetics and pharmacodynamics. Williams and Wilkins, Baltimore, pp 55–66

Swain SM, Whaley FS, Gerber MC et al (1997) Cardioprotection with dexarosozane for doxorubicin containing therapy in advanced breast cancer. J Clin Oncol 15:1318–1332

Swift C (1990) Pharmacodynamics: changes in homeostatic mechanisms, receptor and target organ sensitivity in the elderly. British Medical Bulletin 46(1):38

Ten Tije AJ, Verweij J, Loos WJ, Sparreboom A (2003) Pharmacological effects of formulation vehicles: implications for cancer chemotherapy. Clin Pharmacokinet 42:665–685

Tranchant B (2002) Pharmacology of cytotoxic agents: guidelines for dose adaption. Acts of the 7th International Conference on Geriatric Oncology Cancer in the Elderly, Boston, 27–28 September 2002: 127–128

Vaishampayan U, Parchment RE, Jasti BR, Hussain M (1999) Taxanes: an overview of the pharmacokinetics and pharmacodynamics. Urology 54(6A):22–29

Vestal RE (1997) Aging and pharmacology. Cancer 80:1302–1310

Wildiers H (2007) Mastering chemotherapy dose reduction in elderly cancer patients. E Journal of Cancer 43:2235–2241

Wildiers H, Highley MS, de Bruijn EA et al (2003) Pharmacology of anticancer drugs in the elderly population. Clin Pharmacokinet 42(14):1213–1242

Yancik R (1997) Cancer burden in the aged. Cancer 80:1273–1283

Zagonel V, Pinto A, Monfardini S (1998) Strategies to prevent chemotherapy-related toxicity in the older person. In: Balducci L, Lyman GH, Ershler WB (eds) omprehensive geriatric oncology. Hardwood Academic Publishers, London, pp 481–500

Part IV
Psychosocial Considerations

Chapter 21
Delayed Presentation of Breast Cancer in Older Women

Lindsay J.L. Forbes and Amanda J. Ramirez

Women in the UK have poorer survival rates for breast cancer than many other Western European countries even after taking into account differences in the age distribution of the population. (Berrino et al. 2007). So-called high resolution studies suggest that late stage at diagnosis is largely responsible for the differences in survival rates (Sant et al. 2003). Late stage at diagnosis is almost certainly due to a combination of late presentation by some women and delays in onward referral by some general practitioners. Most delay appears to be due to patient delay (Westcombe et al. 1999), which may be because of late discovery of symptoms or delayed presentation after discovering symptoms.

Delay in discovery or presentation with breast symptoms is particularly common in older women. Many clinicians can tell stories about elderly women presenting with apparently unmissable locally advanced breast cancer that must have been causing symptoms for a considerable period of time. While we know that very late presentation is associated with poor prognosis, what is more controversial is the extent to which less prolonged delays (of weeks to months) in presentation influence survival. This is important because at clinical and policy levels, we need to know how strong our message to check for symptoms and present early should be, and how that message should be delivered. The wrong message, delivered to the wrong audience, could lead to breast clinics crowded with the worried well, which would probably have little effect on breast cancer survival. More importantly, it would increase anxiety, unnecessary investigations, and would incur opportunity costs to health services.

In this chapter, we examine the extent to which women delay presentation with breast cancer symptoms, the risk factors for delayed presentation, the evidence that delay influences survival, and recent work to develop an intervention to promote early presentation in older women with breast cancer.

L.J.L. Forbes (✉)
Adamson Centre for Mental Health, St. Thomas' Hospital, King's College London,
London, UK
e-mail: Lindsay.forbes@kcl.ac.uk

M.W. Reed and R.A. Audisio (eds.), *Management of Breast Cancer in Older Women*,
DOI 10.1007/978-1-84800-265-4_21, © Springer-Verlag London Limited 2011

21.1   What is the Extent of Delayed Presentation in Breast Cancer?

In the developed world, about 50% of women present to primary care within 1 month of discovering symptoms, but between 18 and 35% delay more than 3 months and between 9 and 20% delay more than 6 months (Westcombe et al. 1999; Arndt 2002).

In studies in the UK, USA, Germany, and Denmark, older age has been found to be associated with greater delay in presentation with breast cancer symptoms (Arndt 2002; Ramirez et al. 1999). The most recent population-based study in Germany found that women over the age of 65 were more than three times as likely to delay seeking medical help after symptom discovery as women under 50 (25% vs. 7% delayed more than 3 months) (Arndt 2002). This study excluded women over the age of 80, who may be at even higher risk of delayed presentation.

21.2   Why Do Older Women Delay Presentation with Breast Cancer Symptoms?

Risk factors for delayed presentation for breast cancer symptoms in women of any age include having non-lump symptoms, not disclosing symptoms to others, being prompted by someone else to seek help, and presenting initially with a non-breast symptom (Ramirez et al. 1999; Burgess et al. 1998; Coates et al. 1992). There is limited evidence of an association between lower socioeconomic status and education and delayed presentation (Arndt 2002; Ramirez et al. 1999).

In a UK study of 68 women aged 65 and older, 29 (43%) delayed presentation for more than 3 months, but of those with a non-lump initial symptom, 65% delayed presentation for more than 3 months (Burgess et al. 2006). There is some evidence that older women have particularly poor knowledge of non-lump breast cancer symptoms (Linsell et al. 2008; Grunfeld et al. 2002). There is also some evidence that older women with breast cancer who delay presentation are less likely to attribute their symptoms to cancer than those who do not delay (Burgess et al. 2006).

Besides having poor knowledge of what to look for, several surveys have found that older women have poor knowledge of their personal risk of breast cancer. In a survey of 1,500 women asking in which decade of life a woman is most likely to get breast cancer, more than half stated that age did not matter to risk of breast cancer, and the 40s and 50s were considered the decades in which women were most at risk (Moser et al. 2007). In another large survey, in women aged 67–73, 62% responded that age did not make a woman more or less likely to develop breast cancer (Linsell et al. 2008). Thirty-one per cent of these women correctly identified the lifetime risk of breast cancer as one in nine, the majority believing that the risk was much lower; 50% believed the risk was 1 in 100 or less. In another large survey,

30% of women over 75 reported that they were less likely than the rest of the female population to develop breast cancer (Grunfeld et al. 2002). It is likely that the fact that the NHS Breast Screening Program stops sending routine appointments at age 70 (soon to be increased to 73) may send the inadvertent message that risk is reduced after this age. Media reporting about younger famous women with breast cancer is rarely accompanied by a message emphasizing the relatively low risk of breast cancer in young women.

Even if an older woman does know what to look for, and understands that she is at relatively high risk, if she never touches or looks at her breasts, she is unlikely to detect symptoms that may be very obvious to others even on cursory examination. Little is known about the extent to which women delay detecting symptoms simply because they do not touch or look at their breasts; however, one in five UK women aged 67–73 report that they never touch their breasts (Linsell et al. 2008). Health professionals in the UK rarely encourage older women to check their breasts since the publication of a Cochrane systematic review that found that breast self-examination was associated with no mortality reduction and unnecessary investigations (Kosters and Gotzsche 2003). However, both the trials included in the review recruited women under the age of 67; whether breast checking, or even full breast selfexamination would increase detection rates at an earlier stage and reduce mortality in older women is unknown. After all, the probability of any breast symptom being one of cancer is much higher in this age group (one in three in women aged 65 and over) than in younger women (one in ten) (Nichols et al. 1981).

As well as knowing why to look for breast symptoms, what to look for and how to look for them, a woman with a breast cancer symptom must have the ability to seek help for symptoms. Women in the UK generally have good access to primary care, but they may have barriers which prevent them presenting promptly. Women who delay are more reluctant to bother their general practitioner and they are more likely to express explicit fears about the consequences of a cancer diagnosis and of treatment (Burgess et al. 1998). A qualitative study of older women with breast cancer found that they reported competing priorities, either related to their own or relatives' health (Burgess et al. 2006).

21.3 Do Delays Affect Stage at Diagnosis and Survival?

In a retrospective analysis of 3,000 women with breast cancer attending Guy's Hospital in London between 1975 and 1990, 32% were found to have had symptoms for more than 3 months before presentation (Richards et al. 1999a). These patients had a significantly worse survival than those with shorter duration of symptoms whether survival was measured from the date of diagnosis or from onset of symptoms to control for lead-time bias. Ten years after symptom discovery, survival was 52% for women with delays less than 12 weeks and 47% for those with longer delays. Multivariable analyses indicated that the adverse impact of delay in presentation on survival was attributable to an association between longer delays and more advanced stage.

A subsequent systematic review found 87 reports examining the association between duration of symptoms and survival in breast cancer from the time of diagnosis (Richards et al. 1999b). These reports, published between 1907 and 1996, include more than 100,000 patients. Thirty-eight reports provided 5-year survival figures. Meta-analysis of these found that the odds of death at 5 years was 1.24 (95% confidence interval 1.17–1.30) times higher for women with duration of symptoms of 3–6 months more compared to those with shorter delays. The absolute reduction in survival associated with delaying for 3–6 months compared with less than 3 months was 7%.

The systematic review also found 13 studies including 12,739 patients that people with longer duration of symptoms presented with more advanced stage at diagnosis (Richards et al. 1999b), which supports the hypothesis that the association between delay in presentation and survival is mediated by stage.

21.4   What is the Public Health Significance of Delay in Older Women?

Delay in presentation may be responsible for 900 avoidable deaths in women aged 65 and over each year in England alone, based on the assumptions that 22,000 women aged 65 and over are diagnosed from breast cancer each year (National Statistics 2005), 62% have an initial lump symptom, 28% of women with lump symptoms, and 65% with initial non-lump symptoms delay presentation more than 3 months (Burgess et al. 2006), 80% 5-year survival in those who do not delay presentation, and 73% 5-year survival in those who do (Richards et al. 1999b).

As well as causing avoidable death, delay in presentation is likely to be associated with significant costs to the health service and the quality of life of women with breast cancer because of the need for more intensive treatment if breast cancer is diagnosed at a later stage.

21.5   How Can We Reduce Patient Delay in Presentation?

There is virtually no useful evidence of effectiveness or cost-effectiveness of interventions to promote early presentation in breast cancer. Social marketing campaigns targeting communities aiming to raise cancer awareness have been implemented in the UK, including the West of Scotland Cancer Awareness Project focusing on bowel and oral cancers (NHS Argyle and Clyde 2002) and the Cancer Research UK Sunsmart Campaign, focusing on skin cancer (CR-UK Sunsmart 2003). However, while these campaigns have reported improvements in cancer awareness and health-related behavior following implementation, they have not been evaluated in controlled trials. Their long-term impact on behavior and, crucially, on stage at diagnosis and mortality is unknown and, most importantly for policy-makers, so is their cost-utility compared with other competing interventions. The UK Cancer Reform Strategy 2007 (Department of Health 2007) acknowledged that late diagnosis is a major factor contributing to poor cancer survival in the UK and launched the National Awareness and Early Diagnosis Initiative in November 2008. The UK Department of Health has commissioned community intervention programmes to promote early presentation for breast, bowel, and lung cancer. These will be evaluated by examining effects on a number of outcomes, including presentations for cancer symptoms in primary care and referrals for investigations; however, there are no plans currently to evaluate these using controlled trials.

The King's College London Cancer Research UK Promoting Early Presentation Group has developed an intervention to promote early presentation in older women with breast cancer (Burgess et al. 2008), following the MRC Framework for developing and evaluating complex interventions (Medical Research Council 2008). It consists of a scripted 10 min one-to-one interaction with a health professional, designed to educate older women about breast cancer symptoms and their personal risk of breast cancer, to increase their skills and confidence to be breast aware, and motivation to seek help promptly in the event of discovering a breast change. In addition, women are reminded that although they will no longer be routinely invited for mammograms after the age of 70 (soon to be raised to 73), they are eligible to receive them every 3 years on request. It is supplemented with a booklet that the woman can take home. Table 21.1 summarizes the key messages provided in the interaction and booklet.

During the interaction, a woman's intentions to act are fortified by:

- Encouraging her to complete an action plan about how she will be breast aware and what she will do with a breast change, i.e., go straight to her GP
- A series of statements, in the booklet, describing anticipated positive feelings related to seeking help immediately with a breast change, i.e., relieved, reassured, satisfied
- Regular summary of the key messages

The intervention was designed based on theoretical framework for delayed presentation (Bish et al. 2005), which incorporated elements of health psychology theories, including self-regulation theory (Leventhal 1984), the theory of planned behavior (Ajzen 1991), and implementation intentions (Gollwitzer 1999). We built on these to develop our framework for the intervention to promote early presentation (Fig. 21.1). Based both on our review of the literature and our experience of piloting our intervention, we incorporated additional components linked to promoting behavior change. We increased the emphasis on improving breast cancer awareness via broadening symptom appraisal (Leventhal 1984) and on improving confidence in the ability to perform breast checking and early medical help-seeking (self-efficacy) (Bandura 1977).

Table 21.1 Intervention to promote early presentation of breast cancer

Subject area	Key messages
Risk of developing breast cancer	Education about the lifetime risk of breast cancer in risk of breast cancer with age supported by graphics in the booklet
Knowledge of breast cancer symptoms	Education about the full range of breast cancer symptoms, with emphasis on the non-lump symptoms, supported by photographs of signs of early breast cancer
Confidence to be breast aware and to detect a breast change	Education about how to be breast aware to increase the likelihood of early detection of symptoms, supported by cartoon illustrations in the booklet
	Demonstration and rehearsal of breast checking using a silicone breast model to increase women's confidence to detect a breast change. This is not a tutorial in breast self examination but rather simple guidance in techniques for breast checking
Action in the event of symptom discovery	A strong persuasive recommendation to seek medical attention immediately in the event of discovering a breast change, outlining the benefits of prompt help-seeking
	Suggestions for overcoming barriers to seeking medical help, such as embarrassment and fear about cancer treatments are outlined in the booklet, including cartoon illustrations and affirming quotes from women with breast cancer
Disclosure	Direct recommendation to tell someone close in the event of breast symptom discovery with cartoon illustrations and dialog to model this behavior

The model incorporates techniques designed to maximize the probability of behavior change, including:

- Delivery by a health professional (Jepson 2000)
- Tailoring to the individual (Jepson 2000; de Nooijer et al. 2002)
- Positive approach (Wardle et al. 2003)
- Positive motivational style, positive feedback, verbal persuasion (Rollnick and Miller 1995)
- Action planning (Gollwitzer 1999; Webb and Sheeran 2006)

The intervention is being tested within the NHS Breast Screening Program, with the interaction delivered by trained radiographers. The NHS Breast Screening Program was chosen as a platform for evaluation as it represents an efficient way of reaching large numbers of women aged 67–70; more than 170,000 women of this age attend for

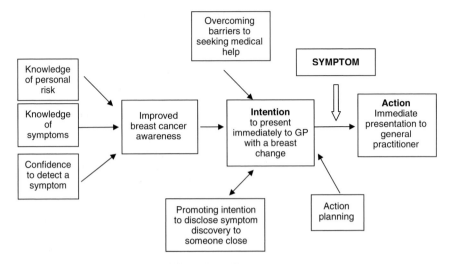

Fig. 21.1 Framework for the intervention to promote early presentation of breast cancer. A woman's knowledge of her personal risk of developing breast cancer, her knowledge of the range of symptoms of breast cancer, and her confidence to detect a breast change are each essential and together sufficient to raise her breast cancer awareness and instigate or strengthen the intention to present immediately in the event of detecting a breast change. Promoting disclosure and overcoming barriers to seeking medical help may influence intention and/or the decision to act, but are neither necessary nor sufficient factors in the pathway to prompt presentation. Action planning is likely to increase the chances of intentions being turned into action if and when a symptom is discovered

the final breast screening appointment to which they are routinely invited each year. The NHS Breast Screening Program also focuses the intervention on older women, who are at a high risk of developing breast cancer, which means that it is unlikely to cause unnecessary health care attendances in younger women at lower risk.

Work to evaluate the intervention within the NHS Breast Screening Program can be seen as "proof of concept": we envisage that if it is shown to be cost-effective in that setting it can be exported to other settings, such as primary care. Furthermore, the principles may guide the development of similar interventions for other cancers with a strong relationship between stage at diagnosis and prognosis.

Preliminary testing of the intervention in a before-and-after study in 292 women aged 67–70 during 2006 showed a significant increase in knowledge of 11 breast symptoms at 6 months post-intervention, a 2.75-fold increase in the odds of women reporting that they check their breasts at least monthly at 6 months, and no adverse events (Burgess et al. In press). There was no increase in Lerman Cancer Worry Score (Lerman et al. 1991) at 6 months post-intervention.

A randomized controlled trial of efficacy comparing the interaction with the radiographer plus booklet plus usual care, the booklet plus usual care vs. usual care alone is currently underway, also within the NHS Breast Screening Program. Usual care consists of a notification that a woman can return every 3 years for further mammographic screening if she wishes, by arrangement, but that she will not be routinely invited any longer. The trial recruited 867 women and has just completed 6 month follow-up; the early results show sustained improvements in breast cancer awareness compared with usual care.

21.6 Conclusion

Delayed presentation in breast cancer – and other cancers – is a major cause of avoidable death in the UK. A scripted one-to-one interaction with a health professional to promote early presentation increases breast cancer awareness compared with usual care. We hypothesize that breast cancer awareness and the clear recommendation to seek medical help promptly for breast symptoms will lead to early presentation, diagnosis at a less advanced stage, improved survival, and reduced NHS costs because of less intensive treatment. The next stage of evaluation needs to demonstrate the cost-effectiveness and cost-utility of the intervention in terms of life-years gained, quality-adjusted life-years gained, and cost per quality-adjusted life-year gained in a randomized controlled trial with stage at diagnosis and mortality as outcomes. As with any trial of an intervention on healthy people aiming to reduce mortality, this trial would have to be very large. However, if cost-effective, the intervention has the potential to save many lives from breast cancer, and would help bring survival from breast cancer in the UK in line with our European counterparts.

References

Ajzen I (1991) The theory of planned behavior. Organ Behav Hum Decis Process 50(2):179–211
Arndt V (2002) Patient delay and stage of diagnosis among breast cancer patients in Germany—a population based study. Br J Cancer 86:1034–1040
Bandura A (1977) Self-efficacy: Toward a unifying theory of behavioral change. Psychol Rev 84(2):191–215
Berrino F, De Angelis R, Sant M, Rosso S, Lasota MB, Coebergh JW et al (2007) Survival for eight major cancers and all cancers combined for European adults diagnosed in 1995–99: results of the EUROCARE-4 study. Lancet Oncol 8(9):773–783
Bish A, Ramirez A, Burgess C, Hunter M (2005) Understanding why women delay in seeking help for breast cancer symptoms. J Psychosom Res 58(4):321–326
Burgess CC, Ramirez AJ, Richards MA, Love SB (1998) Who and what influences delayed presentation in breast cancer? Br J Cancer 77(8):1343–1348
Burgess CC, Potts HW, Hamed H, Bish AM, Hunter MS, Richards MA et al (2006) Why do older women delay presentation with breast cancer symptoms? Psycho-Oncology 15(11):962–968
Burgess CC, Bish AM, Hunter HS, Salkovskis P, Michell M, Whelehan P et al (2008) Promoting early presentation of breast cancer: development of a psycho-educational intervention. Chronic Illn 4(1):13–27
Burgess CC, Linsell L, Kapari M, Omar L, Michell M, Whelehan P et al. (2009) Promoting early presentation of breast cancer by older women: A preliminary evaluation of a one-to-one health professional-delivered intervention. J Psychosom Res. In press (doi:10.1016/j.jpsychores.2009.01.2005

Coates RJ, Bransfield DD, Wesley M, Hankey B, Eley JW, Greenberg RS et al (1992) Differences between black and white women with breast cancer in time from symptom recognition to medical consultation. J Natl Cancer Inst 84(12):938–950

CR-UK Sunsmart. SunSmart Campaign (2003). At: http://info.cancerresearchuk.org/healthyliving/sunsmart/aboutsunsmart/pastcampaigns/?a=5441. Accessed June 2008

de Nooijer J, Lechner L, de Vries H (2002) Tailored versus general information on early detection of cancer: a comparison of the reactions of Dutch adults and the impact on attitudes and behaviors. Health Educ Res 17(2):239–252

Department of Health. Cancer Reform Strategy. Gateway reference 9092. 3–12–2007. London, Department of Health. http://www.dh.gov.uk/prod_consum_dh/groups/dh_digitalassets/documents/digitalasset/dh_081007.pdf. Accessed 22nd September 2009

Gollwitzer PM (1999) Implementation intentions: strong effects of simple plans. Am Psychol 54:493–503

Grunfeld EA, Ramirez AJ, Hunter MS, Richards MA (2002) Women's knowledge and beliefs regarding breast cancer. Br J Cancer 86(9):1373–1378

Jepson R (2000) The effectiveness of interventions to change Health-Related Behaviours: a review of reviews. MRC Social and Public Health Sciences Unit 2000; Occasional Paper No 3

Kosters JP, Gotzsche PC (2003) Regular self-examination or clinical examination for early detection of breast cancer. Cochrane Database Syst Rev (2):CD003373

Lerman C, Trock B, Rimer BK, Jepson C (1991) Psychological side effects of breast cancer screening. Health Psychol 10(4):259–267

Leventhal H (1984) Illness representations and coping with health threats. In: Baum A, Taylor SE, Singer JE (eds) Handbook of psychology and health. Erlbaum, Hillsdale, New Jersey, pp 219–252

Linsell L, Burgess CC, Ramirez AJ (2008) Breast cancer awareness among older women. Br J Cancer 99:1221–1225

Medical Research Council (2008) Developing and evaluating complex interventions: new guidance. Medical Research Council, London. Ref Type: Report

Moser K, Patnick J, Beral V (2007) Do women know that the risk of breast cancer increases with age? Br J Gen Pract 57(538):404–406

National Statistics. Cancer statistics: registrations of cancers diagnosed in 2005. 36. 2008. Newport, Office for National Statistics. Series MB1

NHS Argyle and Clyde. West of Scotland cancer awareness project 2002–2005 (WOSCAP): final report. 2005. Paisley, NHS Argyle and Clyde

Nichols S, Waters WE, Fraser JD, Wheeller MJ, Ingham SK (1981) Delay in the presentation of breast symptoms for consultant investigation. J Public Health 3(3):217–225

Ramirez AJ, Westcombe AM, Burgess CC, Sutton S, Littlejohns P, Richards MA (1999) Factors predicting delayed presentation of symptomatic breast cancer: a systematic review. Lancet 353(9159):1127–1131

Richards MA, Smith P, Ramirez AJ, Fentiman IS, Rubens RD (1999a) The influence on survival of delay in the presentation and treatment of symptomatic breast cancer. Br J Cancer 79(5–6):858–864

Richards MA, Westcombe AM, Love SB, Littlejohns P, Ramirez AJ (1999b) Influence of delay on survival in patients with breast cancer: a systematic review. Lancet 353(9159):1119–1126

Rollnick SR, Miller WR (1995) What is motivational interviewing? Behav Cogn Psychother 23:325–334

Sant M, Allemani C, Capocaccia R, Hakulinen T, Aareleid T, Coebergh JW et al (2003) Stage at diagnosis is a key explanation of differences in breast cancer survival across Europe.[see comment][erratum appears in Int J Cancer. 2003 Dec 20;107(6):1058]. Int J Cancer 106(3):416–422

Wardle J, Williamson S, McCaffery K, Sutton S, Taylor T, Edwards R et al (2003) Increasing attendance at colorectal cancer screening: testing the efficacy of a mailed, psychoeducational intervention in a community sample of older adults. Health Psychol 22(1):99–105

Webb TL, Sheeran P (2006) Does changing behavioural intention engender behaviour change? a meta-analysis of the experimental evidence. Psychol Bulletin 132:249–268

Westcombe AM, Richards MA, Ramirez AJ, Love SB, Sutton S, Burgess C et al (1999) A systematic review of the delay in diagnosis/treatment of symptomatic breast cancer. NHS Research and Development

Chapter 22
Patient Decision Making

Martine Extermann

Decision making in older cancer patients involves several aspects. Some are physician-assessed: objective benefits (e.g., response rate, survival), objective risks, amount of co-morbidity and its impact on treatment choices. Others are patient-assessed: value of the benefits compared to the risks, impact of the cancer, and treatment on the life of the patient compared to other illnesses, events, and life values. One should be aware, however, that the physician's presentation of the options is colored by the physician's own experience: other patients treated with that regimen, other patients with this disease, "look" of the patient, physician's a priori guesses about the willingness of the patient to undergo the treatment. The latter is especially difficult, as, with age, cancer patients become increasingly diverse in their health and life experience. Therefore, besides knowing as much data as possible about cancer and its treatment in the elderly, it is important to gain knowledge about what is known concerning the decision making of older cancer patients. Fortunately, a certain amount of data is available.

22.1 Undergoing Chemotherapy

Research on patient decision making in oncology started around 1990. Slevin and collaborators, a group of British investigators, published in 1990 a vignette study (Slevin et al. 1990). Cancer patients who had received chemotherapy were asked whether they would accept chemotherapy for a benefit in survival (1–100%), life prolongation, and palliation of symptoms. A vignette was describing the treatment and its side effects. The answers of the patients were compared to that of various health professionals and that of matched general controls. The results for a 1% threshold in survival are shown in Fig. 22.1. Results for the two other end-points

M. Extermann (✉)
Senior Adult Oncology Program, H. Lee Moffitt Cancer Center and Research Institute, 12902 Magnolia Drive, Tampa, Florida, 33612, USA
e-mail: martine.extermann@moffitt.org

M.W. Reed and R.A. Audisio (eds.), *Management of Breast Cancer in Older Women*, DOI 10.1007/978-1-84800-265-4_22, © Springer-Verlag London Limited 2011

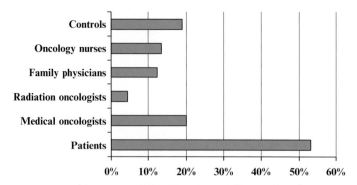

Fig. 22.1 Percentage of patients that would accept a strong chemotherapy for a 1% chance of cure (Slevin et al. 1990)

were matching these results. The median age of these patients was 60 years (range 23–80). Slevin's report does not discuss the impact of age on patients' decisions. Several studies approached that point. A Norwegian study found that patients aged >60 had higher threshold than patients younger than 50 (median for cure: 50 vs. 10%, prolongation 12 vs. 6 months, symptom relief 50 vs. 20%) (Bremnes et al. 1995). A team from Colorado assessed patients aged 65 and older with stage 3 colon cancer for receipt of chemotherapy (Kutner et al. 2000). The factors associated with receipt of adjuvant chemotherapy were: seeing an oncologist, being less than 80, and being married. The patients expressed that the most important issues in their decision were: professional opinion, expected benefit, and family wishes. Whereas physicians rated co-morbidities and literature as important, these items had very little impact on the patient's decision making. An American study retrospectively interviewed breast and colon cancer patients about their treatment decisions and compared patients <65 vs. 65 and older (Newcomb and Carbone 1993). Older women were less likely to have received conservative surgery, radiation, and adjuvant therapy. They also less frequently had a consultation with a medical or radiation oncologist. Regardless of age, the most common reasons for not selecting treatments were physician's recommendations and the patient's desire for more comprehensive treatment. Concern about side effects tended to be more frequently reported by older women. Another study compared the willingness of French and American patients aged 70 and older to undergo chemotherapy (Extermann et al. 2003). Cancer patients and controls from geriatric clinics were presented vignettes of a strong (platinum-taxane-like) and a moderate (weekly vinorelbine-like) chemotherapy. Cancer patients from both countries had a high willingness to accept the chemotherapy (USA: 70.5%, F 73.4% for strong, USA 88.5%, F 100% for moderate). A wide range of benefit thresholds were expressed, and interestingly the type of benefit or the strength of chemotherapy had little impact on the mean expected benefit. As a group, patients tended to fall back on a "2/3 chances of benefit" rule of thumb. For non-cancer controls, cultural differences were apparent, with acceptance rates of USA: 73.8%, F: 34% for strong ($p<0.001$), and USA: 95.2% vs. 67.9% for moderate ($p<0.002$).

22.2 Other Treatment Modalities

Although a large literature exists concerning patient decision making between lumpectomy and mastectomy (with or without reconstruction), only a small portion addressed specifically the influence of age. Several studies did find that the fact of having the choice, rather than the type of surgery itself, had the most impact on patient satisfaction with the surgery and quality of life, without pejorative effect of age. In fact, older women might be more satisfied with their surgery than younger ones (Lantz et al. 2005). The appropriate extent of involvement in the decision (neither more nor less than the patient desired) is also a factor in satisfaction. A study of breast cancer women aged 67 and older specifically found that surgeons trained in surgical oncology, or who treated a high volume of breast cancer patients, more frequently initiated communication with their patients, which was in turn associated with a sense of choice and a greater satisfaction with care (Liang et al. 2002). We are not aware of any study that has addressed the willingness of older cancer patients to undergo radiation therapy.

22.3 Factors Influencing Decisions

As there is a wide variation in willingness to undertake chemotherapy, various factors have been explored as to their impact on decision. As mentioned above, colorectal cancer patients mentioned professional opinion, expected benefit, and family wishes as the most important influencers of their treatment decision. Age, co-morbidity, life expectancy, travel, and tumor characteristics were rarely mentioned, and if so, more likely by patients >80 (Kutner et al. 2000). Physician's opinion was also a strong influencer in Newcomb and Carbone's study (Hirose et al. 2005). In our study, the key influencing factor across patient groups was self-rated health for the acceptance of a moderate chemotherapy (Extermann et al. 2003). For the strong chemotherapy vignette, the only significant association was the presence of a cancer in French patients that was dramatically shifting thresholds of acceptance. A qualitative Swiss study interviewed 21 patients aged 70 and older having undergone chemotherapy (Anchisi et al. 2006). The patients did not consider their age as an obstacle to acceptance of chemotherapy. However, mainly due to fatigue, patients did drop activities during chemotherapy and did not go back to their previous level of functioning. This did not however lead them to retrospectively question their decision. Certain psychological characteristics of the patient might affect the way their health influences their decision making. Chen et al. discovered that co-morbidity, as measured by the cumulative illness rating scale-geriatric (CIRS-G), rather than function, was influencing patients' decision making regarding chemotherapy (Chen et al. 2003). However, in risk-taking patients, co-morbidity had no influence on the willingness to undertake treatment, whereas in risk-adverse patients, increasing co-morbidity was associated with lesser willingness to undertake treatment. Depression significantly influences decision making. In a review of women aged 67–90 from the SEER/Medicare registry, having a diagnosis of depression within 2 years before the breast cancer diagnosis was associated with a lesser likelihood of receiving definitive treatment (59.7 vs. 66.2%) (Goodwin et al. 2004). This difference remained after controlling for age, ethnicity, co-morbidity, and SEER site (city or state). In addition, for similar stage and treatment, depression remained a negative factor for survival.

Most of the studies conducted above were in an academic setting. A study addressed the issue of whether academic patients were representative of a more general population. Silvestri et al. studied patients with metastatic lung cancer from an academic center, a veterans' hospital, and a community practice (Silvestri et al. 1998). Patients treated in the community had the lowest threshold to accept a mild chemotherapy, whereas veterans had the lowest threshold to accept a strong chemotherapy. Therefore, patients treated in academic centers do not appear to be a population with a particularly aggressive stance toward their treatments, as often surmised.

22.4 Cultural Differences

What impact does culture have on patient decision making? One vignette study targeted this question, comparing French and American patients (Extermann et al. 2003). Two sets of vignettes ("platinum-doublet like," and "weekly vinorelbine-like") were presented to patients from a cancer clinic and patients from a geriatric clinic (without cancer) in each country. Geriatric French patients were one-third less likely than American patients to undertake chemotherapy. However, cancer patients on both sides of the Atlantic Ocean were equally willing to take chemotherapy: three quarters would take the strong chemotherapy, and nearly all the moderate chemotherapy. It was more difficult to evaluate the threshold of benefit expected, because as a group, patients tended to fall back on a 2/3 benefit vs. 1/3 risk average, no matter what the options, with wide variations. The main factors influencing a patient's willingness to undergo treatment were self-rated health and, for the non-cancer patients, the country of residence. In French patients, the occurrence of a cancer was a significant influencer as well. A Japanese group conducted a similar study comparing lung cancer patients (all ages) with patients having other respiratory diseases (Hirose et al. 2005). Increasing age raised the threshold of benefit required to accept treatment. Similarly to European patients, the cancer patients were more willing than their non-cancer counterparts to receive chemotherapy.

22.5   Clinical Trials

As older cancer patients are underrepresented in clinical trials, a study explored the willingness of older patients to enroll into them as a possible factor of underrepresentation (Kemeny et al. 2003). This CALGB study found that eligible breast cancer patients were less likely to be offered a clinical trial when they were above 65 years of age (34 vs. 68%, $p=0.0004$). However, once offered the trial older women were as likely as younger ones to accept the offer (50 vs. 54%: $p=$NS).

22.6   Intervention Studies

A randomized study has assessed the impact of a nurse case manager on the decision making and receipt of treatment of older women with breast cancer (Goodwin et al. 2003). Patients were assessed with a comprehensive geriatric assessment, and the goal was "to ensure that the patient was fully informed of her options and that the surgeon and other providers were aware of all matters relevant to ensuring a successful outcome." Women in the intervention group were more likely to receive breast reconstruction surgery, chemotherapy, recover normal arm function, and state they had a real choice in their treatment. Several studies were conducted to implement decision aids, although none to the knowledge of the author specifically targeted older patients. A systematic review of randomized controlled trials was recently published. Overall decision aids significantly increased the choice of breast-conserving surgery (by 25%), knowledge of the patient (by 24%), and might have also decreased decisional conflict and increased satisfaction with the decision-making process (Waljee et al. 2007). In clinical practice, a tool frequently used in the adjuvant setting is Adjuvant! Online (www.adjuvantonline.com). Although this can be useful to pose the decision on objective bases, one should be aware that this is only a decisional model. It has a trend to overestimate the risk of relapse in healthy older women.

22.7   Conclusion

The prominent feature that stems from this review of the literature is that older patients want to have all options presented to them. There appear to be no significant differences with younger patients for surgery choices. Patients might request higher thresholds of effectiveness to accept chemotherapy, but there is a wide variation. When offered participation in clinical trials, eligible older patients are as likely as younger ones to accept. Although large cultural variations may exist in the general population toward cancer treatment from country to country, it appears that in the presence of cancer, older patients react in much more similar ways across the globe. This should be kept in mind when applying the results of trials conducted in other countries.

References

Anchisi A, Anchisi S, Hugentobler V et al (2006) Accepting chemotherapy at the age of 70 and over: between autonomy and ageing. Bull Cancer 93:407–414

Bremnes RM, Andersen K, Wist EA (1995) Cancer patients, doctors and nurses vary in their willingness to undertake cancer chemotherapy. Eur J Cancer 31A:1955–1959

Chen H, Haley W, McEvoy C, Extermann M, Balducci L (2003) Willingness to Accept Risk of Treatment Toxicity in Older Cancer Patients: The Effects of Comorbid Conditions, Functional Disability, Risk Propensity, and Risk Perception. J Am Geriatr Soc 51:S70

Extermann M, Albrand G, Chen H et al (2003) Are older French patients as willing as older American patients to undertake chemotherapy? J Clin Oncol 21:3214–3219

Goodwin JS, Satish S, Anderson ET et al (2003) Effect of nurse case management on the treatment of older women with breast cancer. J Am Geriatr Soc 51:1252–1259

Goodwin JS, Zhang DD, Ostir GV (2004) Effect of depression on diagnosis, treatment, and survival of older women with breast cancer. J Am Geriatr Soc 52:106–111

Hirose T, Horichi N, Ohmori T et al (2005) Patients preferences in chemotherapy for advanced non-small-cell lung cancer. Intern Med 44:107–113

Kemeny MM, Peterson BL, Kornblith AB et al (2003) Barriers to clinical trial participation by older women with breast cancer. J Clin Oncol 21:2268–2275

Kutner JS, Vu KO, Prindiville SA et al (2000) Patient age and cancer treatment decisions. Patient and physician views. Cancer Pract 8:114–119

Lantz PM, Janz NK, Fagerlin A et al (2005) Satisfaction with surgery outcomes and the decision process in a population-based sample of women with breast cancer. Health Serv Res 40:745–767

Liang W, Burnett CB, Rowland JH et al (2002) Communication between physicians and older women with localized breast cancer: implications for treatment and patient satisfaction. J Clin Oncol 20:1008–1016

Newcomb PA, Carbone PP (1993) Cancer treatment and age: patient perspectives. J Natl Cancer Inst 85:1580–1584

Silvestri G, Pritchard R, Welch HG (1998) Preferences for chemotherapy in patients with advanced non-small cell lung cancer: descriptive study based on scripted interviews. BMJ 317:771–775

Slevin ML, Stubbs L, Plant HJ et al (1990) Attitudes to chemotherapy: comparing views of patients with cancer with those of doctors, nurses, and general public. BMJ 300:1458–1460

Waljee JF, Rogers MA, Alderman AK (2007) Decision aids and breast cancer: do they influence choice for surgery and knowledge of treatment options? J Clin Oncol 25:1067–1073

Chapter 23
Culture, Ethnicity, and Race: Persistent Disparities in Older Women with Breast Cancer

Antonella Surbone and Marjorie Kagawa-Singer

23.1 Introduction

The elderly population, arbitrarily defined as adults older than 65 years, is rapidly increasing worldwide, and is changing with regard to physical, psychological, and sociocultural dimensions. In 2005, the World Health Organization in its *International Plan of Action on Aging* established that disease prevention and treatment in the elderly is a global health priority and approved a *Resolution on Cancer Control* worldwide. Sixty percent of all cancers in the western world are diagnosed in people over the age of 65, and two thirds of all cancer mortality worldwide occurs in this age group. Due to longer life expectancy and improved cancer care, cancer in the elderly is also becoming more frequent in developing countries and will be the number one cause of death worldwide by 2010 (World Health Orgnanization 2005a, b, 2008). On April 14, 2008, the IOM issued the document *Retooling for an Aging America: building the Health Care Workforce* that describes geriatric care in terms of a crisis and a challenge in the US (Institute of Medicine 2008). According to the report, the elderly are the fastest growing population segment, now comprising 12% of the U.S. population, and projected to almost double between 2005 and 2030, from 37 to 70 million, with a substantial increase in the number of persons older than 80. Many international agencies and institutions, including the National Institute of Aging, have begun to systematically question existing assumptions and prejudices in geriatric oncology to transform it into an active field of research, education, and organizational changes.

23.2 Impact of Age on Cancer Care

In the US, a 65-year old person has an average life expectancy of 15 years, for the most part to be lived in functionally independent ways, yet the statistics for health care are daunting. The elderly currently account for more than one third of

A. Surbone (✉)
Department of Medicine, New York University, New York, NY, 10016, USA
e-mail: antonella.surbone@nyumc.org

M.W. Reed and R.A. Audisio (eds.), *Management of Breast Cancer in Older Women*, 349
DOI 10.1007/978-1-84800-265-4_23, © Springer-Verlag London Limited 2011

all hospital stays and of prescriptions, more than a fourth of all office visits to physicians in the U.S., and 90% of nursing homecare. The average 75-year old American has three or more comorbidities and takes at least four medications (Institute of Medicine 2008). Delivering optimal geriatric care is, thus, a medical and ethical priority in all aging societies.

Currently, cancer is the second leading cause of mortality worldwide, killing more people than AIDS, tuberculosis, and malaria combined. In 2007, about 8 million people died of cancer, accounting for about 13% of *all* deaths. Globally, the cancer burden doubled from 1970 to 2000 and is expected to double again between 2000 and 2020, and then triple by 2030, when 64% of the 26.4 million people diagnosed with cancer in 2030 will die (World Health Orgnization 2005a, b, 2008). The 2008 WHO World Cancer Report predicts that cancer will soon overtake heart disease as the world's leading mortality cause. Approximately 72% of current cancer deaths occurred in developing countries, and if these trends continue, annual global cancer mortality will rise to about 11.5 million persons by 2030 (World Health O 2005a, b, 2008).

Despite the statistics that show that in developing countries such as the U.S. and Europe, the rate of mortality from cancer is dropping due to earlier diagnosis and better treatments, and now approximately 25 million persons are living with cancer throughout the world, such benefits are not distributed equally across all populations or subgroups within each population group including the elderly (Institute of Medicine 2008). Contrary to the widespread belief that concomitant illnesses and intrinsic age-related frailty are determinant factors for lower survival in elderly cancer patients, the poorer outcomes are mainly due to inadequate delivery of care that the elderly receive. The elderly tend to be diagnosed later in the disease process, are often subjected to less rigorous cancer staging, and are less likely to be treated according to established guidelines, to receive adequate rehabilitative services and palliative care, and to be offered less psychosocial support (Bouchardy et al. 2003; Denmark-Wahnefried Wea 2008). Multiple cultural reasons also account for inadequate treatment based on assumptions by the clinician regarding, for example, beliefs and values of diverse population groups regarding decision-making styles, even though numerous studies show no differences in ability to tolerate surgical, radiation, and chemotherapy treatments between young and older adults in the absence of severe concomitant illnesses (Audisio et al. 2004; Horiot 2007; Lichtman et al. 2007). In addition, older cancer patients are often excluded from the benefits of clinical trials (Surbone 2008).

23.3 Impact of Ethnicity on Cancer Care

Approximately 60% of cases of breast cancer, the most common cancer in women, occur in women older than 65 years. Notably, women of color will comprise the largest segment of the elderly population by 2030 (Institute of Medicine 2008). Breast cancer is the first cause of cancer mortality in Hispanic and Asian American women and the second most common cause in non-Hispanic white, African-American, Pacific Islander, and American Indian/Alaska Native women. The mortality rate is much higher in women of color, and the difference in death rates between African American and non-Hispanic white women has essentially remained the same over time, despite the efforts over the last 40 years to eliminate health disparities (Syme 2008).

Health disparities are defined as "differences in the incidence, prevalence, mortality, and burden of diseases and other adverse health conditions that exist among specific population groups in the United States" (National Cancer Institute 2008). Disparities in cancer outcomes, documented by the Institute of Medicine in 1999 in the *Unequal Burden of Cancer,* occur even among fully insured patients, as reported by a study of African-American women at the 2008 International Meeting of the American Society of Clinical Oncology (Short et al. 2008). Lack of equity involves multiple aspects of breast cancer care, such as longer waits for diagnostic procedures, less presentation of information including treatment options, patient involvement in decision making, enrolment in clinical trials, pain control, and supportive and palliative care, which cumulatively have negative effect on the survival and outcomes and quality-of-life (QoL) in elderly women with breast cancer (Brawley and Freeman 1999).

Although numerous studies focus on the needed policy and institutional changes to address these inequities, one area of investigation of ethnic differences in cancer outcomes that has been overlooked in the equation of factors impacting outcomes is that of cultural variations. Too often culture is used synonymously with race or too poorly conceptualized to be informative regarding health disparities. Little attention is paid to the scientific inaccuracy and lack of precision in the understanding of the impact of culture on the cancer experience, and the lack of understanding and incorporation of its variations in the delivery of cancer care. Yet, culture plays a key role in overcoming health disparities. The purpose of this chapter is to illuminate the triple burden of discrimination for diverse populations of older women due to ageism and sexism, and differential care or racism, which together create added barriers that prevent those elderly women of diverse cultural groups from receiving adequate and fair cancer care. We will better define these issues, elucidate their influence on breast cancer care in older women, and provide guidelines to integrate a more scientific understanding of culture that will help us eliminate the unequal burden of cancer on older minority women (Institute of Medicine 2001).

23.4   Older Age: Biology and Socio-cultural Constructs

The goal of equal access to care and research for elderly cancer patients can only be achieved by first examining the meaning and value that we attribute to aging. In western countries, old age tends to be represented only in terms of decreased productivity, functional impairment, comorbidity, cognitive limitations, and the burden of care placed on the family and/or the health care system (Surbone et al. 2006). This distorted cultural perception of age, known as ageism, negatively influences attitudes toward, and practices of, providing health care to elderly cancer patients. In western societies, the elderly generally are offered fewer opportunities to be involved in their communities, have lower incomes, and are often underserved with respect to health care. Poverty is especially common in the elderly, and when low socioeconomic status combines with cultural factors in older minority patients, leading, for example, to not challenging authority (here doctors), their health status is negatively affected, resulting in increasing morbidity and frailty, while access to medical care and research is dramatically limited (Institute of Medicine 2008).

From a biological standpoint, aging involves a progressive decline in the functional reserve of multiple organs and systems that modulate the person's adaptation to stress (Lipsitz 2004). The word "frailty" is often used improperly to indicate a generic increased vulnerability of elderly patients when compared to younger adults, whereas it technically refers to a specific entity resulting from the interplay of physical, psychological, cognitive, functional, social, and environmental factors (Fried et al. 2004). Comorbidity, disability, and frailty are three distinct entities in elderly patients, which may occur separately or concomitantly and whose multidimensional assessment is necessary to guide clinical decision making in geriatric oncology. For example, the cancer patient's frailty often limits the safety of administration of standard and experimental treatments. Frailty, however, may also result from the patient's underlying cancer, and the degree of frailty can be improved or even reversed by active oncologic treatment (Balducci 2007). Studies show that the frequent undertreatment of elderly cancer patients and their underrepresentation in clinical trials frequently stem from misconceptions about an inevitable correlation between aging, vulnerability, and frailty (Surbone 2008). By contrast, available data suggest that age itself, in the absence of severe concomitant illnesses or psychological, cognitive, or functional impairment, is not an independent risk factor for either increased toxicity or lack of cancer treatment efficacy (Giovannazzi-Bannon et al. 1994).

Furthermore, elderly cancer patients are often considered to be at high risk for diminished QoL and increased psychological stress, yet psychological and psychosocial studies and meta-analyses suggest that elderly cancer patients may adjust and adapt to stressful events better than younger adults by using passive and emotion-focused coping strategies such as distancing, acceptance of responsibility, and positive reappraisal (Folkman et al. 1987; Ganz et al. 2004). Coping with cancer is generally determined by personal experiences, history, beliefs, social relationships, cultural meanings and values, and by the clinical features of the disease itself. From the few studies that have addressed how cancer patients of 75 years of age and older cope with their illness, it appears that the cancer experience is met with more equanimity than younger patients. They exhibit a sense of mastery, one's perceived control over circumstances, and self-efficacy or sense of ability to successfully accomplish tasks or meet age-appropriate goals. This equanimity in the face of the challenges of the cancer and its treatment, including death, appears to be partially a function of the feedback they receive from the social environment (Kotkamp-Mothes et al. 2005), as well as their greater life experience, and internal resources developed through meeting past challenges in life. Not surprisingly, those who have adequate family and social support do better than those who do not (Thome et al. 2003; Hann et al. 2002).

A gap then exists between older cancer patients' physical and psychological coping abilities and their poorer outcomes in terms of cure rates, survival, and QoL. In large part, this gap appears to be influenced by socioculturally biased attitudes toward the elderly. We can eliminate this gap through adequate policy making and individual and collective efforts to create a new culture of geriatric oncology where we do not conflate the different dimensions of aging. For example, while there is a higher prevalence of cognitive dysfunction, depression, and frailty in older cancer patients, poverty, isolation, and lack of social support worsen these disabilities. However, the degree to which these factors impact an individual's physical and emotional ability to undergo rigorous treatment should not be assumed. Objective clinical measurements should be conducted to provide the data required to deliver best cancer treatment, accompanied, when needed, by appropriate ancillary services, such as home assistance or special supportive measures required to maintain and regain adequate QoL in elderly cancer patients (Balducci 2007; Hann et al. 2002).

23.5   Race, Ethnicity, Culture, and Disparities

Considerable variations in the site, incidence, morbidity, and mortality rates of cancers have been documented worldwide as well as within the U.S. according to racial/ethnic groups. Men and women of color in the U.S. fare much worse than non-Hispanic whites. Biology or genetic polymorphisms appear to have minor relationships with the variations, while the major source of variations appears to be lifestyle (Bonham et al. 2005).

Culture has a major influence on lifestyle choices as well as life circumstances or options, as we shall describe and illustrate in this section, but little attention has been focused on this factor. Culture, race, and ethnicity appear to profoundly impact the incidence and prevalence of health disparities, but these concepts are still poorly operationalized, and little explanatory power is provided in research or practice with the current use of these terms. In Table 23.1, we present more scientifically based definitions of these concepts, which affect cancer outcomes along the entire care continuum.

Race is a scientifically unsubstantiated term (Bonham et al. 2005). In the eighteenth century, race was thought to describe subspecies of homo sapiens. The categories were based upon phenotypic characteristics that were assumed to indicate stages of evolutionary development. Scientifically, this has proven to be false, as greater within-group genetic variations exist among the members of the racial categories. These categories function more powerfully as social and political constructs, rather than as biologically-based differences (Williams et al. 1997).

Reflexive use of the US racial/ethnic categories, non-Hispanic whites, Hispanics, African Americans, Asian Americans, Native Americans, and Native Hawaiians

Table 23.1 Key definitions of race, culture, ethnicity and racism

Concept	Definition
Race	Scientific myth that genetic differences separate racially designated groups. – assumed that someone's phenotype predicts their genotype and character
Ethnicity	A subcultural group within a power structure of a multicultural society and self-identified membership in a group formed within a sociohistorical context
Racism	Assertion of power ego-fulfillment, and status by one group at the expense of others based upon skin color (or language) or phenotypic characteristics
Culture	System of beliefs, values, lifestyles, ecologic, and technical resources and constraints that form and are informed by the ecologic niche in which a population has biologically evolved

and Pacific Islanders, without clear scientific rationale, results in three primary problems. First, the stereotypical or racialized assumption is that genetic differences are the primary causes of differences in disease incidence, prevalence, and mortality; second, the first assumption diverts attention from the more malleable social and political causes of disease and intra group variability and vulnerability; and third, this leads to the underestimation of the purpose of culture and thus the assets and strengths that each culture holds for its members.

Ethnicity is a subcultural group within a power structure of a multicultural society, and also constitutes an individual and group's self-identified membership. This identity is formed within sociohistorical circumstances that have defined the relative political and social positions of the various groups. Thus, ethnicity is a subjective sense of individual and group identity by the observer as well as the actor, and importantly, is contextually and geographically based due to social barriers and political circumstances. These social-political forces must be recognized and neutralized in health care delivery models to provide quality care to the elderly from diverse ethnic backgrounds.

Racism is the assertion of power for ego-fulfillment and status by one group at the expense of others based upon skin color or other phenotypic characteristics. The force of racism is institutionally codified in a society and is the compelling factor that shapes health outcomes through biased or differentially administered care (Institute of Medicine 2001) for people of color and the medically underserved at every stage of the cancer continuum: from prevention, screening and early detection to treatment (access and response), rehabilitation and palliative care, and end of life care or survivorship. What is not usually recognized is that the entire research and practice arena of cancer care in the U.S. occurs within a monocultural milieu and transpires unconsciously for and within its members. This mono-cultural European-American framework becomes more visible when patients and families from cultures other than that of the dominant U.S. society try to navigate our health care services. Many of the structural issues, including the social determinants of poorer health outcomes, such as education, occupation, social status, housing, availability of quality services, diet, health literacy, and degree of integration in a community social network, disproportionately affect the elderly in communities of color and among the medically underserved as well (Adler 2008). While most researchers and practitioners recognize these differences, they are less open to acknowledge the forces of sexism, ageism, racism, and ethnocentrism, which comprise the underlying causes of differences among racial/ethnic groups. Unless these issues are more clearly recognized and identified, however, existing disparities will continue to be perpetuated.

23.6 Culture and Health

Cross-cultural differences influence patients' views of illness and suffering, the patient-doctor relationship, trust in institutions and in medical science, and attitudes toward experimental therapies. Culture fundamentally constitutes the milieu in which all human life occurs and it forms the context in which life decisions are made. It is the core organizing system of life used by an individual or group to make sense of the cancer experience and to guide people's lifestyles and that of their social network.

The purpose of culture is to ensure the survival and well-being of its members in an ever changing and chaotic world. Thus, necessarily, cultures are dynamic, responsive, adaptive, and somewhat coherent in system of beliefs, values, and lifestyles that are developed by fellow members to successfully adapt to life within a particular geographic and political location using available technology and economic resources. The variations in these cultural tools function as filters and modulators of input that refract stimuli to interpret the meaning of events and prescribe appropriate behavior to meet them (Kagawa-Singer 1996). This dynamically evolving way of life, including lifestyle patterns, such as diet, marriage rules, gender roles, and means of livelihood, is passed from one generation to the next to ensure their survival and give meaning to life (Kagawa-Singer 2006).

Since all of these factors vary around the world due to geographic, social, and political circumstances and history, cultures differ. Also, since they are adaptive systems, any operationalization of the concept of culture would require measures at every level of a socioecologic model and likely across time. One useful metaphor of culture is the technique of weaving, which is universal, yet the patterns that emerge from each group are culturally identifiable (Kagawa-Singer 1988). The warp and woof or the perpendicularly woven threads of a tapestry are analogous to the two dimensions of culture, integrative and functional. The integrative dimension provides individuals with the beliefs and values that supplies its members meaning in life and a sense of identity. The functional dimension contains the rules for behavior that support an individual's sense of self-worth, and maintains group function and welfare (Jones and Kay 1992). Specific, discrete cultural beliefs and behaviors are like the threads in the tapestry. A single thread of one cultural tapestry can be taken out and compared across cultural groups for its inherent characteristics, but the usefulness and integrity of the thread as representative of the entire tapestry cannot be judged unless seen within the pattern of the entire cultural fabric within which such behaviors were meant to function.

Taken out of context and without its counterpart, a belief or behavior may be misinterpreted or even disregarded as unnecessary or maladaptive, especially if evaluated against the standard for the behavior of focus in another culture. For example, to understand why the medical truth is not disclosed to cancer patients in many countries, it is necessary to appreciate the protective role that family assumes in community-centered cultures, as opposed to those centered on individuals and their rights (Surbone 2006a). Cultural elements are woven into a whole with reciprocal parts in order for the social order to function in an organized, systemic fashion. When members of cultural groups immigrate, however, or technologies and practices are adopted from other cultural groups, the "fit" of these new elements may not necessarily connect in a coherent manner or in a coordinated fashion as a whole or within its subgroups or even within families. Thus, no culture is homogenous or static and dissonance among cultural elements is likely to occur, especially in our globalized society. Stereotypes are, therefore, not only wrong, they are dangerous.

Varying levels of acculturation, assimilation, age, education, income, family structure, gender, wealth, foreign vs. U.S.-born status, and immigrant status also modify the degree to which one's cultural group membership may influence health practices and health status, and importantly, views toward aging and the elderly. In a multicultural society like the United States, each cultural group is contemporaneously undergoing modifications and mixtures that render it different from the original cultural group it grew from and continually changing. Tensions across generations are inevitable, and affect an elder's sense of well-being.

Notably, the majority of the literature on racial/ethnic differences studies the vulnerabilities of nonwestern/European-American cultures. Few studies focus on the protective and health-promoting beliefs and practices of cultural groups other than the dominant Northern European American population that is used as the standard against which all other groups are measured. This bias in research clouds our ability to see equal validity among different cultural strategies to meet life's adversities and understand other social structures based upon gender, age, social status, and levels of authority that may be more beneficial than the European-American cultural practices and lifestyles (Airhihenbuwa et al. 1995). For example, the "Mediterranean" diet is known to protect against different diseases, while most Northern European-American based diets include less healthy processed foods that are low in fibers or vitamins and high in fats or sugars. Unfortunately, the elderly and individuals from groups of color are more likely than more educated, wealthier citizens to consume such foods, as they are relatively inexpensive. In the US, the elderly become increasingly malnourished due to high poverty rates, but this is also occurring in the Mediterranean countries, as they are increasingly unable to afford healthy diets (Huang et al. 2002). Growing levels of poverty in elderly and minorities, thus, may lead to malnourishment, which in turn may severely compromise the fortitude needed to withstand cancer therapies.

23.7 Culture, Aging, and Ethical Norms: Role of Relational Autonomy

While high ethical standards should be applied consistently in all age and ethnic groups, certain ethical issues in geriatric oncology carry special weight, such as the limitation of economic and practical resources of many elderly patients. The influence of social support and family functioning on patient coping and adaptation, gender differences in care giving among elderly patients, and considerations of the emotional and economic contribution of caregivers are all social forces entwined with age, gender, and culture.

The emerging notion of relational autonomy helps us understand and address the complex reality of caring for older minority cancer patients (Surbone 2006a). Traditionally, in Western industrialized countries, ethical considerations in geriatrics and geriatric oncology are connected to the narrow notion of patient autonomy based on the right of fully informed patients to make choices independently, rationally, and freely (Huang et al. 2002; Sherwin 1988). In this view of individual autonomy, patients are considered capable of making decisions about health care and life and death matters, because they are deemed to possess all the instruments necessary to understand their options and the resources needed to choose among a set of options (Sherwin 1988). "Autonomy" is a universal attribute of rational human beings, but the exercise of autonomy is always relational and situational, rather than simply a matter of individual choice (Mahowald 2000). Moreover, internal and external forces are inextricably related with one's state of perceived or actual vulnerability and with varying degrees of interdependency on others (Mahowald 2000; Nussbaum 1993). The notion of relational autonomy in the clinical context involves individual autonomy, but it also acknowledges the relational, cultural, socioe-conomic, and contextual aspects of patients' decision-making (Surbone 2006a). In clinical practice, we repeatedly observe how different factors often prevent patients, even when they are fully informed, from experiencing the freedom of choice implicit in an atomistic notion of ideal autonomy. For example, despite a major evolution in truth telling attitudes and practices of physicians and patients worldwide, cross-cultural differences persist with respect to disclosure of information regarding diagnosis, prognosis and treatment options, and involvement of cancer patients in the decision-making process (Surbone 2006c; Blackhall et al. 1995; Kagawa-Singer and Blackhall 2001). Older women with breast cancer who belong to minority groups tend to be less informed and less respected by their physicians and sometimes their families in their decisional autonomy than they might desire (Maly et al. 2006, 2008).

Patients' decisions about treatment, palliative, and end-of-life care are never based solely on the objective information that they possess. By contrast, cultural values and attitudes, socioeconomic status, education, family, and community support, all affect patients' choices. Similarly, patients' decisions to participate in a clinical trial do not depend only on the information received about the trial, but also on possible barriers to access such as cost, the availability of community resources, such as transportation, and the sense of burden on family and family resources (Surbone 2008; Hutchins et al. 1999).

Table 23.2 Factors that may influence elderly patients' autonomy and decision-making

Internal	Personal past experiences
	Cultural values and attitudes affecting decision-making styles
	Personal stance toward the patient-doctor relationship
	Cognitive impairments affecting mental capacity
	Vulnerability induced by concomitant illnesses
	Psychological stressors related to loss of life roles
	Loneliness or sense of being a burden
External	Information received
	Education
	Socioeconomic status
	Physical, instrumental and social dependence on others
	Family and community support
	Degrees of social integration and social capital
	Available resources (transportation, companionship, home help, others)
	Economic and geographic barriers to access to cancer treatment facilities

Mental capacity, the ability to understand medical information, personal attitudes toward the patient-doctor relationship, decision-making styles, stressors, and vulnerability may also internally shape a person's desire for and ability to exercise autonomy. In the case of older cancer patients, loss of productivity and consequent life roles, degrees of social integration or isolation or of physical and social independence, and presence or absence of family support are among the many factors that shape elderly patients' decision to exercise their autonomy in health care matters (Surbone 2008) (Table 23.2). Older breast cancer patients may be especially subject to such limitations on their autonomy due to their position in their social network.

Despite the presence of factors that may influence older persons' dependency on others, elderly cancer patients retain their ability to exercise their autonomy as long as they are competent. Frank and colleagues (1998) found that cultural variations also impact autonomy due to the salience of relational autonomy in more community-focused cultures. A Korean-American woman declined autonomous decision making for her own care, because she said that that would impose her wishes upon her children who would be left to bear the burden of her decisions. The children were the ones who would live on after her death, and she felt, since death was inevitable in the vignette presented to her, it was up to her children to express their wishes and not her. Efforts to encourage her independent decision making would meet great resistance. Paternalism toward them, even in weak forms, should be avoided. For example, physicians often make unilateral decisions about enrollment in clinical trials on the presumption that older women neither want nor can tolerate aggressive or new therapies, or that they would be less adherent than younger patients (Surbone 2008). Paternalism and unilateral decision making by the physician regarding treatment options are often exacerbated for women of color (Maly et al. 2005). Thus, age and cultural differences raise ethical questions about the degree to which relational autonomy is recognized and integrated into breast cancer care.

23.8   Disparities in Access to Breast Cancer Care and Research in Older Minority Women: Empirical Data

As we have described and analyzed in previous sections, older breast cancer patients are often undertreated because of misconceptions related to ageism. Older minority breast cancer patients face additional discriminatory practices along the continuum of their cancer care, starting with information, screening, diagnosis, treatment, follow-up, and access to state of the art care, which contribute to their higher mortality when compared with affluent, better educated, non-Hispanic white patients (Keating et al. 2007; Li 2005; Smigal et al. 2006; Albano et al. 2007). Delays in diagnosis and underutilization of cancer treatment are frequent in women of color and other minority women, and they are mostly attributable to poor communication between minority patients and oncology professionals, particular beliefs held about health care systems and curative measures, including complementary and alternative treatments, economic barriers and poor social support, and biased attitudes by both the individual health care professional and the structure of the health care system (Shavers and Brown 2002; Richards et al. 1999; Gwyn et al. 2004; Elmore et al. 2005; Kaplan et al. 2004; Struthers and Nichols 2004).

For example, ONE study showed that African-American women living in poor, high crime rate areas of Chicago develop a more aggressive form of breast cancer, do so at a younger age, and are 68% more likely to die of breast cancer than white women (Conzen 2008). Genetic variations account for differences but foremost, this study, like many others, documents that social and cultural factors lead to limited information and access to cancer screening care and research. The consequence of environmental and lifestyle factors potentially affects the biology of breast cancers and their responsiveness to treatments in women of color, which contribute to their poorer outcomes. The stress derived from social isolation and lack of social support may, in fact, lead to disrupted cortisol rhythms while higher fat diet may also contribute to altered estrogen metabolism (Carey et al. 2006).

In the US, mammography rates for black women of age 65–69 years (57%) are lower than for white women (64%). These rates also vary by state, reaching the highest of 74% in Maine and the lowest of 56.9% in Mississippi (Painter and Lavizzo-Mourey 2008). The role of wealth in access to screening mammography was recently established in a group of 4,222 women with Medicaid insurance, showing that wealthier women were more likely to have undergone mammography. The lower mammography rates for poorer women may be due to lack of information, supplemental Medicaid insurance, and transportation. Additionally, women with lower quality health insurance or no insurance go to treatment facilities where they encounter increased difficulties in long waiting times for screening or seeing a doctor for treatment. Often these women are working or have major caregiving responsibilities at home and are unable to spend many hours waiting for scheduled appointments (Williams et al. 2008). Minority women may also differ in their approach to screening and cancer detection, due to psychosocial and cultural factors, such as fears and anxiety older age or various degrees of fatalism or resignation the complexity of the health care system and frustration with its fragmented services (Ramirez et al. 1999; Kerner et al. 2003). Black women, due to less education and/or over commitment of time, may also overestimate their actual screening rates, thereby having fewer screening tests than recommended for their age (Maly et al. 2008).

While over 50% of all breast cancer patients appear to be ill informed about the risks and benefits of treatment options, an analysis of SEER registry data on 1,132 patients, coupled with a survey of 277 surgeons, showed that almost two-thirds of African-American women and Latinas were unaware of their survival odds and of the surgical treatment options (i.e. breast conserving surgery and mastectomy), (Hawley et al. 2008). A 2002 Commonwealth report suggested that African-American, Hispanic, and Asian American breast cancer patients reported being offered less information and treatment options than those made available to non-Hispanic white women (Collins et al. 2002).

A 2007 study assessed the types of therapies received by over 143,000 Medicare recipients for breast, colon, rectal, and prostate cancer from 1992 to 2002 (Gross et al. 2008). They found that black patients were consistently less likely than whites to receive standard treatments. Among breast cancer patients, black women were 7% less likely than whites to have received radiation therapy after lumpectomy, an omission known to increase the risk of local recurrence. The study revealed no improvement in racial disparities in cancer treatment in the period studied, and attributed most of the inequities to institutional and societal factors, rather than individual racism (Gross et al. 2008).

Other researchers have also reported lower administration of radiation therapy to black women, and a study of 626 breast cancer patients who had undergone mastectomy showed that older and minority patients were less likely to have had breast reconstruction, or even a proper discussion with their oncologists about this therapeutic option (Bleicher et al. 2008). Physicians' gender and medical training also seems to determine the quality of care received by breast cancer patients, as shown in a SEER-based study of nearly 30,000 women of 65 years and older, 75% of whom had been treated with breast conserving surgery. Patients of US-trained female physicians were more likely to have received radiation therapy, a finding that may suggest differences in patients' preferences or in doctors' medical training, but also in physician-patient interactions or (Hershman et al. 2008).

According to US Food and Drug Administration, drugs should be studied in all age groups for which they will be used to properly assess their risks and benefits (Services UDoHaH 1994). Yet, of about 80,000 clinical trials performed yearly in the US for different diseases, only 25% of participants are 65 years or older, and between 1995 and 1999, only 10% belonged to African-American, Asian-Pacific Islanders, Hispanic and Native American groups, despite comprising although they comprise 25% of the population (Newman et al. 2008). The under-representation of elderly and minority breast cancer patients in medical and surgical clinical trials has been widely documented (Murthy et al. 2004; Stewart et al. 2007; O'Brien 2007; Gross et al. 2005a). Low socioeconomic status in older women and women of color in particular is also associated with major barriers to participation in clinical trials. This low rate of participation may, in turn, contribute to the racial disparities.

Clinical trials are the most reliable research method for establishing the efficacy of new medical, surgical, or radiation therapies while rejecting unsafe or ineffective ones, and for confirming or discounting the benefits of existing treatments by enabling accurate comparisons among them. Yet, while over 60% of cancers occur in patients older than 65 and 35% in patients older than 75, in western countries, only 10% of the patients older than 65 are enrolled in clinical trials (Surbone 2008) A case-controlled study comparing participants in NCI cooperative group breast cancer trials with a population-based sample of breast cancer patients obtained from the linked SEER-Medicare data base aged 65 years or more showed that enrollment in clinical trials was inversely proportional with residence in areas of high poverty, high unemployment rates, and Medicaid insurance (Gross et al. 2005b). The under-representation of older breast cancer patients and those in under-represented minority populations in clinical trials impairs our ability to generalize research findings to this important segment of the population. Furthermore, lack of data and evidence with respect to new anticancer therapies perpetuates the frequent use of substandard treatments in older breast cancer patients (Kumar et al. 2007).

Accrual to psycho-social research on QoL and interventions to improve adjustment of breast cancer survivors is also lower for older and minority patients. In a 2008 German study of 170 breast cancer patients to whom interventions on QoL-related aspects, such as pain therapy, sports activities, nutrition, and social counseling were provided, only 11% of breast cancer patients enrolled were 70 years or older, though 27% of the general breast cancer population in the same German region belonged to this age group (Klinkhammer-Shalke et al. 2008). Aziz and Rowland conducted the first review of the literature on cancer survivorship among ethnic groups of color and found that between 1966 and 2002, only 65 articles had been published, compared to over 50,000 studies on primarily non-Hispanic white groups. Subgroup analyses by ethnic groups were not reported in these studies. These studies focused on physiologic sequelae, psychosocial needs, health services issues, and patterns and quality of care, and found significant differences compared to non-Hispanic whites. The number of studies per ethnic group, however, is insufficient to provide enough support for practice recommendations, except to note the differences and encourage further exploration by clinicians with their patients and their families.

23.9   Cultural Competence and Health Disparities

Cultural competence can contribute to reducing disparities. We define cultural competence as a learnable skill that enables the clinician to respectfully elicit from the patient and the family the information needed to make an accurate diagnosis and negotiate mutually satisfactory goals for treatment (Kagawa-Singer and Kassim-Lakha 2003). This requires that the clinicians have knowledge about the various cultures that are represented in their practice and also the openness required to be "students" of the patient and family to learn how the potential values of that cultural group may or may not influence their goals and decision-making wishes. Clinicians would then be better able to ask the right questions and integrate their knowledge and understanding to develop credibility with their patients and families. They could, thus, establish and sustain a relationship of trust, acceptance, and mutual respect for each other's values, beliefs, and practices that is necessary to successfully negotiate the goals for acceptable and appropriate action.

Cultural information must be used as the basis for generating hypotheses regarding individuals, not stereotypes. For some patients, their natal culture may be salient. For others, it may not. Respect and trust are built through dialog, which is essential to accurately assess the impact of culture and other social and economic factors on the treatment plan.

Cultural competence also includes developing skills that enable health professionals to provide culturally competent quality care to patients also during brief discordant medical encounters. Formal teaching and training of patient-centered approaches to cross-cultural care, based on assessing core cross-cultural issues, exploring the meaning of illness to the patient, determining their lived social context, and negotiating adherence to recommendations and treatments, are being implemented in many countries, including the US (Kagawa-Singer and Kassim-Lakha 2003). A 2003 survey mailed to 3,435 US medical residents evaluated their preparedness to deliver culturally competent care. Of the 2047(60%) residents who replied, 93% believed that cultural competence was moderately or very important. Yet, 24% reported that they lacked adequate skills to identify cultural customs relevant to medicine and 33–50% had received no instructions after medical school. Furthermore, 41% of general practitioners and 83% of surgeons were never evaluated for cultural competence during their residency (Weissman et al. 2005). Many respondents expressed particular concerns about dealing with specific aspects of cross-cultural care, including health beliefs at odds with western medicine (25%), issues related to new immigrants (25%), and religious beliefs affecting medical treatment (20%). The major barriers to delivering cross-cultural care were felt to be lack of time, role models, ongoing training, and evaluation (Weissman et al. 2005).

Patient-centered care and cultural competence are means to improve the quality of cancer care for all patients and to foster equal access to cancer care and research (Institute of Medicine 2001; Institute of Medicine 2007). Individual cultural competence alone, however, is not sufficient to eliminate health care disparities. Individual skills must be accompanied by the implementation of culturally-competent health-care systems. This requires policy making and institutional commitment to expand cultural knowledge to assess cross-cultural relations and their dynamics within all cancer care facilities and to adapt oncology services to meet the culturally unique needs of patients or groups of patients (Betancourt et al. 2003).

For example, African-American older women are more likely than white women to have comorbidities, such as diabetes and hypertension, which may limit their breast cancer treatment options. Culturally sensitive interventions, targeted at minority women with the aim to improve life styles and foster early detection and treatment of concomitant illnesses, as well as encourage screening and early detection of breast cancer, may significantly contribute to reduce the gap in the quality of cancer treatment that they may receive. Women of color are known to have higher rates of mastectomies as opposed to breast conserving surgery, even when their breast cancer characteristics and stage would allow for either one, with expected similar recurrence rates, and Latino women tend to conform to family centered decision-making styles when treatment options are discussed. Yet a recent survey of 995 patients with nonadvanced breast cancer shows that many Latino women reported great dissatisfaction with their choices and would have liked to have been better informed and more involved by their doctors in their decision-making (Maly and Silliman 2003).

In fact, whether discrimination is perceived or real, it drives differences in health outcomes, and culturally sensitive and competent communication with oncology patients and their families is key to providing optimal cancer care (Surbone 2006b). As disparities are multifactorial in origin, individual and institutional cultural competence is part of a multidimensional strategy to reduce discriminatory attitudes and practices, which also includes culturally and linguistically appropriate programs of patient advocacy and education, and involves local communities in discussing and developing health care policies for minority and underserved breast cancer patients.

23.10   Conclusion

The approach to older breast cancer patients should be based on sound evidence, rather than on cultural myths, biases, or prejudices related to ageism or sexism. The distorted cultural perception of age that dominates most western societies, known as ageism, has, in fact, a major influence on our attitudes toward, and practices of, providing health care to elderly patients. Older persons in contemporary western societies tend to have reduced opportunities to be involved in their communities, to have lower incomes, and to be underserved with respect to health care. Ageism sexism and racism combined, lead older women of color with breast cancer to receive differential information and less than standard cancer care.

The correlation between aging and low socioeconomic status further impacts on the health status of older patients and their access to care and research studies including clinical trials. Poverty is especially common in elderly women, and socioeconomic factors combined with cultural ones in ethnic minorities in western countries render their access to breast cancer care extremely difficult. Gender differences also play a major role with access to medical care, as well as health status. For example, older breast cancer patients tend to be underdiagnosed and undertreated because they are often the care givers in their families and communities, carrying multiple responsibilities that limit, both culturally and structurally, their availability to take care of themselves,

While providing solutions to the needs of older minority women is a matter of political and health policy choices, some of the socioeconomic and cultural barriers that prevent older minority women from having equal access to breast cancer prevention, diagnosis, treatment, supportive and palliative care, as well as clinical and psycho-social services, can already be understood and overcome in daily oncology practices. Education of patients and oncology care professionals about the impact of frequent misunderstandings related to ageism and cultural differences on treatment outcomes should go hand in hand with eliminating all residual forms of paternalism that professionals often adopt toward older patients. Individual racism or bias is less common than institutional and societal racism, and individual physicians and cancer professionals could acquire through education and training sufficient cultural competency to overcome many of the existing barriers to the standard of cancer care. Many studies show that the first step in cultural competency is for health professionals to recognize their own cultural biases that often lead to stereotyping and/or discriminatory approaches to older minority breast cancer patients. While minority patients tend to report better experiences when doctors share their ethnicity or cultural background, being culturally competent in culturally discordant clinical encounters is possible. Then, both the patient and physician are able to appreciate and respect the different health values of each other and work toward mutually agreeable goals of treatment. Effective educational and training programs, coupled with specific and reliable outcome measures to evaluate the impact of teaching cultural competence in the clinical context, are therefore needed in oncology programs worldwide. This, in turn, could help reduce persisting inequalities in the quality of care delivered to older minority breast cancer patients.

23.11   Summary

In this chapter we investigate the impact of culture, ethnicity, and race on the phenomenon of disparities in access to standard and experimental oncology care for older women. We start by exploring salient aspects of the relationship between aging, illness, and culture, as they relate to health and health disparities. Subsequently, we discuss the meaning of age as both a biologic reality and a sociocultural construct, and we analyze those factors that contribute to age-based discrimination in health care. Old age and culture, overlooked but powerful influences on cancer incidence and treatment, are interdependent variables that require recognition of diverse disciplinary knowledge, such as medicine, psychology, anthropology, philosophy, sociology, and political science. Research on health disparities has grown over the last 40 years, and yet the inequity in outcomes among the ethnic populations in the U.S. has not decreased.

Society and healthcare practitioners continue to view and treat elderly patients on the basis of ageism and consequently, incorrect assumptions of uniform frailty, treatment intolerance, and cognitive impairment. This distorted appraisal limits the adequacy of care, research, and education in geriatrics. On the contrary, the elderly population is physiologically, psychologically, socially, and culturally heterogeneous, and available data suggest that age itself, in the absence of severe concomitant illnesses or psychological, cognitive, or functional impairment, is not an independent risk factor for either increased toxicity or lack of cancer treatment efficacy.

After an in-depth review of published data on disparities in diagnosis and treatment of breast cancer in older women, we describe how cultural competence in geriatric oncology, in both its individual and systemic dimensions, could enhance the quality of cancer care and reduce health disparities.

We conclude by presenting evidence-based recommendation in favor of a culturally competent and sensitive approach to older women with breast cancer, and by indicating potential areas of future research and scholarly work that will lead us to provide equal access to quality care to older patients. Individual elderly patients should be approached on the basis of sound evidence rather than on cultural myths, biases, or prejudices related to ageism, sexism, and racism. Our chapter is intended as a contribution toward a new culture of geriatric oncology, which is possible only through a rational and humane reappraisal of the sociocultural meaning of older age.

23.12 Online Sources

23.12.1 Cancer Health Disparities

- American Association of Clinical Oncology: www.asco.org/healthdisparities
- National Cancer Institute: http://www.cancer.gov/cancertopics/types/disparities
- National Cancer Institute Center for Cancer Health Disparities: http://crchd. cancer.gov/
- U.S. Department of Health and Human Services, Health Resource and Service Administration:
  http://www.healthdisparities.net/hdc/html/collaboratives.topics.cancer.aspx

23.12.2 Survivorship

- American Cancer Society, People Living With Cancer:http://www.cancer.org/docroot/MBC/content/MBC_4_1X_Living_With_Cancer.asp
- American Society of Clinical Oncology: http://www.PLWC.org
- People Living with Cancer and Complementary and Alternative Medicine: http://nccam.nih.gov/news/2003/100103.htm
- BBC – Living With Cancer: http://www.bbc.co.uk/health/conditions/cancer/index.shtml
- National Cancer Institute: Facing Forward: Life After Cancer Treatment http://www.cancer.gov/cancertopics/life-after-treatment

- National Coalition for Cancer Survivorship: http://www.canceradvocacy.org/
- The Lance Armstrong Foundation:
  http://www.livestrong.org/site/c.khLXK1PxHmF/b.2660611/k.BCED/Home.htm

23.12.3   Ethnic Specific Breast Cancer Information and Support

- Native Americans: http://www.fnbreastcancer.bc.ca/
- Breast Cancer Resource Directory of North Carolina:
- http://bcresourcedirectory.org/directory/05-african_american.htm
- Cancer Connection, Florence, Massachusetts: http://www.cancer-connection. org/links
- Asian American Resources: http://www.apiahf.org/programs/cdp/aapicancerre- sources.htm

References

Adler NR (2008) US disparities in health: descriptions, causes, and mechanisms. Annu Rev Public 29:235–252

Airhihenbuwa C, Kumanyika S, Agurs TD, Lowe A (1995) Perceptions and beliefs about exercise, rest, and health among African-Americans. Am J Health Promot 9(6):426–429

Albano J, Ward E, Jemal A, Anderson R, Cokkinides V, Murray T, Henley J, Liff J, Thun M (2007) Cancer mortality in the United States by education level and race. J Natl Cancer Inst 99(18):1384–1394

Audision et al. (2004): The surgical management of elderly cancer patients; recommendations of the international society of geriatric oncology (SIOG) surgical task force. Eur J Cancer 40(7):1832–1843

Aziz NM, Rowland JH. Cancer survivorship research among ethnic minority and medically underserved groups. Oncol Nurs Forum. Jun 2002;29(5):789–801.

Balducci (2007): Aging, frailty and chemotherapy. Cancer Control 14:7–14

Betancourt J, Green AR, Carrillo JE, Ananeh-Firempong O (2003) Defining cultural competence: a practical framework for addressing racial/ethnic disparities in health and health care. Public Health Rep 118(4):293–302

Blackhall LJ, Murphy ST, Frank G, Michel V, Azen S (1995) Ethnicity and attitudes toward patient autonomy. JAMA 274(10):820–825

Bleicher R, Abrahamse P, Hawley ST, Katz SJ, Morrow M (2008) The influence of age on the breast surgery decision-making process. Ann Surg Oncol 15(3):854–862

Bonham VL, Warshauer-Baker E, Collins FS (2005) Race and ethnicity in the genome era. Am Psychol 60(1):9–15

Bouchardy et al. (2003): Undertreatment strongly decreases prognosis of breast cancer in elderly women. J Clin Oncol Bouchardy et al. (2003): 21:3580–3587

Brawley OW, Freeman HP (1999) Race and outcomes: is this the end or the beginning for minority health research? J Natl Cancer Inst 91(22):1908–1909

Carey et al. (2006): Race, breast cancer subtypes, and survival in the Carolina breast cancer study. JAMA 295(21):2492–2502

Collins KS, Hughes DL, Doty MM, Ives BL, Edwards JN, Tenney K (2002) Diverse communities, common concerns: assessing health care quality for minority Americans. The Commonwealth Fund, New York

Conzen SD (2008) Nuclear receptors and breast cancer. Mol Endocrinol 22(10):2215–2228

Demark-Wahnefried Wea (2008) Elderly cancer survivors improve ability at daily functions with home-based intervention, AACR San Diego, CA, USA. April 12. http://www.medicalnewsto-day.com/articles/130017.php

Elmore J, Nakano CY, Linden HM, Reisch LM, Ayanian JZ, Larson EB (2005) Racial inequities in the timing of breast cancer detection, diagnosis, and initiation of treatment. Med Care 43(2):141–148

Folkman S, Lazarus RS, Pimley S, Novacek J (1987) Age differences in stress and coping processes. Psychol Aging 2(2):171–184

Frank G, Blackhall LJ, Michel V, Murphy ST, Azen SP, Park K.A discourse of relationships in bioethics: patient autonomy and end-of-life decision making among elderly Korean Americans. Med Anthropol Q. 1998 Dec;12(4):403–23.

Fried et al. (2004): Untangling the concepts of disability, frailty, and comorbidity: implications for imporved targeting and care. J Gerontol 59(3):255–263

Ganz PA KL, Stanton AL, Krupnick JL, Rowland JH, Meyerowitz BE et al (2004) Quality of life at the end of primary treatment of breast cancer: first results from the moving beyond cancer randomized trial. J Natl Cancer Inst 96(5):376–387

Giovannazzi-Bannon et al. (1994): Treatment intolerance of elderly cancer patients entered onto phase II clinical trials: an Illinois Cancer Center study. J Clin Oncol 12(11):2447–2452

Gross, Herrin, Wong, & Krumholz. (2005): Enrolling older persons in cancer trials: the effect of sociodemographic, protocol, and recruitment center characteristics. J Clin Oncol 23(21):4755–4763

Gross C, Filardo G, Mayne ST, Krumholz HM (2005b) The impact of socioeconomic status and race on trial participation for older women with breast cancer. Cancer 103(3):483–491

Gross C, Smith BD, Wolf E, Andersen M (2008) Racial disparities in cancer therapy: did the gap narrow between 1992 and 2002? Cancer 112(4):900–908

Gwyn K, Bondy ML, Cohen DS et al (2004) Racial differences in diagnosis, treatment, and clinical delays in a population-based study of patients with newly diagnosed breast carcinoma. Cancer 100(8):1595–1604

Hann D, Baker F, Denniston M et al (2002) The influence of social support on depressive symptoms in cancer patients: age and gender differences. J Psychosom Res 52(5):279–283

Hawley S, Fagerlin A, Janz NK, Katz SJ (2008) Racial/ethnic disparities in knowledge about risks and benefits of breast cancer treatment: does it matter where you go? Health Serv Res 43(4):1366–1387

Hershman D, Buono D, McBride RB et al (2008) Surgeon characteristics and receipt of adjuvant radiotherapy in women with breast cancer. J Natl Cancer Inst 100(3):199–206

Horiot (2007): Radiation therapy and the geriatric oncology patient. J Clinc Oncol 25(14):1930–1935

Huang MH, Schocken M, Block G et al (2002) Variation in nutrient intakes by ethnicity: results from the Study of Women's Health Across the Nation (SWAN). Menopause 9(5):309–319

Hutchins et al. (1999): Under-representation of patients 65 years of age or older in cancer treatment trials. N Engl J Med 341(27):2061–2067

Institute NC. Health disparities defined. http://crchd.cancer.gov/definitions/defined.html. Accessed 5 Dec 2008

Institute of Medicine (2001) Crossing the quality chasm: a new health system for the 21st century. National Academy Press, Washington, DC

Institute of Medicine. Unequal treatment: confronting racial and ethnic disparities in health care. http://www.iom.edu/?id=16740. Accessed 22 Jul 2007

Institute of Medicine (2008) Retooling for an aging America: building the health care workforce. committee on healthcare workforce for older Americans. The National Academies Press, Washington, DC

Jones & Kay (1992): Instrumentation in cross-cultural research. Nurs Res 41(3):186–188

Kagawa-Singer M (1988) Bamboo and oak: Differences in adaptation to cancer between Japanese-American and Anglo-American patients [Unpublished dissertation]. Los Angeles: Anthropology, University of California

Kagawa-Singer M (1996) Cultural Systems Related to Cancer. In: McCorkle R, Grant M, Frank-Stromberg M, Baird SB (eds) Cancer nursing: a comprehensive textbook, 2nd edn. W. B. Saunders Company, Philadelphia, PA, pp 38–52

KMS (2006): Population science is science only if you know the population. J Cancer Educ suppl 21(1):S22–S31

Kagawa-Singer M, Blackhall LJ (2001) Negotiating cross-cultural issues at the end of life: "You got to go where he lives.". Jama 286(23):2993–3001

Kagawa-Singer M, Kassim-Lakha S (2003) A strategy to reduce cross-cultural miscommunication and increase the likelihood of improving health outcomes. Acad Med 78(6):577–587

Kaplan C, Crane LA, Stewart S, Juarez-Reyes M (2004) Factors affecting follow-up among low-income women with breast abnormalities. J Womens Health (Larchmt) 13(2):195–206

Keating N, Landrum MB, Guadagnoli E, Winer E, Ayanian J (2007) Surveillance testing among survivors of early-stage breast cancer. J Clin Oncol 25(9):1074–1081

Kerner J, Yedidia M, Padgett D et al (2003) Realizing the promise of breast cancer screening: clinical follow-up after abnormal screening among Black women. Prev Med 37(2):92–101

Klinkhammer-Shalke M, Koller M, Ehret C et al (2008) Implementing a system of quality-of-life diagnosis and therapy for breast cancer patients: results of an exploratory trial as a prerequisite for a subsequent RCT. Br J Cancer 99(3):415–422

Kotkamp-Mothes N, Slawinsky D, Hindermann S, Strauss B (2005) Coping and psychological well being in families of elderly cancer patients. Crit Rev Oncol Hematol 55(3):213–229

Kumar et al. (2007): Treatment tolerance and efficacy in geriatric oncology: a systematic review of phase III randomized trials conducted by five National Cancer Institute-sponsored cooperative groups. J Clin Oncol 25(10):1272–1276

Li C (2005) Racial and ethnic disparities in breast cancer stage, treatment, and survival in the United States. Ethn Dis 15(2 suppl 2):S5–S9

Lichtman et al. (2007). International society of geriatric oncology chemotherapy taskforce: evaluation of chemotherapy in older patients-an analysis of the medical literature. J Clin Oncol 25(14):1832–1843

Lipsitz L (2004) Physiological complexity, aging, and the path to frailty. Sci Aging Knowl Envir: pe 16

Mahowald M (2000) Genes, women, equality. Oxford University Press, New York, Oxford

Maly RC LB, Silliman RA (2003) Health care disparities in older patients with breast carcinoma: informational support from physicians. Cancer 97(6):1517–1527

Maly RC UY, Leake B, Silliman RA (2005) Mental health outcomes in older women with breast cancer: Impact of perceived family support and adjustment. Psycho-Oncology 14(7):535–545

Maly RC, Umezawa Y, Ratliff CT, Leake B (2006) Racial/ethnic group differences in treatment decision-making and treatment received among older breast carcinoma patients. Cancer 106(4):957–965

Maly R, Stein JA, Umezawa Y, Leake B, Anglin MD (2008) Racial/ethnic differences in breast cancer outcomes among older patients: effects of physician communication and patient empowerment. Health Psychol 27(6):728–736

Murthy V, Krumholz HM, Gross CP (2004) Participation in cancer clinical trials: race-, sex-, and age-based disparities. JAMA 292(8):922

Newman L, Roff NK, Weinberg AD (2008) Cancer clinical trials accrual: missed opportunities to address disparities and missed opportunities to improve outcomes for all. Ann Surg Oncol 15(7):1818–1819

Nussbaum M (1993) Sen, AK. The Quality of Life. Claredon Press, Oxford

O'Brien T (2007) Health care disparity : an overlooked problem in phase I oncology trials. J Clin Oncol 25(21):3182–3183

Painter M, Lavizzo-Mourey R (2008) Aligning forces for quality: a program to improve health and health care in communities across the United States. Health Aff (Millwood) 27(5):1461–1463

Ramirez A, Westcombe AM, Burgess CC, Sutton S, Littlejohns P, Richards MA (1999) Factors predicting delayed presentation of symptomatic breast cancer: a systematic review. Lancet 353(9159):1127–1131

Richards M, Westcombe AM, Love SB, Littlejohns P, Ramirez AJ (1999) Influence of delay on survival in patients with breast cancer: a systematic review. Lancet 353(9159):1119–1126

Shavers V, Brown ML (2002) Racial and ethnic disparities in the receipt of cancer treatment. J Natl Cancer Inst 94(5):334–357

Sherwin S (1988) A relational approach to autonomy in health care. In: The feminist health care ethics research network, the politics of women's health: exploring agency and autonomy. University Press, Philadelphia, PA, pp 19–44

Short L, Fisher MD, Whal P, Kelly M, White S, Rodriguez NA, Lawless GD, Brawley OW (2008) Evaluation of treatment patterns and disparities in commercially insured patients newly-diagnosed with breast cancer. J Clin Oncol ASCO Annual Meeting Proceedings (Post-Meeting Edition) 26(15 S):6593

Smigal et al. (2006). Trends in breast cancer by race and ethnicity: update 2006. CA Cancer J Clin 56(3):168–183

Stewart et al. (2007). Participation in surgical oncology clinical trials: gender-race/ethnicity, and age-based disparities. Ann Surg Oncol 14(12):3328–3334

Struthers & Nichols (2004): Utilization of complementary and alternative medicine among racial and ethnic minority populations: implications for reducing health disparities. Annu Rev Nurs Res 22:285–313

Surbone (2006): Telling truth to patients with cancer: what is the truth? Lancet Oncol 7:944–950

Surbone A (2006b) Cultural aspects of communication in cancer care. In: Stiefel F (ed) Communication in cancer care. Recent results in cancer research. vol 168. Springer, Heidelberg, pp 91–104

Surbone A (2006) Truth telling and ethical issues: an overview. Paper presented at: UICC World Cancer Congress, Washington, DC, USA, 8–12 July 2006

Surbone (2008): Ethical considerations in conducting clinical trials for elderly cancer patients. Aging Health 4:253–260

Surbone A, Kagawa-Singer M, Terret C, Baider L. The illness trajectory of elderly cancer patients age across cultures: SIOG position paper. Ann Oncol, 2006; 18(4):633–638.

Syme SL (2008) Reducing racial and social-class inequalities in health: the need for a new approach. Health Aff (Millwood) 27(2):456–459

Thome et al. (2003). The experience of older people living with cancer. Cancer Nurs 26(2):85–96

US Department of Health and Human Services (DHHS) (1994) Guidelines for industry. Studies in support of special populations: Geriatrics. Rockville, MD: Food and Drug Administration

Weissman J, Betancourt J, Campbell EG, Park E (2005) Resident physicians' preparedness to provide cross-cultural care. JAMA 294(9):1058–1067

Williams D, Yan Y, Jackson JS, Anderson NB (1997) Racial differences in physical and mental health: socioeconomic status, stress and discrimination. J Health Psychol 2(3):335–351

Williams B, Lindquist K, Sudore RL, Covinsky KE, Walter LC (2008) Screening mammography in older women. Effect of wealth and prognosis. Arch Intern Med 168(5):514–520

World Health O (2005a) Resolution on Cancer Control WHA58.22. World Health Organization, Geneva

World Health O (2005b) International plan of action on ageing: report on implementation. Fifty-Eight World Health Assembly, Geneva

World Health O (2008) World Cancer Report 2008. International Agency for Research on Cancer, Lyon

Chapter 24
Supportive, Palliative and End-of-Life Care for Older Breast Cancer Patients

Elaine Cachia, Ruth Broadhurst, and Sam H. Ahmedzai

24.1 Introduction

Breast cancer is predominantly a disease of older women, but the bias towards inclusion of younger patients and exclusion of older ones in clinical studies has led to a relative paucity of specific data on their well-being. In this chapter, therefore, much of the evidence reviewed will be generic to all ages of patients, but whenever age-related changes are known, these will be highlighted. The authors feel justified in this inclusive approach, as the key messages about supportive, palliative, and end-of-life care are still poorly recognized by many professionals, even those providing excellent surgical and oncological care for both younger and older women.

What has been increasingly acknowledged, is that the provision of high-quality cancer care is much more than just making a diagnosis and aiming to "cure" the patient by surgery and maximal adjuvant therapies. The scope of anticancer interventions has changed dramatically in recent years, so that patients can now be offered sequential hormonal manipulations and targeted biological therapies such as trastuzumab, long after the cytotoxic drug regimens have lost effect or their side effects become unacceptable. The concept of "cancer survivorship" has gained acceptance, but it has also changed inherently to include patients living with, as well as beyond, cancer for many years (Fig. 24.1). Thus the new aim of the oncological team should be refocused on supporting more patients to live the rest of their lives WITH cancer, and not abandon those who have failed to achieve a remission (Ahmedzai 2004). With older women who develop breast cancer, the biological impact of the malignancy needs to be seen in the context of the ageing body and mind, with the co-morbidities that come with surviving to the sixth decade and beyond (Satariano and Silliman 2003). For such patients, the cancer may even seem relatively insignificant in comparison to the burden of their other diseases; or for some, their need to care for an equally ageing and dependent male partner. The term

S.H. Ahmedzai (✉)
Academic Unit of Supportive Care, University of Sheffield, Beech Hill Road,
Sheffield, South Yorkshire, S10 2RX, UK
e-mail: s.ahmedzai@sheffield.ac.uk

M.W. Reed and R.A. Audisio (eds.), *Management of Breast Cancer in Older Women*,
DOI 10.1007/978-1-84800-265-4_24, © Springer-Verlag London Limited 2011

Sheffield Model of supportive care
Treating the cancer, patient and family

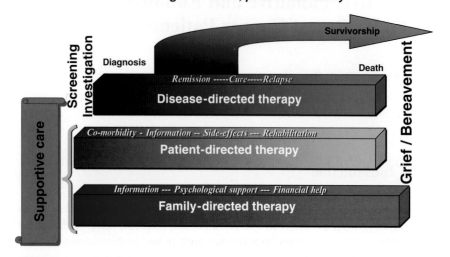

Fig. 24.1 The Sheffield model of supportive care in cancer

which encompasses this range of medical and nonmedical issues is "holistic needs"—this will be clarified below.

In this emerging oncological scenario, issues of quality of life can become as prominent and possibly more relevant to the patient's personal objectives, as the traditional medical endpoints of response and survival. The transition of the patient from oncological care to "terminal" care, which used to be thought of as the domain predominantly of the general practitioner or hospice, is also changing. The cancer team needs to be aware of the changing definitions of "supportive," "palliative," and "end of life" care. These are not euphemistic synonyms of each other – they have come to have specific meanings and are often undertaken by different professional groups.

The science underlying our understanding of symptoms – especially of pain— and how to palliate them, has also undergone a revolution in recent years. However, unlike in oncology, where laboratory discoveries are rapidly translated into clinical studies and then into working guidelines, palliative treatments are slow to be researched in the clinic; thus both guidelines and teaching of new knowledge in palliation often lag behind the scientific evidence. It is likely, therefore, that the surgeon or oncologist who trained more than a decade ago will be relatively unaware of new thinking on the causation of symptoms, and even newly qualified practitioners may be unfamiliar because of the patchy way that these topics are taught at undergraduate or postgraduate levels. Very few countries yet recognize palliative medicine as a legitimate specialty or subspecialty. Even in a "harmonized" region such as the European Union, compared to the trend toward standardization of oncological services, there are large-scale variations in the breadth and depth of palliative care provision and state funding.

24.2   Definitions of Holistic Care in Cancer

"Holistic" is a term that is often used in healthcare, but is poorly understood or interpreted by many healthcare professionals as well as the public. Although it originally signified widening the focus of attention on the "whole" rather than the component parts, in healthcare it has effectively come to mean ensuring that psychological, social, spiritual (or existential) and other nonclinical aspects of the patient's life are considered as being valid and important, alongside the more obvious medical and nursing issues.

In the context of cancer management, holistic care is a very appropriate concept because malignancy affects the patient—and her family and others close to her—in many more ways than the purely medical perspective can embrace. Co-morbidities acquired through life, such as chronic respiratory, cardiac, and arthritic conditions, may already have imposed significant limitations on the patient's well-being and lifestyle (Satariano and Silliman 2003). In later life, many women will have established families and have expectations and even duties of care for grandchildren as well as ageing partners. A truly holistic approach to cancer care is thus very difficult for any one team or service to achieve, because of inherent limitations on their staffing, experience, and resources. Usually, this can be realized by the patient being cared for by a range of services both within and outside the traditional healthcare settings, e.g., patient self-help groups, complementary therapy centers, hospices and, increasingly, Internet-based resources. Nevertheless, it is appropriate for cancer teams to evaluate their own role in the overall management of patients, putting the medical investigations and management into perspective of the patient's own stage in life and her expectations and choices.

There has been much confusion over the terms "palliative care," "palliation," "terminal care," "end of life care," "care of the dying," and so on. Because these are not precise biomedical concepts, it is likely that there will never be exact definitions for them which are as specific as those for staging, response, or progression of disease itself. International variations in the level of provision of holistic care, as well as nuances of meaning attached to these words in different languages and cultures, mean that it can be hard to compare services across regions of the world.

The World Health Organisation (WHO) issued a new definition of palliative care in 2002: "Palliative care improves the quality of life of patients and families who face life-threatening illness, by providing pain and symptom relief, spiritual and psychosocial support from diagnosis to the end of life and bereavement.

Palliative care provides relief from pain and other distressing symptoms

- Affirms life and regards dying as a normal process
- Intends neither to hasten or postpone death
- Integrates the psychological and spiritual aspects of patient care
- Offers a support system to help patients live as actively as possible until death
- Offers a support system to help the family cope during the patients illness and in their own bereavement

- Uses a team approach to address the needs of patients and their families, including bereavement counselling, if indicated;
- Will enhance quality of life, and may also positively influence the course of illness
- Is applicable early in the course of illness, in conjunction with other therapies that are intended to prolong life, such as chemotherapy or radiation therapy, and includes those investigations needed to better understand and manage distressing clinical complications." (WHO 2002)

The difficulty of such a comprehensive definition and description is that is can be almost too broad a concept for busy cancer clinicians to hold in mind, as they are struggling with the advancing disease and are trying to balance another round of anticancer treatment with diminishing returns, against increasing frailty of the patient. It is not surprising, therefore, that in many oncology settings, patients are treated "actively" (that is, with disease-modifying therapies) until it is very late and the patient resists—and then she is referred back to the GP or to a local hospice or palliative care service for what is assumed to be "nonactive," symptom-modifying treatments. In reality, when patients are transferred suddenly from acute anticancer management to end-of-life services, the transition is psychologically devastating for many. This dichotomous view of cancer care is no longer valid or helpful to the patient and family.

For this reason, the concept of "supportive care" has rapidly been gaining acceptance. Initially, this term was used rather specifically for medical interventions that supported the patient to undergo more and more intensive anticancer treatments without toxicity. Thus, blood and platelet transfusions, hematopoietic growth factors, antiemetics, antibiotic and antifungal regimens were the early tools of supportive care. In recent years, there has been a shift in emphasis in which some have argued that supportive care should embrace not only those therapies, but other interventions aimed at relieving symptoms and preserving functioning and quality of life at all stages of disease—not just in the final stages, where palliative care is focused (Ahmedzai 2001).

The Multinational Association for Supportive Care in Cancer (MASCC) has defined supportive care as: *"The prevention and management of the adverse effects of cancer and its treatment. This includes physical and psychosocial symptoms and side effects across the entire continuum of the cancer experience including the enhancement of rehabilitation and survivorship."* (MASCC website)

In the UK, the National Institute for Clinical Excellence (NICE) also offered a definition of supportive care in its guidance for cancer patients in 2004: *"[supportive care] . . . helps the patient and their family to cope with cancer and treatment of it—from pre-diagnosis, through the process of diagnosis and treatment, to cure, continuing illness or death and into bereavement. It helps the patient to maximise the benefits of treatment and to live as well as possible with the effects of the disease. It is given equal priority alongside diagnosis and treatment."* (NICE 2004)

Taking these two definitions of supportive care, it is evident that the *concept* of supportive care differs from palliative care in that it:

- Starts earlier in the disease, actually from the time of diagnosis
- Embraces both symptom-modifying and disease-modifying objectives
- Continues after cancer is in remission, i.e., into "survivorship"

In *practice*, supportive care differs from palliative care by:

- Being managed by a much broader, often "virtual," team (sometimes called a "comprehensive cancer care team") than the traditional palliative care service offers
- Taking place alongside anticancer disease management, often through joint clinics and shared care in hospital wards, rather than as a dichotomous two-stage process

To put it another way, supportive care exists in parallel with disease-modifying anticancer treatments and even beyond, into long-term survivorship; while palliative care is a subset of supportive care, focusing almost exclusively on the advanced stages of disease until death and bereavement. To provide supportive care in a timely way, its professionals need to be well-integrated in the oncology service. Palliative care services, on the other hand, are usually separate from oncology but need to liaise with them as well as with primary care.

Because supportive care is a relatively new concept compared to palliative care, models of how it can function are still developing and are likely to evolve further as the medical armamentarium of oncology itself develops, e.g., by the growing use of biological therapies and drugs such as bisphosphonates, which can palliate but also modify the disease process (Smyth 2007; Ahmedzai 2004; Rabow et al. 2004; Porta-Sales et al. 2008). Figure 24.2 shows the "Sheffield model" of supportive care in relation to oncology and palliative care.

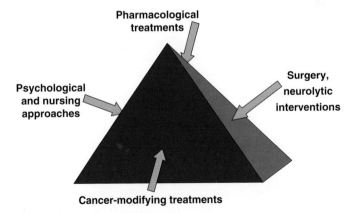

Fig. 24.2 The pyramid model of symptom palliation of pain

The terms "end of life care" and "terminal care" are still interpreted variably in different settings. In general, they should be used for patients who are acknowledged to be in the most advanced stage of disease, usually (but not exclusively) when anticancer treatments have run out of options, and for whom the focus of care is allowing the patient to spend maximum time with her family. In breast cancer, for some patients this period will last a few weeks or months at most; for others, owing to the variable type of disease progression and unpredictable responses to late applied therapies, it may continue for a year or more. It should be noted that supportive care teams and those palliative care teams which do accept patients long before they are "dying," often use the terms "end of life care" and "terminal care" to signify when the patient has actually reached the last few days of life.

24.3 Assessment of Holistic Needs

The UK's NICE guidance for supportive and palliative care in cancer (2004) emphasized probably for the first time in a national document, the importance of making a "holistic assessment" of the patient's needs. What is meant by this term has been clarified by more recent work by various groups, but there is as yet, by no means a global standard for how this is to be done, in comparison to the classification of histology or the staging of disease extent (Richardson et al. 2005). Some of the assessment methods have focused, rather predictably, on patients in the more advanced stages, because that is usually when palliative care services which have the resources to make such assessments, first come into contact with the patient (Barresi et al. 2003). Other needs assessment approaches have tried to be more inclusive and applicable earlier upstream, as well as applying in long-term remission and survivorship (Wen and Gustafson 2004).

An example of a new tool for assessing holistic needs in cancer (and also noncancer) patients, at any stage of disease, is the Sheffield profile for assessment and referral for care (SPARC) (Ahmed et al. 2009). This has been rigorously developed and validated psychometrically, to provide a screening for several dimensions of holistic needs regardless of the disease or stage of disease. The domains that SPARC covers are shown in Table 24.1. Another tool which is also being taken up

Table 24.1 Changing aims of oncology

Original aims	Modern aims
Diagnosis	Prevention
Cure	Early and accurate diagnosis
Palliation	Cure
	Prolonging life
	Palliation
	Rehabilitation
	End-of-life care

Table 24.2 Domains of holistic needs screened by sparc[a] and distress thermometer[b]

Domain	SPARC	Distress thermometer
Professional contacts made	✓	✗
Physical symptoms	✓	✓
Psychological needs	✓	✓
Religious and spiritual issues	✓	✓
Sexual issues	✓	✓
Family and social issues	✓	✓
Housing and transportation issues	✗	✓
Issues around treatment	✓	✓
Help with personal affairs	✓	✗
Need to talk with professionals	✓	✗
Information needs	✓	✗

[a]Sheffield Profile for Assessment and Referral for Care (Ahmed et al. 2009)
[b]Ref Bulli 2008

by cancer services is the "Distress Thermometer." This is basically a single-item visual analogue scale (VAS) which, when used with an accompanying problem checklist, can elicit a range of physical and psychosocial issues affecting the patient (Bulli et al. 2009). The range of problems picked up this approach is shown in Table 24.2, to contrast with those assessed by SPARC.

It is important to recognize that these tools are not meant to be diagnostic – rather, they indicate the presence (and with SPARC, the severity) of a problem area which ideally needs to be explored further with the patient and probably her family. The tools are meant to be completed by the patient, perhaps with assistance for the very old or those who are frail, but acted on by a multidisciplinary team. In practice, it is usually the specialist nurse based in the cancer team who will be responsible for administering the needs assessment and acting on the results. These measurements should be done at specific points in the disease process—soon after diagnosis, after completion of primary treatment, at intervals during later treatment and in follow-up and more frequently when the disease is progressive (Richardson et al. 2005).

An aspect of assessment that is usually overlooked is attempting to make a more precise estimation of the patient's prognosis. This is less relevant in the new supportive care model, because patients are considered for supportive therapies regardless of the stage of disease and estimated prognosis, compared to the traditional palliative care model where referral to the service will depend on someone—usually the oncologist or a general practitioner – making a prognosis of a short lifespan. Unfortunately, clinicians are notoriously unreliable at making prognoses in cancer and other life-limiting diseases, often erring on the side of being overoptimistic. This can lead to significant delays in referring patients to appropriate palliative and end-of-life care services – often such teams complain of being sent patients when it is "too late" for them to have a useful impact on the patient's and family's well-being.

The "Palliative Prognostic Index" has been developed to overcome this problem in unreliable prognostication (Stone et al. 2008). The prognosis is computed from simple scoring for performance status, oral intake, presence of edema, dyspnea at rest, and delirium. Although not always accurate, it has been shown in different settings and cultures to have a positive predictive value of between 80 and 91%, a sensitivity between 56 and 83% and a specificity between 85 and 94%. The routine incorporation of prognostic scoring systems such as this, together with a validated holistic needs assessment, would mean that many more cancer patients could receive the appropriate levels of supportive and palliative care, at the right time in their lives.

The relevance of this was shown in a survey of all patients (cancer and noncancer) admitted to a UK university hospital, who met specific criteria for inclusion under the scope of palliative or end-of-life care. (Gott et al. 2001) It was found that ward-based doctors and nurses identified roughly similar numbers of patients who they thought should be referred to the hospital palliative care team—but on inspection, they were identifying quite different patients, for different professional and personal reasons. It is interesting that the concordance of medical and nursing views about referral grew larger as the estimated prognosis was shorter. The need for standardization of whom and when to refer patients for supportive and palliative care is therefore amply clear (Ahmed et al. 2004).

24.4   What Are the Clinical Issues for Older Women with Breast Cancer?

Although the term "quality of life" in cancer has been in use for a long time, it was when it became an endpoint in clinical trials that the science of measuring it became established. As a result of the last two decades of "quality of life" research, we now understand much more about the clinical problems faced by breast cancer patients at all stages of their disease. An extensive review of "quality of life" literature in breast cancer yielded 477 studies covering nearly 30 years from 1974 to 2007 (Montazeri 2008). It revealed that the main instruments used are the EORTC QLQ-C30 with its breast cancer module EORTC QLQ-BR23, and the FACIT-G with its breast cancer module FACIT-B. In general, FACIT tools are used extensively in USA while EORTC tools are used in Europe, Canada, and many other countries. They are broadly similar in approach and cover similar domains, namely selected physical symptoms, multiple aspects of functioning, and global "quality of life" assessment.

The most commonly reported symptoms in breast cancer were pain, fatigue, arm morbidity, and postmenopausal symptoms. A particular aspect of functioning which is often overlooked in the clinic, but which these tools did pick up, was sexuality. The literature review also found that, in common with other cancers that have been studied, patient's self-rated quality of life in advanced stages of disease (but not in early stage disease) was an independent predictor of survival. In particular, physical symptoms such as pain, loss of appetite, and overall physical health have prognostic value, but psychological and social aspects of quality of life do not.

The START trial in the UK assessed quality of life in patients with breast cancer who were randomized to different radiation therapy regimens (Hopwood et al. 2007). An analysis of 2,208 patients who were entered examined the effects of age and clinical factors on quality of life, measured using EORTC QLQ-C30 and BR-23. The mean age of the sample was 57 years (range 26–87); poorer quality of life was found in both younger and older extremes, for different domains. Chemotherapy affected most "quality of life" domains negatively, especially for body image, sexual functioning, and breast and arm symptoms. Mastectomy was associated with more body image concerns, while wide local excision surgery had more arm symptoms. Interestingly, endocrine therapy did not affect quality of life. With respect to age, it was younger women (<50 years) who had the greatest "quality of life" impairment in respect of anxiety, body image, and breast symptoms. Age had no effect on the reporting of depression.

Another large UK trial (PRIME) assessed the effect of omitting radiation therapy from the management following breast-conserving therapy in older women aged over 65 years (Prescott et al. 2007). Although overall quality of life was not improved by the omission of radiation treatment, there were short-term benefits in terms of fatigue, insomnia, and endocrine effects. Issues regarding transport for treatment also caused some concern for these older women. In contrast, patients in follow-up expressed more worries about recurrence if they had not had radiation treatment. Cosmetic results were better in those who did not have radiation, but interestingly this did not seem to be an important issue for this group of patients. The health economic analysis accompanying this study showed identical health values with greater cost associated with treatment, suggesting that, at least for the first 15 months, radiation treatment was not cost-effective for this older age group.

In overview, the literature indicates that it is younger women with breast cancer who have the greater psychological adjustment problems. Research on psychological function suggest that older females adjust more easily both postsurgery and at one year postdiagnosis than younger females with breast cancer. In a US study of 304 women enrolled in a trial of psychosocial telephone counseling immediately after treatment, it was found that women under 50 years had significantly greater "quality of life" disturbance with respect to emotional well-being, depression, breast cancer specific concerns, and disease-specific intrusive thoughts (Wenzel et al. 1999). There were no age differences for sexual dysfunction or body image differences.

However, women who are older at the time of diagnosis of breast cancer are more likely to suffer decreased physical function, physical and emotional role function, vitality, and social function, compared with nonbreast cancer females. (Kroenke et al. 2004) It is noteworthy that physical decline will occur in all elderly females and much of the deterioration observed in breast cancer studies may simply be age-related.

As patients move in to "survivorship," their concerns shift from the more physical to ones about the future. In a study of 321 long-term (5 years+) older cancer survivors (mean age 72 years) attending a major US cancer center, 41% of the sample had breast cancer (Deimling et al. 2006). The main concerns expressed by these patients were—cancer coming back (31% of patients), symptoms indicate recurrence of cancer (36%), developing another type of cancer (30%), and future diagnostic tests (36%). It was noteworthy that older breast cancer survivors had generally fewer concerns of these types than patients with colorectal or prostate cancers. Increasing age itself was a weak but significant correlate for a reduced level of concern about symptoms indicating recurrence, developing another cancer and cancer-related health worries.

A more recent Dutch study has confirmed the findings about breast cancer patients' concerns about recurrence (van den Beuken-van Everdingen et al. 2008). A cohort of 136 patients (mean age 59 years), of whom most had completed their primary curative treatment within the last 6 months, were given the Dutch language version of the "concerns about recurrence scale" (CARS). Moderate-to-high levels of fear of recurrence were found in 56% of subjects: worries about health and death were the most prominent. Pain was a strong predictor of fear. However, the prevalence of fear about health, death, and role functioning decreased significantly with increased age. In contrast, women with a higher education level expressed more fears.

A resource which is increasingly used by cancer patients with raised levels of anxiety about their illness is the worldwide web and Internet-based information and support services. One US study reported that eight months after diagnosis, the top three information sources used by women with breast cancer were books (64%), the Internet (49%), and videos (41%). However, at follow-up (16 months after diagnosis), the most frequently cited information source was the Internet (40%), followed by books (33%), and the American Cancer Society (17%). The study found that women continued to use the Internet as a means of gathering information even after their treatment ended. Significant unique predictors of Internet use were more years of formal education and younger ages. Cancer stage was not a significant predictor of Internet use (Satterlund et al. 2003).

In another study of breast cancer patient usage of the Internet, 42% used it for medical information. Internet users differed from nonusers on income level, educational level, and by race/ethnicity. After controlling for the other predictors, Internet users had a higher income ($OR = 3.10$; 95% $CI = 1.09$–8.85) and tended to be more educated ($OR = 2.59$; 95% $CI = 0.87$–7.74) than nonusers. There was also a suggestion that those of non-White ethnicity were less likely to use the Internet ($OR = 0.39$; 95% $CI = 0.14$–1.11). Increasing age, length of time since diagnosis, and breast cancer stage had no effect (Fogel et al. 2002a). In another study by the same group, 188 breast cancer Internet users were interviewed. Forty-two percent used the Internet for medical information related to breast health issues and did so for an average of 0.80 h per week. The Interpersonal Support Evaluation List and the UCLA Loneliness Scale, with results controlled for covariates, showed that Internet use for breast health issues was associated with greater social support and less loneliness than Internet use for other purposes or nonuse. Thus breast cancer patients may obtain these psychological benefits with only a minimal weekly time commitment (Fogel et al. 2002b).

Recent research with other cancer types has given further insight into the uses and benefits of Internet information and support. In one study of 175 mixed cancer patients, Internet use, either directly or via friend or family, was widespread and reported by patients at all stages of cancer care, from early investigations to follow-up after treatment. Patients used the Internet to find second opinions, seek support and experiential information from other patients, interpret symptoms, seek information about tests and treatments, help interpret consultations, identify questions for doctors, make anonymous private inquiries, and raise awareness of the cancer. Patients also used it to check their doctors' advice covertly and to develop an expertise in their cancer. This expertise, reflecting familiarity with computer technology and medical terms, enabled patients to present a new type of "social fitness" (Ziebland et al. 2004).

This conclusion was supported by another very recent Dutch study in mixed cancer patient Internet users, which showed that some patients are becoming more demanding of what electronic communications can do for them. Of the 261 (75%) patients who responded, 60% used the Internet by themselves, 9% via others, whereas 31% did not use the Internet. High education, young age, and high socioeconomic status were all independently positively associated with Internet use. Of the patients with complaints but prediagnosis, 41% searched the Internet for information about cancer daily to several times a week. After diagnosis, during treatment, and at follow-up, this was, respectively, 71%, 56%, and 4%. Although patients preferred to get reliable information from the website of their oncologist (88%), hospital (70%), or Dutch Cancer Society (76%), websites that are completely financed and created by pharmaceutical industry were mentioned most as the source of information. Patients who used the Internet to find information about cancer felt themselves to be better informed about their disease (72%); only 3% thought that consulting the Internet increased the frequency of visiting their doctor, whereas 20% felt that information from the Internet influenced the treatment decision made by their doctor. Most patients who used the Internet stated that they would like to be able to access their own medical file (79%) or test results (81%) if possible (van de Poll-Franse and van Eenbergen 2008).

24.5 Symptoms and Principles of Their Palliation

It is beyond the scope of this chapter to provide an in-depth coverage of all the specific symptoms which may arise for older women with breast cancer. Instead, we will make general points about the approach to understanding and tackling symptoms, and about the principles underlying a modern scientific approach to palliating them. Some key symptoms will be discussed to illustrate this approach, but for details on the specific management of individual symptoms, the reader is directed to the many comprehensive accessible textbooks and pocketbooks of palliative medicine and therapeutics of palliation (Twycross and Wilcock 2002; Twycross and Wilcock 2008a, 2008b; Watson 2009).

Symptoms are essentially bodily sensations that cause distress to the individual to varying extents. Many sensations that are experienced in normal everyday life are seen as temporary inconveniences if they are attributable to a known cause and disappear when the cause is removed, e.g., breathlessness on running for a bus or climbing up several flights of stairs, aching muscles after a heavy gym workout or skiing, or nausea associated with travel sickness. These sensations may become worrying or bothersome to the person if:

- The cause is not clear, e.g., breathlessness at rest.
- The sensation is associated with a possible sinister cause, e.g., pain arising in a person with previous cancer.
- The intensity of the sensation is out of keeping with the known or putative cause.
- The person is psychologically distressed for other reasons.

In a person who has recently been diagnosed and treated for cancer, it is easily possible for what might have been previously regarded as normal or transient sensations, to take on a new disturbing significance. Thus, when assessing a patient with cancer who expresses symptoms, it is important to take a few minutes to understand the context of that symptom in the person's life at that time.

Often the symptom is self-evidently related to overt pathology or an iatrogenic cause, e.g., pain arising from a pathological fracture of a limb bone or pain persisting in the wound days after recent surgery. When the cause is within the body and unseen to the patient, it is important to share medical information and explanations, as often ignorance and imagination can lead to a heightened sense of concern and may even exaggerate the intensity of the symptom. Reassurance is very powerful in symptom management, but it must not be gratuitous or a replacement for effective intervention if that is possible. As previously mentioned, co-morbidity is a common occurrence in older people with cancer and so it is important to determine whether a "new" symptom is actually associated with coexisting nonmalignant disease. This may be especially difficult to diagnose if the symptom shares features of both cancer and noncancer disease—for example, back pain in a patient with age-related osteoporosis or degenerative vertebral disease who later develops vertebral bone metastases; or breathlessness in a patient with COPD and new evidence of malignant pleural effusion.

Detailed assessment is central to good symptom management. If the patient has completed a holistic needs assessment tool such as SPARC, many symptoms will already have been identified and scored for their degree of bother or concern. Key aspects of a symptom which are useful to characterize are listed in Table 24.3. It takes only a few minutes to evaluate these and failing to do so can lead to weeks or longer of misplaced reassurance and wrong or potentially harmful interventions. With older people, in particular those with cognitive impairment, special care must be taken to ensure that they understand the questions. The assessment of pain has probably been the most developed in this context (see below). An important question in assessing a new or deteriorating symptom is—"What treatments have been used for similar symptoms in the past, and how helpful/harmful were they?" Asking

Table 24.3 Key aspects of assessing symptoms

Topic	Example/relevance
Time of onset	Is this actually a chronic con-morbid problem?
Provoking factors	Incident pain caused by skeletal metastasis
Relieving factors	Comfortable positions, helpful self-treatments
Site of symptom	Pain, itching, swelling, etc.
Spread or radiation	Dermatomal distribution of nerve root pain
Impact on functioning	How much does it restrict activity?
Current medical treatments	Detailed list of drugs; check for interactions and incompatibilities
Previous medical treatments	Avoid reusing unhelpful or harmful treatments
Preferences for medication and procedures	Oral or patch? Willingness to be admitted for procedure?
Check with family caregiver	Patient is uncommunicative, e.g., cognitively impaired or withdrawn
Review	Check on symptom and response to intervention after suitable time – modify to start new intervention if not improved or intolerable side effects

this question can avoid re-presenting inappropriate or potentially dangerous treatments to a person. Unfortunately it is not uncommon for older people to have vague or unreliable memories of previous drugs or other interventions. It is helpful then to ask a family carer or the patient's GP if hospital notes are not available.

A symptom only arises in the consciousness of a person when it has been processed in the brain (Dalal et al. 2006). Functional magnetic resonance imaging (fMRI) and positron emission tomography (PET) have given fascinating insights in the past decade into the topography of symptom perception in the human brain, and also how intrinsic neuronal mechanisms and pharmacological manipulations can modulate these (Apkarian et al. 2005). It has been shown, for example, that experimentally induced pain in volunteers is correlated to a high degree with oxygenated blood flow changes in key areas of the higher brain such as the primary and secondary somatosensory, insular, anterior cingulate, and prefrontal cortices. Experimentally induced breathlessness (air hunger) has similarly been found to cause activation on fMRI in the anterior cingulate and insula, but also activates other areas in the operculum, cerebellum, amygdala, thalamus, and basal ganglia (Evans et al. 2002). The science of neuroimaging of symptoms is still developing, but may present great prospects for increasing our understanding of how symptoms are generated in the consciousness and how pharmacological and other interventions—including the "placebo response"—can impinge on these (Colloca and Benedetti 2005; Borsook and Becerra 2006).

How much should a patient be clinically investigated to elucidate a symptom? This is sometimes a difficult question, for example, if the patient is objectively well and in remission from cancer and it may be thought that pursuing a "symptom" with extensive tests may heighten unnecessary anxiety. However, unresolved fears about a perceived symptom may itself raise anxiety levels which could potentially aggravate even pathologically based symptoms. A typical situation is an ambulant patient, several months after completing chemotherapy, who starts to have dyspepsia, nausea, and intermittent vomiting. This may bring back memories of severe chemotherapy emesis and the patient may become very anxious and even phobic about returning to hospital. If simple blood tests exclude hepatic or renal impairment and hypercalcemia, then a difficult choice may be to give reassurance with a prokinetic antiemetic such as domperidone, or to proceed to an upper gastrointestinal endoscopy. With the latter option, if acid-related gastritis or frank peptic ulceration is found, this can be treated specifically and the symptoms should resolve promptly. If the endoscopy is negative, at least the patient can be reassured and referred for psychological help such as relaxation training, or she can be prescribed a mild anxiolytic such as lorazepam to be taken when the tension builds up.

Another difficult scenario with respect to investigation of symptoms is when the patient may be very ill and approaching the terminal stage. Such a patient may become progressively more breathless, so that she is increasingly immobilized and become chair- and bed-bound. If she is at home, the choice is to treat the dyspnea symptomatically which may include sedation—or to arrange for hemoglobin, oxygen saturation, chest radiograph, and possibly ultrasound if pleural or pericardial effusion is clinically suspected. Taking a blood test is easy and undemanding of the patient—most individuals, even when terminally ill, would consent to blood tests (Meystre et al. 1997). Being moved to hospital for the imaging tests may seem to professionals to represent a significant burden to the patient, but many would still agree to this if the potential gain were made clear. The crucial step before ordering investigations is to make a thorough clinical evaluation of the patient. If then, potentially treatable conditions such as effusions or even pulmonary embolism are raised in the differential diagnosis, an honest discussion should take place with the patient, her family, and preferably her family doctor. It would be unreasonable and poor medical practice to assume that any of these serious medical conditions are established and untreatable and to start sedating the patient without her understanding and agreement.

It is useful to have a formal evaluation of symptoms at all stages of breast cancer and the tools mentioned above, such as SPARC or the Distress Thermometer may be especially helpful as they pick up the psychological and social consequences as well as the symptom itself (Ahmed et al. 2009; Bulli et al. 2009). At the least, patients should be asked to rate the symptoms in question on a 0–10 numerical scale. This is quite intuitive for most people, but it is important to ensure that the patient is using '0' as no symptom and '10' as the worst possible intensity of the symptom. Verbal scales such as "none-mild-moderate- severe" may seem easier to use conversationally but are less sensitive to change and there may be considerable interindividual differences in personal interpretations of these levels (Jensen et al. 2002). The least useful assessment method clinically is the written visual analogue scale: this may be hard for older people and those with cognitive impairment to perform and it should be confined to the setting of clinical studies.

Once a symptom has been evaluated and diagnosed and treatment is being planned, it is important to keep the patient fully informed. Compliance with medical management with drugs is likely to be higher and safer if the patient has a good understanding of the reasons for each new drug treatment and has been given a written summary of the drugs and how they should be taken. With respect to the older patient, the treatment plan needs to take into account the known biological changes that occur with respect to effects of ageing on physiological systems and the ability to metabolize drugs as well as reduced capacity of older people to withstand adverse effects such as sedation and cardiovascular events (Goodlin 2004).

The effect of ageing influences all physiological bodily systems and this requires drug selection and correction of drug dosage. The pharmacokinetics of many drugs changes with age and this reduces the tolerance of normal tissues. Absorption may be decreased in the elderly while the progressive reduction of total body water and decrease of plasma protein concentration leads to a decreased volume of distribution with consequently increased serum concentrations and potential for toxicity of drugs. Drug excretion via the kidneys also declines with age. Hepatic metabolism that is affected by age is mainly via the p-450 cytochrome enzymes while glucuronidation is rarely influenced (Turnheim 2003; Monfardini 2002).

24.6 Key Symptoms and Psychosocial Well-Being

Although there are relatively few studies on the natural history of symptoms and well-being in older breast cancer patients, controlled clinical trials in which "quality of life" measures such as the EORTC or FACT scales, or in earlier studies the Rotterdam Symptom Checklist, have provided some insight into the symptom burden in these highly selected populations. However, in recent years the growth of interest in long-term survivorship has led to a surge of new studies in symptoms, well-being, and quality of life in cancer patients which have started to shed light on the influence on age (Stava et al., 2006; Perkins et al. 2007; Mehnert and Koch 2008; Zebrack et al. 2008; Ballinger and Fallowfield 2009).

24.6.1 Arm Morbidity and Lymphedema

A common finding in breast cancer studies is the occurrence of arm morbidity which includes pain and lymphedema. Overall about 30% of breast cancer patients have metastatic spread to the axilla and again overall 30% will develop secondary lymphedema; this figure rises to 56% if there has been axillary lymph-node dissection (Morrell et al. 2005; Moseley et al. 2007). A population-based telephone survey of 1,338 older breast cancer patients (aged 65–89 years) showed that up to 4 years following surgery, altogether 14% had arm lymphedema; this broke down to 7% for those who had undergone sentinel lymph-node biopsy and 21% who had axillary lymph-node dissection (Yen et al. 2009). However, the number of lymph nodes removed and the presence of lymph-node metastasis was more predictive of future lymphedema than the type of surgery.

Early studies (before 2000) served the purpose of highlighting this area of concern for patients, but they have been heavily criticized for methodological flaws (Poole and Fallowfield 2002). One review found only 6 out of 15 to be robust enough to analyze and even in these there was a high variation in prevalence of lymphedema (6–43%), pain (12–51%), reduced range of movement of the arm (2–51%), and decreased muscle strength (17–33%) (Rietman et al. 2003). Another recent systematic review again found weaknesses in the research, with only six out of ten studies having a control group (Kligman et al. 2004). It is clear that lymphedema not only causes pain and restriction of movement but brings significant psychological and social impact (McWayne and Helney 2005). The former consists of general distress and frustration at loss of functioning and impaired body image. Obese women (BMI >25) are more likely to report distress. Lack of information about lymphedema was found to be a predictor of subsequent anxiety and depression. Social sequelae include restrictions in interacting with family and friends as well as loss of independence and inability to work, do household tasks and hobbies. The visible disfigurement leads to avoidance of certain types of clothing and this is especially a problem in the summer. The presence of arm pain is itself a significant predictor of psychological and social morbidity.

The findings from these literature reviews were confirmed in a recent exhaustive study of 128 women with breast cancer (mean age 58 years, 64 with lymphedema) which used the FACTB "quality of life" questionnaire for breast cancer, an ad hoc 52-item symptom checklist, and 18-item questionnaire on skin/arm condition, an 11-item depression scale, and a 37-item short form of the profile of mood states (POMS) tool, as well as detailed measurement of lymphedema using a bioelectric impedance device (Ridner 2005). Women with lymphedema scored worse for quality of life and those with >10% difference in arm size reported more symptoms of arm discomfort, loss of confidence, fatigue, and psychological distress. BMI was a covariate for all significant outcomes. A "symptom cluster" was identified consisting of alteration in limb sensation, loss of confidence in body, decreased physical activity, and psychological distress. Neither the literature reviews nor this questionnaire study identified specific risk factors for lymphedema with respect to age of the patient.

It is beyond the scope of this chapter to detail the management of arm lymphedema: several techniques have been described ranging from limb elevation and simple limb exercises to compression garments (graduated compression over limb), compression bandaging, pneumatic pumps around limb to encourage fluid drainage proximally, manual lymphatic drainage using light massage and complex physical therapy including manual lymphatic drainage, compression bandaging, skin care, and limb exercises (Twycross et al. 2000; Harris et al. 2001; Moseley et al. 2007). It is useful to teach partners as well as patients to perform daily massage. Pharmacological approaches are generally unsuccessful; there is no evidence that diuretics are helpful. An important practical point for clinicians is that a difference of 2.0 cm between arms at any of the recommended points could warrant referral for specific lymphedema management (Harris 2001).

24.6.2 Fatigue

Cancer-related fatigue is defined by the US National Comprehensive Cancer Network as "a persistent, subjective sense of tiredness related to cancer or cancer treatment that interferes with usual functioning"(NCCN web address). In most surveys of cancer patients, regardless of the stage of disease, fatigue (also referred to as "weakness," "tiredness," or "asthenia") is the most prevalent symptom (Winters-Stone 2008).

Fatigue is caused and modified by multifactorial etiology, psychological factors, and patients' perceptions. The pathophysiology of fatigue is not fully understood. It can be caused directly by the tumor, either through peripheral mechanisms such as raised energy expenditure or by central mechanisms such as dysregulation of the hypothalamic-pituitary-adrenal axis or serotonin metabolism (Bower et al. 2005). Both of these mechanisms may ultimately be related to high circulating levels of cytokines which are produced as a host response to cancer. Surgery, chemotherapy, radiation therapy, and even the new biological treatments for cancer can have short- and long-term effects that generate fatigue. For example, doxorubicin is now understood to have a direct negative effect on skeletal muscle as well as its known cardiotoxicity effect (van Norren et al. 2009). Pathophysiological factors that contribute to the development of fatigue include anemia, fever, infections or metabolic complications, as well as sedative drugs for symptom control that can produce secondary fatigue (Ahlberg et al. 2003; Rao and Cohen 2004). Hypothyroidism was found in 14% of older breast cancer patients and as this was not directly related to irradiation of the thyroid area, it probably represents a co-morbid effect of ageing (Smyth 2007).

A US study of 48 breast cancer survivors (mean age 68 years, range 60–89) with a mean time 7.5 years from diagnosis, found that 48% experienced fatigue (Winters-Stone et al. 2008). The key factors correlated with fatigue were age, lower extremity muscle strength, and physical activity levels. Surprisingly, the age correlations were all inverse, i.e., older women reported less fatigue than younger women.

In a study of advanced British cancer patients, it was found that the prevalence of fatigue amongst patients with solid tumors was as high as 75% when compared with a control group of age and sex-matched volunteers without cancer (Stone et al. 1999). In this palliative care study the severity of fatigue was unrelated to age, sex, diagnosis, presence or site of metastases, anemia, dose of opioid or steroid, any of the hematological or biochemical indices (except urea), nutritional status, voluntary muscle function, or mood.

There are several fatigue assessment tools that have been tested for reliability and are valid in cancer populations, e.g., Piper Fatigue scale, the Brief Fatigue Inventory, Schwartz Cancer Fatigue Scale, and the Multidimensional Fatigue Inventory. Of note, none of these scales have been specifically validated in elderly cancer patients. Two scales that could be useful in the elderly cancer patient are the Brief Fatigue Inventory, which has nine items; and the Schwartz Fatigue Scale, which has only six items (Rao and Cohen 2004; Winters-Stone et al. 2008).

The management of fatigue should include treating the cause where possible, to remove or modify potential etiologies and the correction of metabolic and electrolyte disturbances, and symptomatic or palliative treatment with pharmacological and nonpharmacological interventions (Mock 2004). Easy-to-understand information and education of patients about their disease and treatment is also crucial so that patients know what to expect as disease progresses and can adopt management strategies and adhere to treatments (Ahlberg et al. 2003).

Correction of anemia with blood transfusion may bring short-term relief but longer-term benefits have been shown in several studies of mixed cancer types using the growth factor erythropoietin (Mock 2004). However, blood transfusions carry significant medical risks and both they and erythropoietin are expensive options. Moreover, the majority of patients with cancer-related fatigue are not usually significantly anemic.

A recent Cochrane review of drug treatment for the management of cancer related fatigue supports the use of psychostimulants. Side effects may be dose limiting and for methylphenidate include nervousness, irritability, agitation and sometimes cardiac side effects such as arrhythmia and tachycardia. (Minton et al. 2008) On the other hand, there is no evidence for the use of steroids in fatigue.

Whereas in the past the preferred nonpharmacological treatment for fatigue was to take rest, it is now known that inactivity is likely to be counterproductive as it leads to muscle wasting and a loss of cardio-respiratory fitness (called de-conditioning), generating increased fatigue. There have been several studies of exercise programs in cancer patients, both during and after treatment. A Cochrane review and meta-analysis of 28 studies including 2,083 patients (majority breast cancer—16 studies with 1,172 participants) showed a statistically significant net benefit of exercise compared to control (Cramp and Daniel 2008). More recently, another Cochrane review of exercise focusing just on breast cancer patients receiving adjuvant therapy analyzed nine studies involving 452 women (Markes et al. 2006). The meta-analyses showed that for cardiorespiratory fitness ($n=207$) there was a statistically significant improvement of exercise vs. control, but for fatigue ($n=317$) the improvement was not significant. Adverse effects of lymphedema and shoulder tendonitis were noted in two trials, indicating the potential harm even from non-pharmacological therapeutic modalities. There are insufficient data from these studies so far to know if there is a specific benefit of exercise for older patients. A qualitative British study of 29 older breast cancer survivors (mean age 67 years, range 59–86) involving interviews and focus groups identified that these women preferred activities that were gentle, tailored for their age and cancer-related abilities, holistic, included other breast cancer survivors, and with an understanding instructor (Whitehead and Lavelle 2009).

24.6.3   Pain

Despite it being less prevalent a symptom in cancer than fatigue, pain has a much higher prominence in the minds of patients, professionals, and in the literature. Cancer pain in particular has a rapidly growing evidence base, although this is not as well-developed in terms of large, multicenter randomized controlled clinical trials as with oncology treatments. There are so many comprehensive texts and reviews of cancer pain that this section will focus on just the key issues relating to assessment and specific management in breast cancer. Once again, the data on older patients are sparse and much of the current knowledge of cancer pain management is admittedly based on extrapolation from studies in cancer and noncancer pain in younger samples (McGuire 2004).

Measurement of symptoms has already been discussed above but it is worth adding a little more here about pain assessment. This field has advanced enormously from the first attempt to categorize pain into five groups in the 1930s, to the introduction of psychophysical methods in the 1940s, the 10 cm VAS in the 1950s, the McGill Pain Questionnaire in the 1970s, and the use of standardized measures of "total pain relief" (TOTPAR), "summed pain intensity difference" (SPID), and "number needed to treat" (NNT) in the 1990s (Noble et al. 2005). Whereas for research studies and short-term pain changes the 10 cm VAS is sensitive and reliable, in everyday clinical situations the 0–10 numerical scale or the mild-moderate-severe verbal scales are more appropriate (Williamson and Hoggart 2005). In general, a report of "mild" pain corresponds to 1–4 on a 0–10 point scale, "moderate" corresponds to 5–6 and "severe" corresponds to 7 and over (Serlin et al. 1995). If older cognitively impaired patients are unable to verbalize about the nature, location, or intensity of pain, behavioral methods or surrogates should be used (Collett et al. 2007; Ahmedzai and Ahmed 2008 = http://www.connectingforhealth.nhs.uk/engagement/clinical/doas). Thus with training, the monitoring of facial expressions, changes in activity levels, and even nonspecific verbalizing can help the doctor or nurse to build up a picture in the elderly patient with dementia about how much pain is being experienced.

Training of staff to recognize and make a record about pain was an issue raised by a US study comparing breast cancer patients' self-reports of pain using a 0–10 numerical scale, in two healthcare settings, on the same day (Reyes-Gibby 2003). Out of 63 patients in the study, 51% had differing levels of pain in an out-patient breast clinic and an out-patient chemotherapy suite; 38% reported a pain score difference of four or more out of ten on the same day. Although pain may indeed vary in intensity within a day, e.g., because of incident pain or delays in medication, this finding suggests that the way that staff approach patients and elicit pain scores from them may influence they way the express symptoms.

"Cancer pain" may in fact be directly related to the primary, locally invasive, or metastatic disease process, or it can arise from diagnostic and surgical procedures, or from side effects and toxicities of therapies (McGuire 2004). In breast cancer, the overall prevalence has been reported as high as 70%, with 62% of patients having functional impairment caused by pain (Saxena and Kumar 2007). In elderly patients, reports of the prevalence of overall cancer pain range from 25 to 50% in US nursing homes. It is important to recall that, especially with older patients, pain arising from co-morbid conditions can play an important part in the overall "pain experience." A Norwegian survey of oncology outpatients ($n = 1549$) found that 53% had only cancer pain, 25% had noncancer pain, and 22% had both cancer and noncancer pain. Age did not influence the type of pain but males were more likely to have only cancer pain. Pain severity was comparable for all groups but interference by pain in daily activity was highest in the combined pain group.

Pain arising from breast cancer surgery has received attention in recent years. An early survey had shown that of 408 breast cancer patients who completed a questionnaire, 43% had suffered from postmastectomy pain syndrome (Smith et al. 1999) It was noteworthy that increasing age was significantly associated with reduced postsurgical pain (65% with pain in 30–49 year group, 40% in 50–99 year group, and 26% in group over 70 years). In the short term, some cases of postmastectomy pain may be associated with persisting axillary hematoma following axillary surgery, which may not be clinically obvious (Blunt and Schmiedel 2004). For pain up to 30 days following breast surgery, younger age, being unmarried, and having greater preoperative anxiety were found to be significant predictors (Katz et al. 2005) A classification has been devised of the types of neuropathic pain syndromes following breast cancer surgery, which should be useful for future studies in this area (Jung et al. 2003). This identifies three main types of pain: phantom breast pain (reported prevalence 17–44%); intercostobrachial neuralgia, including postmastectomy pain syndrome and ipsilateral axillary or arm pain (14–68% depending on type of surgery); and neuroma pain, including scar pain (23–49%).

It is presently accepted that the Brief Pain Inventory is the best way to assess cancer pain and especially its impact on daily living within formal studies. Using the BPI as well as the EORTC QLQ-C30 "quality of life" questionnaire, a recent large-scale Dutch study of 1,429 cancer patients showed that 55% had experienced pain in the past week and in 44% it was moderate or severe (van den Beuken-van Everdingen et al. 2007). This level of pain was present throughout the disease trajectory: the prevalence of moderate to severe pain was 43% in those currently or recently having curative anticancer treatment, 41% who had curative treatment more than 6 months ago, 43% currently receiving palliative treatment, and rose to 70% for whom anticancer treatment was no longer feasible. Breast cancer patients formed 265 of the study sample and these had a significantly higher odds ratio (1.57, CI1.01–2.46) of reporting moderate to severe pain. Age and gender were not significant predictors of pain.

This study also used a "pain management index," which computes the adequacy of pharmacological treatment for pain based on pain score and type of analgesic being used. It was found that pain management was "inadequate" for the level of pain in 42% of subjects. A recent literature review of 26 cancer pain surveys which used a pain management index revealed that treatment was inadequate in 43% of patients studied (Deandrea et al. 2008). Factors associated with a poor pain management index included studies performed in Europe or Asia and countries with national income per capita of <$40,000 per year and a care setting that was not specific for cancer. Age was not a predictor for pain undertreatment.

The importance of pain interference measurement, as captured using the BPI, was underscored in an in-depth prospective US study of 1,124 women with metastatic breast cancer followed up for one year (Castel et al. 2007). This showed, among many other important findings that younger age predicted for greater risk of reaching 7/10 on the BPI pain intensity score, and for reaching all of the scores from 3–7/10 on the pain interference score. However, the authors pointed out that while half of their study sample was aged below 57 years, in reality only 20% of the US breast cancer patients are in this age group, so highlighting the bias inherent in clinical studies.

Breast cancer readily metastasizes to bone, especially in the vertebral spine and in the long bones such as the femur. These metastases are associated with increased levels of pain and also pain interference with mobility and activities of daily living. Radiation therapy is the mainstay of bone pain palliation and breast cancer is responsive to this modality. A Cochrane review of 11 trials involving 3,435 patients, of single fraction vs. multifraction radiotherapy, has concluded that the overall pain responses were 60 and 59% respectively (Sze 2004). However, the patients who received single fraction treatment were more likely to need re-treatment later (22 vs. 7%) and they had a higher pathological fracture rate (3 vs. 2%). The incidence of spinal cord compression was the same for both regimens. It has been estimated that although the response to bone irradiation may increase up to 3 months from treatment, the best time to measure optimal response in terms of pain and reduced analgesia requirements is at two months (Li et al. 2008).

The role of bisphosphonates in the management of skeletal metastases is described in Chap. 18. Bisphosphonates have two important roles in bone pain palliation: they stabilize bone osteolysis and so prevent bone instability and fractures, and they specifically reduce bone pain. The efficacy of bisphosphonates against bone pain has been investigated in several trials and has been demonstrated for pooled studies of breast cancer using oral ibandronate ($P=0.001$), I.V. ibandronate ($P=0.0006$), oral clodronate ($P=0.01$), and pamidronate ($P <0.001$) (Aapro et al., 2008). In a prospective placebo-controlled study in breast cancer, zolendronate consistently reduced BPI composite pain scores at each evaluation carried out throughout a 12-month period ($P <0.05$). It is recommended that in elderly patients receiving bisphosphonates, special attention is paid to rehydration and that creatinine clearance rather than serum creatinine should be monitored.

Surgical and other interventional approaches are also relevant in the management of bone pain in breast cancer patients. Surgical fixation of fractures or unstable long bones may reduce pain and restore mobility even in older subjects (Samsani et al. 2004). Vertebral augmentation comprises techniques of cement vertebroplasty and balloon kyphoplasty which were originally developed for osteoporotic compression fractures and spinal pain, but which are now being successfully in cancers which metastasize to the vertebrae (Siemionow and Lieberman 2007). There are few formal studies of these techniques in cancer patients, especially with subjective evaluations. However, early results show that loss of height can be stabilized and pain is reduced and in some studies, aspects of quality of life have shown improvement. The largest group of cancer patients studied so far has been multiple myeloma, although breast cancer patients have also been included. It is likely that as surgeons and interventional radiologists learn these techniques these procedures will be more commonly used.

Pain management using drugs is a large subject in its own right and the reader is advised to consult the many textbooks and journals of palliative medicine for the latest recommendations in this rapidly advancing field. Cancer pain control has been dominated for two decades by the initially very influential World Health Organisation's (WHO) cancer pain program, which emphasized the three-step ladder approach (WHO 1996). In the past decade, there have been increasing criticisms of this rather simplistic, "one-size-fits-all" approach, which was admittedly originally designed for increasing the availability and usage of opioids in the developing world (Meldrum 2005). The 3-step concept of "nonopioid" for mild pain, moving to a "weak opioid" for moderate pain and a "strong opioid" for severe pain has been challenged on its lack of formal validation, its omission of interventional techniques, and recent studies which have shown that bypassing "step 2" by moving straight to so-called strong opioids can be safe and more effective (Ferreira et al. 2006; Eisenberg et al. 2005).

There have been calls for a more rational, evidence- and mechanism-based model for cancer pain control to replace the outdated empirical WHO 3-step ladder (Burton and Hamid 2007; Ahmedzai and Boland 2007 b). A modern approach to chronic pain management is based on the new understanding of cancer pain as essentially an inflammatory event mediated by cytokines, chemokines, and excitatory neurotransmitters and characterized by peripheral and central sensitization (Holdcroft and Power 2003). Thus the so-called "adjuvant" analgesics as described as optional in the WHO ladder (antidepressants, anticonvulsants, etc.) need to be seen as primary analgesics which sometimes are more important than the opioid drugs. Recent preclinical and clinical studies have also drawn attention to the considerable short- and long-term toxicities of opioids, which are subject to considerable genetic variability in terms of their effectiveness and metabolism between individuals (Ahmedzai and Boland 2007a; Benyamin et al. 2008).

An alternative model to the two-dimensional WHO ladder is the three-dimensional pyramid, in which all relevant modalities of pain management in cancer are shown as equal—cancer-directed treatments (including chemotherapy, hormonal and biological therapies, radiation therapy, bisphosphonates); surgical and interventional approaches (including vertebral augmentation, orthopedic surgery, neurolytic blocks, and spinal drug delivery); analgesic drugs (including NSAIDs, opioids, other nonopioid neuro-modulating drugs); and psychological, nursing and complementary therapy approaches (Ahmedzai 2001; Burton et al. 2004) (Fig. 24.2). For modern comprehensive cancer pain management, the patient should be offered a combination of modalities according to the cause of the symptom, the stage of disease, and the patient's performance status, and taking into account her preferences and history of adverse effects.

24.7 Management of the End of Life

Even though the survival time for breast cancer is steadily increasing, the majority of younger patients will die from this disease. With older patients, however, the cause of death may be more difficult to attribute to the cancer or its late effects, because of the increasing significance of co-morbid conditions with advancing age. In a large-scale Canadian trial of extended adjuvant endocrine therapy using letrozole vs. placebo after five years of tamoxifen, 5,170 breast cancer patients were followed for a median of 3.9 years (range 0–7 years) (Chapman et al. 2008). During this period of follow-up, 256 deaths occurred, of which 102 were from breast cancer, 50 from other malignancies, 100 from other causes, and four from unknown causes. Deaths arising from nonbreast cancer causes were therefore the majority (60%) and accounted for 48% of those dying aged below 70 years compared to 72% for those who were aged 70 years or over. Older age carried an increased risk of dying from all three types of causes. At baseline, the presence of cardiovascular disease was significantly associated with increased risk of death from other causes ($p=0.002$); and baseline osteoporosis was significantly associated with increased risk of dying from another malignancy ($p=0.05$). Another risk factor for death in this follow-up period was the presence of lymph node involvement ($p <0.001$); this effect was valid for all ages, but the 5–year survival was lowest for those with positive nodes and aged over 70 years.

This study has been stressed as it carries an important message about the terminal stage of breast cancer in older people. Even if she is dying from breast cancer and its metastatic spread as the primary pathology, it is very likely that the patient will be carrying a burden of other conditions and late effects of previous treatments. The approach to the care of the dying older breast cancer patient should therefore be based on holistic principles, that is, with a broad focus on overall health and psychosocial concerns and symptoms, and not just narrowly on the consequences of breast cancer.

An early international study of 1,640 patients with advanced cancer being cared for in hospices was one of the first to evaluate symptom prevalence at this stage of disease (Vainio and Auvinen 1996). Breast cancer patients accounted for 186 of the sample. They reported one of the highest levels of pain prevalence in the study (60%) as well high level of weakness (57%). In contrast breast cancer patients had the lowest prevalence of weight loss; cachexia is usually not seen in this disease, partly because of the masking effects of the adipose weight gain from hormonal medication.

A US single center study also examined a large cohort of advanced cancer patients admitted to a palliative care service (Walsh et al. 2000). Of 1,000 patients, 9% had breast cancer. Of note in this study was the finding that older patients (>65 years) had lower prevalence of several somatic and psychological symptoms compared to younger patients: pain reports (for all cancers) were 80% and 88%, respectively; nausea was 32 vs. 40%; sleep problems were 43 vs. 54%; anxiety was 19 vs. 29%; depression was 36 vs. 46%.

Pain may become more significant in the terminal stages, but it should be managed according to the same multimodal approach as described above. In the very ill patient, there will be less scope for cancer-directed treatments such as radiation therapy, and it is worth noting that although a single fraction of radiation is likely to be effective for bone pain, the maximal effective will occur at two months. Patients with a very short estimated prognosis will therefore be unlikely to see the benefits of the extra trouble to attend for this. On the other hand, interventional approaches for pain such as vertebroplasty for acute vertebral collapse or neurolytic blockade can give almost instant relief, providing the patient is fit enough to attend hospital.

In the last weeks or days of life, the emphasis in pain management moves to less interventional and a greater reliance on nonoral routes of medication, such as transdermal patches, rectal and subcutaneous infusions (Plonk and Arnold 2005). In many countries there is now a move toward defining "end of life care pathways," which are essentially guidelines for advising doctors and nurses on how to make these adjustments for medication for the dying patient and how to withdraw unnecessary treatments (Bookbinder et al. 2005; Mirando et al. 2005). It is important to recognize that clinicians need training and experience in order to know when to place a progressively ill patient onto an end-of-life care pathway; and also, occasionally, to know how to recognize when the disease has reached a plateau or possibly even improved and that the patient should be taken off the pathway.

Apart from pain, other difficult symptoms at the end of life include dyspnea, delirium, and in some cases of locally progressive breast cancer, fungating tumors. The latter problem has been poorly researched, partly because it is uncommon and tends to occur late in disease. Fungating malignant wounds are caused by infiltration of the tumor in the skin and this may be locally advanced, recurrent, or metastatic. These wounds may be associated with pain and irritation, odor, copious exudate, risk of bleeding, and an unsightly appearance. This may have an impact on the psychological state of the patient and thus the patient feels isolated and depressed.

The management of fungating malignant wounds is complex and challenging. A small proportion of patients may achieve complete healing following surgical excision. However, because this complication usually arises in late stage disease, treatment is usually palliative and can include radiotherapy and chemotherapy to reduce tumor size, exudate, and malodor. A Cochrane review identified only two suitable trials including a total of 63 patients for analysis and concluded that there was insufficient evidence to give clear guidelines for this problem (Adderley and Smith 2007).

Infection and odor control is achieved by managing local bacterial colonization with wound cleansing and debridement and the use of local antimicrobial agents (Seaman 2006). Local debridement can be performed by gently scrubbing the necrotic areas with gauze saturated with saline or wound cleanser. Another topical antimicrobial agent is Iodosorb gel, iodine complexed in a starch copolymer. This product contains slow-release iodine and has been shown to decrease bacterial counts in wounds without cytotoxicity.

Malodor from a fungating tumor can be a devastating complication as it can restrict the patient's social contact. The use of topical metronidazole to control wound odor is well-supported. Topical therapy is available either as crushed tablets or gel form. Systemic metronidazole should not be used for local bacterial colonization and should be reserved for treatment of clinical wound infection. Another approach for malodor is to use a dressing that acts like a filter and absorbs the odor-forming chemicals liberated from the wound. Charcoal dressing is a powerful deodorizer and is also able to absorb bacterial spores. Honey dressing is another option. Honey is effective in reducing bacterial colonization as it is a supersaturated sugar solution with a low water activity and high osmolarity which means that there is little water available to support the growth of bacteria and yeasts, hence reducing the formation of malodor. Silver dressing can be used as silver interacts with wound fluids and releases ionic silver into the wound bed where it binds to tissue proteins and causes structural changes in the bacterial cell wall. Silver ions also bind to and denature bacterial DNA and RNA, thereby inhibiting replication. Furthermore, silver enhances wound healing and silver sulphadiazine cream (Flamazine) has been found effective in controlling capillary bleeding and this may be useful in fungating wounds (Hampton 2008).

Dyspnea in cancer is the end result of many pathways of pathophysiological changes that occur in patients who have thoracic involvement; co-morbidities (e.g., COPD or heart disease); muscle wasting due to cachexia; deconditioning associated with restricted mobility; and the effects of ageing. It is important to distinguish dyspnea clinically from other types of abnormal breathing pattern, especially tachypnea associated with increased metabolic rate such as with fever; air hunger associated with metabolic acidosis, e.g., diabetic ketosis; hyperventilation associated with panic disorders; Cheyne-Stoke respiration when breathing can appear to be increased and labored, alternating with periods of hypopnea or even apnea (Cachia and Ahmedzai 2008).

The approach to dyspnea management in cancer includes, as with the pain pyramid, cancer-directed treatments, surgical interventions, pharmacological and nonpharmacological approaches. Pleural and pericardial effusions bring a poor prognosis, as does evidence of the patient having pulmonary thromboembolism or lymphangitis carcinomatosa. In an ambulant patient who suddenly develops these complications, there is scope for hospitalization and investigations prior to paracentesis or anticoagulation. If the patient is already very ill and confined to bed, it is unlikely that such interventions will be helpful and could themselves place an extra burden of distress on the patient and her carers. Opioids, benzodiazepines and other sedatives have been shown to have beneficial effects on dyspnea in cancer patients in several small studies (Viola et al. 2008; Currow and Abernethy 2007). Nebulized furosemide has recently been shown in small studies of both cancer and noncancer patients to relieve breathlessness, through a poorly understood mechanism involving bronchial wall receptors. Nonpharmacological interventions for dyspnea include the use of oxygen, but only if there is good evidence from skin oximetry that there is desaturation at rest or on exertion (Cachia and Ahmedzai 2008).

For both increasing terminal pain and dyspnea, there has been a tendency to use higher and higher doses of opioids, often by subcutaneous infusions using a syringe driver. It is now thought that rapidly increasing doses of opioids can themselves be associated with tolerance and hyperalgesia, as well as running the risk of sedation (Benyamin et al. 2008; Glare et al. 2006). It is more helpful to use smaller doses of opioids and utilize alongside, than small doses of benzodiazepines and other agents such as low-dose haloperidol for reducing anxiety and fear (Navigante et al. 2006).

The use of such treatments in a terminally ill patient for palliative intention, which may induce sedation as an unwanted side effect, is not to be confused with the recently introduced concept of "palliative sedation" (Bilsen et al. 2006; Hasselaar et al. 2009). This term covers the deliberate induction of sedation, to varying but potentially reversible levels of depth, in order to relieve the patient from intractable and very distressing symptoms. The literature on palliative sedation also makes the distinction between this technique and euthanasia, or physician-assisted dying: in these, the "therapeutic" aim, which is legal in a very small number of countries, is solely to hasten death itself. In the Netherlands, euthanasia has been legal for the longest time but when restrictions were introduced there has been a tendency for practitioners to resort to "palliative sedation" for essentially the same ends, thus confusing the issues to an unhelpful degree.

It is beyond the scope of this chapter to go into further detail on the ethical and legal ramifications of sedation and assisted dying: the reader is invited to refer to the emerging literature dedicated to this field (Broeckaert 2004; Seymour et al. 2007). As a sociological observation, it is clear that there is increasing popular support in some countries for assisted dying to be legalized, which is in keeping with the secular trend in Westernized societies for a demand for greater public choice in healthcare and lifestyle decisions. On the other hand, in many countries physicians are still opposed to this move. A recent survey of 41,125 individuals in 33 European countries found a broad spread of attitudes toward the acceptance of euthanasia (Cohen et al. 2006). Using a single item question, scores ranged from one extreme toward acceptance in the Netherlands, Denmark, France, and Sweden, to resistance in Romania, Turkey, and Malta. Great Britain appeared exactly halfway in the range of European opinions on this topic.

Other less confrontational ethical decisions that face patients and professionals in advanced cancer include the withdrawal of treatments for infections and the use of clinically assisted (or "artificial") hydration or nutrition (Ford et al. 2005). There are neither clear medical nor ethical grounds for blanket rules for these topics: the decision has to be made individually, depending on the clinical circumstances and, above all, the patient's own views and preferences, if they are known. For this reason, cancer patients are increasingly advised to make and write down their advanced decisions on the withdrawal and use of specific treatments at the end of life. These include the preferred place of terminal care and eventually of death: the two may not be the same as many people would like to spend as long time as possible in their preterminal illness at home with their family, but prefer to be in the security of a hospital or hospice in the final days or hours. Recent qualitative studies are shedding new light on this poorly understood area of healthcare decision-making (Thomas 2005).

24.8   Needs of Carers and Dependents

This chapter has focused closely on the needs of the older breast cancer patient. It should be acknowledged that the families of these patients may also have health and social care needs (Smith 2004). In many countries women are living longer than men and so it is not uncommon for the elderly breast cancer patient to be living singly, having lost a partner. If the husband is alive, he may well be elderly too and have several co-morbid conditions and general effects of ageing that prevent his acting well as a caregiver, as compared to the reverse situation with an older male cancer patient and a female spouse caregiver. There is a broad range of responses to the need to provide care for a partner with cancer, from being a burden if the caregiver is himself frail and ill, to being seen as raising self-esteem and giving a special purpose to life (Haley 2003).

Stresses on carers may come from providing personal care, providing emotional support, helping to manage symptoms and treatment including the administration of medications, dealing with the growing uncertainties of the prognosis and the fear of death, watching helplessly as the patient suffers from pain or other distressing terminal symptoms. In addition, caregivers may experience stress within their families if there is lack of support from others and if caring for the patient upsets the individual's daily routine and lifestyle. If the cancer patient is elderly, then the caregiver may have to cope with extra issues of fatigue, sleep disruption, and impaired mobility. At the same time, the male partner may have his own health problems and may neglect his own welfare.

A longitudinal study of breast cancer patients found that caregivers were actually usually younger than the patient: half of them were a spouse or partner, about a third were female relatives (a sister or daughter), and the rest were friends (Grunfeld et al. 2004). The perceived burden of care was the strongest predictor of caregivers' actual anxiety and depression.

As the disease progresses, the caregiver is usually drawn into decisions regarding care and end-of-life choices, which may be stressful (Haley 2003). The time of death may come as a relief both for the suffering patient and the stressed carer; or the death may usher in a new phase of prolonged loneliness and depression. There is an increased risk of long-term psychological morbidity in bereavement if the patient was seen to be suffering exhaustively and the carer himself had mental distress during the terminal illness.

Other social consequences of caring for an older cancer patient include the possibility of giving up employment or hobbies and social contacts; and the added costs of transport to hospital for appointments and admissions. For these reasons, it is important that social and financial help is provided as soon as it is appropriate for the caregiver under stress. If there are not other family members, then social services, hospices, or other charities may be able to provide financial or practical help in the home and with hospital visits. Respite care, i.e., admission of the patient to give the carer a necessary break, is often helpful but because of increasing admission costs, this facility is becoming less feasible in many countries.

Older patients may have adult children in their early middle ages who have their own children, who may experience distress at seeing their grandmother deteriorate and eventually die. While adult family members may be able to receive psychological support from hospice and bereavement services, these may not always be able to accommodate children. A website which is dedicated to teenagers who have a parent with cancer may also provide support for those with progressively ill grandparents: this support comes in the form of easily understood medical information and the on-line edited sharing of stories and experiences between children going through similar experiences (riprap.org.uk).

References

Aapro M, Abrahamsson PA, Body JJ, Coleman RE, Colomer R et al (2008) Guidance on the use of bisphosphonates in solid tumours: recommendations of an international expert panel. Annals of oncology 19:420–432

Adderley UJ, Smith R (2007) Topical agents and dressings for fungating wounds (abstract). Cochrane database of systematic reviews 2

Ahlberg K, Ekman T, Gaston-Johansson F et al (2003) Assessment and management of cancer-related fatigue in adults. Lancet 362(9384):640–650

Ahmed N, Bestall JC, Ahmedzai SH, Payne SA, Clark D, Noble N (2004) Systematic review of the problems and issues of accessing specialist palliative care by patients, carers and health and social care professionals. Palliat Med 18:525–542

Ahmed N, Bestall JC, Payne SA, Noble B, Ahmedzai SH (2009) The use of cognitive interviewing methodology in the design and testing of a screening tool for supportive and palliative care needs. Support Care Cancer 17(6):665–673

Ahmedzai SH (2001) Window of opportunity for pain control in terminally ill. Lancet 357(9265): 1304–1305

Ahmedzai SH (2004) The nature of palliation and its contribution to supportive care. Supportive care in respiratory disease. Oxford University Press, Oxford

Ahmedzai SH, Ahmed N (2008) Assessment of chronic pain in adults and older children. Report for Do Once and Share Programme of National Programme for IT, Department of Health, England

Ahmedzai SH, Boland J (2007a) Opioids for chronic pain: molecular and genomic basis of actions and adverse effects. Curr opin support palliat care 1:117–125

Ahmedzai SH, Boland J (2007b) The total challenge of cancer pain in supportive and palliative care. Curr opin support palliat care 1:3–5

Apkarian AV, Bushnell MC, Treede RD, Zubieta JK (2005) Human brain mechanisms of pain perception and regulation in health and disease. Eur J Pain 9:463–484

Ballinger RS, Fallowfield LJ (2009) Quality of life and patient-reported outcomes in the older breast cancer patient. Clin Oncol 21:140–155

Barresi MJ, Shadbolt B, Byrne D, Stuart-Harris R (2003) The development of the Canberra symptom scorecard: a tool to monitor the physical symptoms of patients with advanced tumours. BMC Cancer 3(32):1–9

Benyamin R, Trescot AM, Datta S, Buenaventura R, Adlaka R et al (2008) Opioid complications and side effects. Pain phys 11:S105–S120

Bilsen J, Norup M, Deliens L, Miccinesi G, van der Wal G et al (2006) Drugs used to alleviate symptoms with life shortening as a possible side effect: end-of-life care in six European countries. J pain symptom manage 31(2):111–121

Blunt C, Schmiedel A (2004) Some cases of severe post-mastectomy pain syndrome may be caused by an axillary haematoma. Pain 108:294–296

Bookbinder M, Blank AE, Arney E, Wollner D, Lesage P et al (2005) Improving end-of-life care: development and pilot-test of a clinical pathway. J pain symptom manage 29(6):529–543

Borsook D, Becerra LR (2006) Breading down the barriers: fMRI applications in pain, analgesia and analgesics. Mol pain 2:30

Bower JE, Ganz PA, Aziz N (2005) Altered cortisol response to psychologic stress in breast cancer survivors with persistent fatigue. Psychosom Med 67:277–280

Broeckaert B (2004) Palliative care nursing – principles and evidence for practice. In: Payne S, Seymour J, Ingleton C (eds) Ethical issues at the end of life – a very short introduction. Open University Press, UK

Bulli F, Miccinesi G, Maruelli A, Katz M, Paci E (2009) The measure of psychological distress in cancer patients: the use of distress thermometer in the Oncological Rehabilitation Center of Florence. Support Care Cancer 17(7):771–779

Burton AW, Hamid B (2007) Current challenges in cancer pain management: does the WHO approach still have relevance? Expert Rev Anticancer Ther 7(11):1501–1502

Burton AW, Rajagopal A, Shah HN, Mendoza T, Cleeland C et al (2004) Epidural and intrathecal analgesia is effective in treating refractory cancer pain. Pain med 5(3):239–247

Cachia E, Ahmedzai SH (2008) Breathlessness in cancer patients. Eur J Cancer 44:1116–1123

Castel LD, Abernethy AP, Li Y, DePuy V, Saville BR, Hartmann KE (2007) Hazards for pain severity and pain interference with daily living, with exploration of brief pain inventory cut-points, among women with metastatic breast cancer. J pain symptom manage 34(4):380–392

Chapman JAW, Meng D, Shepherd L, Parulekar W, Ingle JN et al (2008) Competing causes of death from a randomized trial of extended adjuvant endocrine therapy for breast cancer. J Natl Cancer Inst 100:252–260

Cohen J, Marcoux I, Bilsen J, Deboosere P, van der Wal G, Deliens L (2006) European public acceptance of euthanasia: socio-demographic and cultural factors associated with the acceptance of euthanasia in 33 European countries. Soc Sci Med 63(3):743–756

Collett B, O'Mahony S, Schofield P, Closs SJ, Potter J, Guideline Development Group (2007) Concise guidance to good practice: No. 8, The assessment of pain in older people, National guidelines. Report of Royal College of Physicians, British Geriatrics Society and The British Pain Society

Colloca L, Benedetti F (2005) Placebos and painkillers: is mind as real as matter? Nat Rev Neurosci 6(7):545–552

Cramp F, Daniel J (2008) Exercise for the management of cancer-related fatigue in adults – review. Cochrane Libr 4:1–32

Currow DC, Abernethy AP (2007a) Pharmacological management of dyspnoea. Curr opin support palliat care 1:96–101

Dalal S, del Fabbro E, Bruera E (2006) Symptom control in palliative care-part 1: oncology as a paradigmatic example. J palliat med 9(2):391–408

Deandrea S, Montanari M, Moja L, Apolone G (2008) Prevalence of undertreatment in cancer pain – a review of published literature. Ann Oncol 19:1985–1991

Deimling GT, Bowman KF, Sterns S, Wagner LJ, Kahana B (2006) Cancer-related health worries and psychological distress among older adult, long-term cancer survivors. Psycho-oncology 15:306–320

Eisenberg E, Marinangeli M, Birkhahn J, Paladini A, Varrassi G (2005) International Association for the Study of Pain. Pain Clinical Updates – *International association for the study of pain*. Time to modify the WHO analgesic ladder? 13(5): 1–4

Evans KC, Banzett RB, Adams L, McKay L, Frackowiak RSJ, Corfield DR (2002) BOLD fMRI identifies limbic, paralimbic, and cerebellar activation during air hunger. J Neurophysiol 88:1500–1511

Ferreira KASL, Kimura M, Teixeira MJ (2006) The WHO analgesic ladder for cancer pain control, twenty years of use. How much pain relief does one get from using it? Support Care Cancer 14:1086–1093

Fogel J, Albert SM, Schnabel F, Ditkoff BA, Neugut AI (2002a) Internet use and social support in women with breast cancer. Health Psychol 21(4):398–404

Fogel J, Albert SM, Schnabel F, Ditkoff BA, Neugut AI (2002b) Use of the internet by women with breast cancer. J Med Internet Res 4(2):E9

Ford PJ, Fraser TG, Davis MP, Kodish E (2005) Anti-infective therapy at end of life: ethical decision-making in hospice-eligible patients. Bioethics 19(4):379–392

Glare P, Walsh D, Sheehan D (2006) The adverse effects of morphine: a prospective survey of common symptoms during repeated dosing for chronic cancer pain. Am J Hosp Palliat Care 23(3):229–235

Goodlin SJ (2004) Care of the older patient with pain. Curr Pain Headache Rep 8:277–280

Gott CM, Ahmedzai SH, Wood C (2001) How many inpatients at an acute hospital have palliative care needs? Comparing the perspectives of medical and nursing staff. Palliat Med 15:451–460

Grunfeld E, Coyle D, Whelan T et al (2004) Family caregiver burden: results of a longitudinal study of breast cancer patients and their principal caregivers. CMAJ 170(12):1795–1801

Haley WE (2003) Family caregivers of elderly patients with cancer. Understanding and minimising the burden of care. Support Oncol 1(2):25–29

Hampton S (2008) Malodorous fungating wounds: how dressings alleviate symptoms. Br J Commun Nurs 13(6):S31-2, S34, S36 passim

Harris SR, Hugi MR, Olivotto IA, Levine M (2001) Clinical practice guidelines for the care and treatment of breast cancer: 11. Lymphedema. CMAJ 164(2):191–199

Hasselaar JG, Verhagen SC, Vissers KC (2009) When cancer symptoms cannot be controlled: the role of palliative sedation. Curr Opin Support Palliat Care 3(1):14–23

Holdcroft A, Power I (2003) Recent developments: Management of pain. BMJ 326:635–639

Hopwood P, Haviland J, Mills J, Sumo G, Bliss JM (2007) The impact of age and clinical factors on quality of life in early breast cancer: an analysis of 2208 women recruited to the UK START Trial (standardisation of breast radiotherapy trial). Breast 16:241–251

Jensen MP, Chen C, Brugger AM (2002) Postsurgical pain outcome assessment. Pain 99:101–109

Jung BF, Ahrendt GM, Oaklander AL, Dworkin RH (2003) Neuropathic pain following breast cancer surgery: proposed classification and research update. Pain 104:1–13

Katz J, Poleshuck EL, Andrus CH, Hogan LA, Jung BF et al (2005) Risk factors for acute pain and its persistence following breast cancer surgery. Pain 119:16–25

Kligman L, Wong RKS, Johnston M, Laetsch NS (2004) The treatment of lymphedema related to breast cancer: a systematic review and evidence summary. Support Care Cancer 12:421–431

Kroenke CH, Rosner B, Chen WY et al (2004) Functional impact of breast cancer by age at diagnosis. J Clin Oncol 15:1849–1856

Li KK, Hadi S, Kirou-Mauro A, Chow E (2008) When should we define the response rates in the treatment of bone metastases by palliative radiotherapy? Clin Oncol 20:83–89

Markes M, Brockow T, Resch K L. (2006) Exercise for women receiving adjuvant therapy for breast cancer. Cochrane Database of Systematic reviews 18(4):CD005001

McGuire DB (2004) Occurrence of cancer pain. J Natl Cancer Inst Monographs 32:51–56

McWayne J, Helney SP (2005) Psychologic and social sequelae of secondary lymphedema - a review. Am Cancer Soc 104:457–466

Mehnert A, Koch U (2008) Psychological comorbidity and health-related quality of life and its association with awareness, utilization, and need for psychosocial support in a cancer register-based sample of long-term breast cancer survivors. J psychosomatic res 64:383–391

Meldrum M (2005) The ladder and the clock: Cancer pain and public policy at the end of the twentieth century. J pain symptom manage 29(1):41–54

Meystre CJN, Burley NMJ, Ahmedzai S (1997) What investigations and procedures do patients in hospices want? Interview based survey of patients and their nurses. BMJ 315:1202–1203

Minton O, Stone P, Richardson A, et al. (2008) Drug therapy for the management of cancer related fatigue. Cochrane Database Syst Rev 1: CD006704

Mirando S, Davies DP, Lipp A (2005) Introducing an integrated care pathway for the last days of life. Palliat Med 19:33–39

Mock V (2004) Evidence-based treatment for cancer-related fatigue. J Natl Cancer Inst Monographs 32:112–118

Monfardini S (2002) Prescribing anti-cancer drugs in elderly cancer patients. Eur J Cancer 38(18):2341–2346

Montazeri A (2008) Health-related quality of life in breast cancer patients: a bibliographic review of the literature from 1974 to 2007. J Experimental Clin Cancer Res 27:1–31

Morrell RM, Halyward MY, Schild SE, Ali MS, Gunderson LL et al (2005) Breast cancer-related lymphedema. Mayo Clin Proc 80(11):1480–1484

Moseley AL, Carati CJ, Piller NB (2007) A systematic review of common conservative therapies for arm lymphoedema secondary to breast cancer treatment. Ann Oncol 18(4):639–646

Multinational Association for Supportive Care in Cancer (MASCC). (2009) Definition of supportive care. http://www.mascc.org/content/20.html Last accessed on 29 May 2009

National Comprehensive Cancer Network (2004) Cancer related fatigue: clinical practice guidelines in oncology. NCCN 2004

Navigante AH, Cerchietti LCA, Castro MA, Lutteral MA, Cabalar ME (2006) Midazolam as adjunct therapy to morphine in the alleviation of severe dyspnea perception in patients with advanced cancer. J pain symptom manage 31(1):38–47

NICE : *National Institute for Clinical Excellence* (2004) *Improving supportive and palliative care for adults with cancer.* London, UK: National Institute for Clinical Excellence

Noble B, Clark D, Meldrum M, ten Have H, Seymour J, Winslow M, Paz S (2005) The management of pain, 1945–2000. J pain symptom manage 29(1):14–21

Perkins EA, Small BJ, Balducci L, Extermann M, Robb C, Haley WE (2007) Individual differences in well-being in older breast cancer survivors. Crit Rev Oncol Hematol 62:74–83

Plonk WM, Arnold RM (2005) Terminal care: the last weeks of life. J palliat med 8(5):1042–1054

Poole K, Fallowfield LJ (2002) The psychological impact of post-operative arm morbidity following axillary surgery for breast cancer: a critical review. Breast 11:81–87

Porta-Sales J, Gomez-Batiste X, Pascual-Lopez A (2008) Acute palliative medicine units. In: Walsh D (ed) palliative medicine. Elsevier, Philadelphia, pp 208–212

Prescott RJ, Kunkler IH, Williams LJ, King CC, Jack W, van der Pol M et al (2007) A randomised controlled trial of postoperative radiotherapy following breast-conserving surgery in a minimum-risk older population. The PRIME trial. Health Technol Assess 11:31

Rabow MW, Dibble SL, Pantilat SZ, McPhee SJ (2004) The Comprehensive Care Team. A controlled trial of outpatient palliative medicine consultation. Arch Intern Med 164:83–91

Rao A, Cohen HJ (2004) Symptom management in the elderly cancer patient:fatigue, pain and depression. J Clin Oncol 32:150–157

Reyes-Gibby CC, McCrory LL, Cleeland CS (2003) Variations in patients' self-report of pain by treatment setting. J pain symptom manage 25(5):444–448

Richardson A, Medina J, Richardson A, Sitzia J, Brown V (2005) Patients' needs assessment tools in cancer care: principles & practice. Kings College London. Worthing and Southlands Hospitals NHS Trust

Ridner SH (2005) Quality of life and a symptom cluster associated with breast cancer treatment-related lymphedema. Support Care Cancer 13:904–911

Rietman JS, Dijkstra PU, Hoekstra HJ, Eisma WH, Szabo BG, Groothoff JW, Geertzen JHB (2003) Late morbidity after treatment of breast cancer in relation to daily activities and quality of life: a systematic review. EJSO 29:229–238

Samsani SR, Panikkar V, Venu KM, Georgiannos D, Calthorpe D (2004) Breast cancer bone metastasis in femur: surgical considerations and reconstruction with Long Gamma Nail. EJSO 30:993–997

Satariano WA, Silliman RA (2003) Comorbidity: implications for research and practice in geriatric oncology. Crit rev ocnol/hematol 48:239–248

Satterlund MJ, McCaul KD, Sandgren AK (2003) Information gathering over time by breast cancer patients. J Med Internet Res 5(3):E15

Saxena AK, Kumar S (2007) Management strategies for pain in breast carcinoma patients: current opinions and future perspectives. Pain Pract 7(2):163–177

Seaman S (2006) Management of malignant fungating wounds in advanced cancer. Semin Oncol Nurs 22(3):185–193

Serlin RC, Mendoza TR, Nakamura Y, Edwards KR, Cleeland CS (1995) When is cancer pain mild, moderate or severe? Grading pain severity by its interference with function. Pain 61:277–284

Seymour JE, Janssens R, Broeckaert B (2007) Relieving suffering at the end of life: practitioners' perspectives on palliative sedation from three European countries. Soc Sci Med 64(8): 1679–1691

Siemionow K, Lieberman IH (2007) Vertebral augmentation in osteoporosis and bone metastasis. Curr Opin Support Palliat Care 1:323–327

Smith P (2004) Working with family care-givers in a palliative care setting. In: Payne S, Seymour J, Ingleton C (eds) Palliative care nursing – principles and evidence for practice. Open University Press, UK

Smith WCS, Bourne D, Squair J, Phillips DO, Chambers WA (1999) A retrospective cohort study of post mastectomy pain syndrome. Pain 83:91–95

Smyth JF (2007) Disclosing gaps between supportive and palliative care – the past 20 years - editorial. Support Care Cancer 16:109–111

Stava CJ, Lopez A, Vassilopoulou-Sellin R (2006) Health profiles of younger and older breast cancer survivors. Cancer 107(8):1752–1759

Stone P, Hardy J, Broadley K et al (1999) Fatigue in advanced cancer: a prospective controlled cross-sectional study. Br J Cancer 79(9–10):1479–1486

Stone CA, Tiernan E, Dooley BA (2008) Prospective validation of the palliative prognostic index in patients with cancer. J Pain Symptom Manage 35(6):617–622

Sze WM, Shelley M, Held I, Mason M (2004). Palliation of metastatic bone pain: single fraction versus multifraction radiotherapy. Cochrane Database of Systematic Reviews 2002, Issue 1. Art. No.: CD004721. DOI: 10.1002/14651858.CD004721.

Thomas C (2005) The place of death of cancer patients: can qualitative data add to known factors? Social Sci Med 60:2597–2607

Turnheim K (2003) When drug therapy gets old: pharmacokinetics and pharmacodynamics in the elderly. Exp Gerontol 38(8):843–853

Twycross R, Wilcock A (eds) (2002) Symptom management in advanced cance, 3rd edn. Radcliffe Medical Press, Abingdon

Twycross R, Wilcock A (eds) (2008a) Hospice and palliative care formulary USA, 2nd edn. Palliativedrugs.Com Ltd, Nottingham

Twycross R, Wilcock A (eds) (2008b) Palliative Care Formulary, 3rd edn. Radcliffe Medical Press, Abingdon

Twycross R, Jenns K, Todd J (eds) (2000) Lymphoedema. Radcliffe Medical Press, Abingdon

Twycross R, Wilcock A, Charlesworth S, Dickman A (eds) (2003) Palliative care formulary, 2nd edn. Radcliffe Medical Press, Abingdon

Vainio A, Auvinen A (1996) Prevalence of symptoms among patients with advanced cancer: an international collaborative study. J pain symptom manage 12(1):3–10

van de Poll-Franse LV, van Eenbergen MC (2008) Internet use by cancer survivors: current use and future wishes. Support Care Cancer 16(10):1189–1195

van den Beuken-van Everdingen MHJ, de Rijke JM, Kessels AG, Schouten HC, van Kleef M, Patijn J (2007) High prevalence of pain in patients with cancer in a large population-based study in The Netherlands. Pain 132:312–320

van den Beuken-van Everdingen MHJ, Peters ML, de Rijke JM, Schouten HC, van Kleef M, Patijn J (2008) Concerns of former breast cancer paints about disease recurrence: a validation and prevalence study. Psycho-Oncology 17:1137–1145

van Norren K, van Helvoort A, Argilés JM, van Tuijl S, Arts K, Gorselink M, Laviano A, Kegler D, Haagsman HP, van der Beek EM (2009) Direct effects of doxorubicin on skeletal muscle contribute to fatigue. Bri J Cancer 100:311–314

Viola R, Kiteley C, Lloyd NS, Mackay JA, Wilson J et al (2008) The management of dyspnea in cancer patients: a systemic review (review article). Support cancer care 16:329–337

Walsh D, Donnelly S, Rybicki L (2000) The symptoms of advanced cancer: relationship to age, gender, and performance status in 1, 000 patients. Support Care Cancer 8:175–179

Watson M, Lucas C, Hoy A, Back I (eds) (2009) Oxford handbook of palliative care 2nd edition. Oxford University Press, Oxford

Wen K-Y, Gustafson DH (2004b) Needs assessment for cancer patients and their families – review. Health Qual Life Outcomes 2:1–12

Wenzel LB, Fairclough DL, Brady MJ, Cella D, Garrett KM et al (1999) Age-related differences in the quality of life of breast carcinoma patients after treatment. Cancer 86(1): 1768–1774

Whitehead S, Lavelle K (2009) Older breast cancer survivors' views and preferences for physical activity. Qual Health Res 19:894–906

WHO, World Health Organization (1996) Cancer pain relief 2nd edition. WHO, Geneva

Williamson A, Hoggart B (2005) Pain: a review of three commonly used pain rating scales. J clin nursing 14:798–804

Winters-Stone KM, Bennett JA, Nail L, Schwartz A (2008) Strength, physical activity, and age predict fatigue in older breast cancer survivors. Oncol nursing forum 35(5):815

Yen TWF, Fan X, Sparapani R, Laud PW, Walker AP, Nattinger AB (2009) A contemporary, population-based study of lymphedema risk factors in older women with breast cancer. Ann Surg Oncol 16:979–988

Zebrack BJ, Yi J, Petersen L, Ganz PA (2008) The impact of cancer and quality of life for long-term survivors. Psycho-oncology 17:891–900

Ziebland S, Chapple A, Dumelow C, Evans J, Prinjha S, Rozmovits L (2004) How the internet affects patients' experience of cancer: a qualitative study. BMJ 328(7439):564

Index